The Psychotherapeutic Stance

Carsten René Jørgensen

The Psychotherapeutic Stance

With Foreword by Anthony Bateman

Springer

Carsten René Jørgensen
Aarhus, Risskov/Skejby, Denmark

ISBN 978-3-030-20436-5 ISBN 978-3-030-20437-2 (eBook)
https://doi.org/10.1007/978-3-030-20437-2

This Springer imprint is published by the registered company Springer Nature Switzerland AG
The registered company address is: Gewerbestrasse 11, 6330 Cham, Switzerland

To Vibeke, Mathilde and Johanne

To the anonymous patients who, despite their past experiences of severe betrayal and transgressions from others, have shown me so much trust by inviting me into their world, so that we could work together to enhance our shared psychological understanding and their quality of life.

This book has undergone a scientific review process, where two independent scholars have reviewed and commented on the authors manuscript.

Foreword

Psychotherapy works! This book outlines the evidence for this assertion and argues strongly that the therapeutic relationship and therapist attitude are key factors contributing to favourable outcomes from psychotherapy, which for many mental health conditions are better than medication. Whilst psychotherapists might cherish their techniques, name and protect their acronymic models of psychotherapy, and believe that their carefully crafted interventions are key to change, the author of this books argues that this misses the point. It is the relationship developed with the client that is the effector of change and not valued techniques. If this is the case it is important to know why this should be and what aspects of the relationship and the therapist are important. This is the subject of this book.

We know that there are good and bad therapists in terms of achieving satisfactory symptom relief and behavioural change for a patient. Yet we do not know which characteristics of a therapist are advantageous to which patient. Some therapists may be good at treating some 'types' of patients and not others. An intriguing finding in a recent longitudinal analysis of clinical outcomes not only found that the therapist is the greatest source of variance in outcomes, but also reported that therapists' effectiveness tends to diminish as their experience increases (Goldberg et al. 2016). The disparate and counter-intuitive range of findings in this area have contributed to a lively debate about the common factors of effective psychotherapy (Wampold and Imel 2015). So what are we to make of this? To explain the significance of the psychotherapeutic relationship and the absence of evidence about the importance of specific techniques in effecting change, it is necessary to go back to reconsider mental health/ill-health, reformulate psychotherapy itself, and understand the relationship between them. This is where the reader will be amply rewarded by reading this book. I will argue here that the central change process of psychotherapy for any individual with mental distress is the generation of a trust in the world, known as epistemic trust, which allows learning from others (Fonagy et al. 2015).

Mental ill-health is commonly considered as the presence of a pathological mental process. Yet it might equally be better conceptualised as the absence of a protective process, namely psychological resilience. The notion that psychopathology may arise from a loss of resilience has gained traction over the past few years. One proposed framework (Kalisch et al. 2015) describes resilience as a cognitive process. A potentially stressful stimulus is perceived and mentally represented by the individual. The mental representation is then appraised using higher-order cognition, and understood using a range of psychological mechanisms and phenomena, including executive function, attention, general intelligence, and self-awareness. The capacity for appraisal determines the emotional response of the individual—that is, their resilience. Thus, according to this formulation, resilience is the outcome of the top-down cognitive appraisal of a stressful stimulus. The external and social factors that have been associated with resilience such as social support or a secure attachment history affect resilience either directly or indirectly, in that they shape the individual's appraisal approach, or minimize exposure to stressors. This is not to deny the role of socio-environmental factors in determining an individual's resilience, or the importance of interventions at a social or community level; it is to suggest that the mechanism by which these social factors affect an individual's resilience is via their impact on the individual's appraisal style. The appropriate functioning of higher-order cognition crucially depends on appropriate judgements about social contexts. The mechanism effecting this judgement is known as mentalizing.

Psychotherapy can be conceptualised as an organised, structured social interaction which generates an attachment interaction based on reciprocal attachment patterns of the patient and therapist. Treatment requires participants to understand the mental states of each other and gradually recognise how mis-understanding mental states in oneself and others impacts on interpersonal interaction and may lead to symptoms. An essential component of this process is mentalizing.

Mentalizing describes a particular facet of the human imagination: an awareness of mental states in oneself and in other people, particularly in explaining their actions. It involves perceiving and interpreting the feelings, thoughts, beliefs, and wishes that explain what people do. This entails an awareness of someone's circumstances, their prior patterns of behavior, and the experiences to which the individual has been exposed. The emphasis on imagination and the inherent lack of certainty in relation to mental states leads to one of the ideas underpinning a mentalizing clinical approach: an *inquisitive stance*. The inquisitive stance is a style of interaction characterized by an expectation that one's mind may be influenced, surprised, changed, and enlightened by learning about another's mind. To some extent, this is a common component of all psychotherapy and may be part of how the therapeutic relationship brings about change (Bateman and Fonagy 2016). Mentalizing is the interpersonal "workhorse" of the social imagination: it is the aspect of social cognition that enables us to make sense of the behavior of ourselves and others, making cooperative and adaptive interaction possible. Failures in mentalizing will lead to a loss of resilience, that is a reduction in the appraisal capacities of the individual, with the inevitable consequences for mental well-being; contrariwise, enhancing mentalizing through psychotherapy will reinstate mental equilibrium.

Mentalizing develops in the context of attachment relationships which are the prototype of our later relationships (Bowlby 1979). Attachment is a biological process which activates cortical and sub-cortical brain structures in response to stress in social relationships (Coan 2010; Virticka and Vuilleumier 2012). Secure attachment enhances the function of the pre-frontal cortex when managing social interaction allowing the person to understand their own mental states and those of others accurately, buffering stress and minimizing the development of symptoms. In contrast insecure attachment, common in the general population at 40%, but twice that in clinical populations (Bakermans-Kranenberg and Van Ijzendoorn 2009), reduces the reserve of the prefrontal processing system and is associated with ineffective mentalizing, more so if combined with disorganized attachment process. In this context, attachment processes are activated but then fail to protect the individual from stress, leaving them vulnerable, unable to use social interaction to regulate their emotions and calibrate their experiences through others. The result is social isolation, distress, and symptoms.

So all psychotherapies share a common core—developing an alliance, working with attachment process, and enhancing mentalizing and facilitating development of epistemic trust. Only then will the individual be able to manage themselves in their social world. In this formulation of psychotherapy, therapist and patient 'fit' in terms of interpersonal process becomes important. Indeed mental health staff need to feel 'secure' in themselves if they are to treat vulnerable and insecure patients. This does not mean all mental health professionals and therapists have to demonstrate secure attachment processes as individuals; it means they have to be supported, trained, supervised, and open to learning. Otherwise they will fail to help a patient to manage insecurities, improve their mentalizing capacities, and adapt their attachment style.

We all have our working theories about ourselves; we could call them personal narratives, or our imagined self, a model of who we feel that we are, and why we feel we are the way we are, based on the evidence arising from our subjective experience. These *dominant* narratives tend to shape the way we mentalize ourselves: they are a kind of heuristic for making sense of our actions. For most of us, at any moment there is one predominant working theory—that is, the most obvious straightforward way of describing oneself. We also all have more *subdominant* narratives; these are the understandings of ourselves that are more nuanced or complex, and are hidden from the normal shorthand we might use to describe ourselves. The dominant narrative is in the foreground, but behind it is a range of subdominant narratives.

For example, a patient might have the dominant narrative "I need to be liked, and to achieve that, I defer to you" but the subdominant narrative might be "I'm tired of trying to work out what people want." The recognition of these subdominant narratives within an attachment process is a particularly potent way of establishing epistemic trust; in this example, the therapist might do this by saying something like: "I have noticed just how hard you work to make sure you meet all the needs of the people around you have; you know, in your shoes I would just get exhausted trying to meet every expectation anyone might have of me." This is a well-crafted empathically validating statement giving an individual a sense of being understood, that is 'mentalized' by the therapist. If someone feels that they are understood by another, in other words that person is able to mentalize them, they will be more inclined to learn from that person. This dynamic creates a special role for mentalizing in psychotherapy.

It is only through the experience of having one's—very individual—mind accurately and tolerably reflected back within an attachment process that primes people to open their minds to absorbing new knowledge about themselves and about the world, whether this information comes from within the clinical setting or from the social context. Without this, individuals cannot calibrate their feelings and thoughts and consequently become trapped within them, leading to inevitable psychological distress.

Effective mentalizing is valuable to the extent that it helps to keep minds open, allowing sincere curiosity which in turn generates epistemic trust, enabling new learning. Mentalizing does this by (a) improving the coherence of my perception of myself, (b) improving my capacity to perceive your perception of me, and (c) improving my capacity to match the two. Acquiring profound insight into myself is of little use if there is a mismatch between how you, my therapist, perceives me and how I see myself. I will feel distrustful and misunderstood. Similarly, I might be able to learn a lot about perceiving others, but in terms of my own psychological and social functioning, I will still have severe limitations if I cannot perceive myself accurately. Further, I can have a picture of myself and a picture of your view of me, but if these are, for example, at radically different levels of sophistication, the dissonance will inhibit effective social communication.

Whilst the facilitation of mentalizing is an essential component of what makes psychological therapies effective (Allen et al. 2008), this is not the end of the change process (Fonagy et al. 2017). Improved mentalizing may be important because it enables the individual to achieve a more fundamental social goal, which is to be able to enhance benefits he/she derives from social experience, to improve his/her functioning in cooperation (and in competition) with other individuals and social groups. It allows individuals to take advantage of felicitous circumstances, say someone appreciating their personal achievement and showing admiration simply because they are open to learning from others elsewhere. They know who to believe and who to be wary of. Trust in ourselves and the world becomes balanced—we trust in ourselves and yet question ourselves; we are uncertain of and circumspect about others but we accept what we learn from them until proven wrong.

So, mentalizing make sense as a change process in therapy only in terms of reintegrating the patient into the large, complex, ever-moving stream of human social communication. This is the fundamental aim of the therapeutic relationship. An emphasis on mentalizing or therapeutic insight in isolation from the imperatives of wider social functioning is meaningless. But whilst mentalizing is a critical part of the therapeutic process, it is only the beginning. To be effective, therapies must also have a systemic function: they must equip the individual to adapt to and benefit from the wider social environment.

A comprehensive model of effective treatment is predicated on the belief that treatment can work only if it involves recognition of, and response to, the patient's needs and perceptions. It is only through identifying, acknowledging, and appreciating the individual's mental state, beliefs, and complex subjectivity that the process by which the individual can begin to learn from the mind of the therapist can be stimulated. Therapy opens epistemic trust, making social communication and cooperative alignment with other minds possible, through the recursive experience of recognizing one's own mind as accurately represented in someone else's. This alignment can bring perspective, constraint, and modification to our wilder expressions of the social imagination. It is a calibrating mechanism through which we put things in their rightful place. Therapeutic interventions are effective because they open perspectives and enable the person to access social learning experiences, which then feed back (Benish et al. 2011) in a "virtuous cycle" that enhances social understanding and communication. The apparently counterintuitive finding that more experienced therapists might have less effective outcomes (Goldberg et al. 2016) might arise from the fact that less experienced therapists are more able to see the individual patient in all their subjective complexity rather than as a "walking diagnostic prototype". They, themselves, are freer and see the person rather than the disease, which is, of course, the heart of all psychotherapy.

London, UK Anthony W. Bateman, M.A.

References

Allen, J. G., Fonagy, P., & Bateman, A. (2008). *Mentalizing in clinical practice*. Washington, DC, APPI.

Bakermans-Kranenberg, M. J., & Van Ijzendoorn, M. H. (2009). The first 10,000 adult attachment interviews: Distribution of adult attachment representations in clinical and non-clinical groups. *Attachment and Human Development, 11*(3), 223–263.

Bateman, A., & Fonagy, P. (2016). *Mentalization based treatment for personality disorders: A practical guide*. Oxford: Oxford University Press.

Benish, S. G., Quintana, S., & Wampold, B. E. (2011). Culturally adapted psychotherapy and the legitimacy of myth: A direct-comparison meta-analysis. *Journal of Counselling Psychology, 58*, 279–289.

Bowlby, J. (1979). The making and breaking of affectional bonds. *British Journal of Psychiatry, 130*, 201–210, 421–431.

Coan, J. A. (2010). Adult attachment and the brain. *Journal of Social and Personal Relationships, 27*, 210–217.

Fonagy, P., Gergely, G., Jurist, Elliot L., & Target, M. (2002). *Affect regulation, mentalisation and the development if the self.* The Other Press.

Fonagy, P., Luyten, P., Allison, E., & Campbell, C. (2017). What we have changed our minds about: Part 2. Borderline personality disorder, epistemic trust and the developmental significance of social communication. *Borderline Personal Disorder and Emotional Dysregulation, 4*, 9.

Fonagy, P., Luyten, P., & Allison, E. (2015). Epistemic petrification and the restoration of epistemic trust: A new conceptualization of borderline personality disorder and its psychosocial treatment. *Journal of Personality Disorders, 29,* 575–609.
Goldberg, S. B., Rousmaniere, T., & Miller, S. D. (2016). Do psychotherapists improve with time and experience? A longitudinal analysis of outcomes in a clinical setting. *Journal of Counselling Psychology, 63,* 1–11.
Kalisch, R., Muller, M. B., & Tuscher, O. (2015). A conceptual framework for the neurobiological study of resilience. *Behavioral Brain Science, 38*, e92.
Virticka, P., & Vuilleumier, P. (2012). Neuroscience of human social interactions and adult attachment style. *Frontiers of Human Neuroscience,* 6, 212.
Wampold, B. E., & Imel, Z. E. (2015). *The great psychotherapy debate: The evidence for what makes psychotherapy work.* Hillsdale: Laurence Erlbaum Associates.

Anthony W. Bateman M.A., is one of the founders (with Peter Fonagy) of mentalization based psychotherapy. He is consultant psychiatrist and psychotherapist and MBT Consultant to the Anna Freud National Centre for Children and Families, Visiting Professor University College London and Visiting Affiliate Professor at Copenhagen University.

Contents

Chapter 1
Introduction

> Although many practitioners and the public may be comforted by the notion that they are offering or receiving an empirically supported psychotherapy that works best, the fact is that success of treatment appears to be largely dependent on the client and the therapist, not on the use of "proven" empirically based treatment treatments (Lambert 2013a:8).

> The therapy relationship makes substantial and consistent contributions to psychotherapy outcome independent of the specific type of treatment. The therapy relationship accounts for why clients improve (or fail to improve) at least as much as the particular treatment method. (…) Efforts to promulgate best practices or evidence-based practices (EBPs) without including the relationship are seriously incomplete and potentially misleading (Norcross and Wampold 2011:423).

> It is because of you that I feel human. It is because of you that I now feel I have a right to be in the world—my father always gave me the opposite feeling (woman with a borderline personality disorder to her therapist).

What does it mean to relate to a patient in a psychotherapeutic manner? What does it mean to apply psychotherapeutic thinking to an issue? What does it means to bring oneself into play in a psychotherapeutic manner and to meet the patient and his or her difficulties with a dynamic-relational psychotherapeutic stance or attitude? I have grappled with these questions for many years without necessarily always being consciously aware of it. They have come up in connection with my teaching and counselling of psychology students, psychologists, doctors in training as psychiatric specialists and many different staff groups in residential and treatment institutions for people with psychological disorders. Similarly, I have asked myself, what is the unique thing that I do when I work with long-term individual psychotherapy? What, essentially, sets my work apart from what a good friend, partner, parent or colleague might provide? In this book, I will attempt to find an answer to these questions, all of which concern what it means to take a psychotherapeutic stance in a treatment process. A stance towards the patient that is reflected, emotionally involved, curious—and virtually the polar opposite to an instrumental, technocratic relationship.

C. R. Jørgensen, *The Psychotherapeutic Stance*,
https://doi.org/10.1007/978-3-030-20437-2_1

Psychotherapy Works

After decades of research into the effect of psychotherapy we can say with certainty that psychotherapy works for the vast majority of psychological disorders, regardless of severity. It has been estimated that the average patient who receives psychotherapeutic treatment fares better than 80% of patients who are not offered psychotherapy (Wampold and Imel 2015:94). With many disorders, psychotherapy is as least as effective as medication, and the effect is often more persistent (Wampold 2013). On the other hand, it has also been argued that the treatment effect in clinical practice is presumably a little lower than in the outcome studies that typically inform these general assessments (Lambert 2013b:204)—in part because therapists in clinical practice often have fewer resources and treat patients with more severe, more complex and more complicated disorders, and in part because one third or more of patients in treatment do not show any significant improvement, and as many as 5–10% are worse at the completion of treatment than before they began in psychotherapy (Lambert 2013a, b:192, 2007:1). The efficacy of psychotherapy is not unlimited, and there is still room for improvement.

If we compare patients who complete psychotherapeutic treatment with patients assigned to a waiting list, it is estimated that about 65% of patients in treatment will improve, compared to some 35% of the waiting-list patients during the same period (Lambert 2013b:176). Thus, being on a waiting list can in some cases have a positive effect in itself, presumably stemming from the patients' expectations of receiving help and their sense of having established contact with a therapist and a treatment institution. Besides, some patients with less severe disorders often improve over time more or less spontaneously, without having received professional help. One should, however, expect considerable variation depending on diagnosis, severity of disorder, duration of treatment and the therapist's skill. The duration and intensity of psychotherapy will often vary depending on the severity of the disorder that is targeted by the treatment; moreover, the treatment of, especially, patients with more complex psychological disorders, such as severe personality disorders, may require specialized skills from the therapist. Further, the risk that the patient fails to improve or even deteriorates after treatment is greater for more severely affected patients (Lambert 2007:7). Generally, however, psychotherapy *is* effective. What we know less about, although we do are not completely in the dark, is *why* psychotherapy works—the exact factors that make psychotherapy effective.

In recent decades, numerous studies have thus documented the efficacy of psychotherapy. That vast majority of these studies compare the outcomes of certain treatment models or methods; alternatively, they compare a new treatment method with a somewhat vaguely described 'treatment as usual', TAU, that has commonly been used to treat patients with certain disorders or diagnoses. Generally, these studies show that psychotherapy is effective, but, just as importantly, they also show that, with very few exceptions, there are no significant differences in effect among the many different psychotherapeutic treatment methods, which enjoy varying degrees of recognition. This becomes especially clear if one reviews the meta-analyses of treatment outcomes that have been published in recent decades (see Chap. 6).

An Excessive Focus on Technique

If we consider the history of psychotherapy—starting with Sigmund Freud and Joseph Breuer, who took the first steps in developing 'the talking cure' in the late 19th century, moving on to Carl Rogers and Rollo May, who initiated the development of, respectively, experience-oriented and existentialist humanistic therapy in the 1950s, further on to Aaron Beck's presentation of a new method for cognitive treatment of depression in the 1970s and finally to the present day, with its myriad psychotherapeutic models—it is remarkable to note how the focus is aimed increasingly at developing therapeutic techniques and specific models for the treatment of specific psychological disorders. Moreover, it becomes clear that the field is increasingly dominated by a sometimes less than fruitful competition between specific treatment models; a competition focused on determining which specific treatment method is the most effective for a given disorder. This despite our very limited success in finding clear differences in the efficacy of the various qualified treatment models.

For decades, the prevailing perception of psychotherapy has been—and still largely remains—that its key, effective component is the specific techniques, the specific method, applied by the therapist. From this view it follows logically that we should strive to refine and spread these methods and techniques and to develop (new) specific methods and techniques for treating each of the large and growing number of psychological disorders listed in our authorized diagnostic classification systems (DSM-5, ICD-11). In a natural extension of this perception of psychotherapy vast resources have been allocated to examining and, not least, comparing the outcomes of specific treatment methods and teaching therapists to apply the methods. Similarly, the healthcare sector, including psychiatric care and clinical psychology, has become increasingly focused on identifying and implementing what, in this perception of psychotherapy, counts as evidence-based methods for the treatment of specific disorders. Clinical guidelines specify how patients with a given disorder (diagnosis) should be treated, and in some settings there is a more or less explicit requirement for therapists to apply certain standardized psychotherapeutic methods in the treatment of patients with specific disorders (diagnoses).

There are many good, as well as less good, reasons driving this development. It will be obvious to most people that, as much as possible, the treatment we offer to people with psychological disorders should have a scientific basis and a documented effect. Psychotherapy in the psychiatric sector and in other public institutions should be carried out by authorized practitioners with the best possible basic education and psychotherapy training. Psychotherapists should have adequate training and receive ongoing supervision in their therapeutic work, and in some cases it is helpful if they specialize in working with patients with certain specific issues. The key question, however, is what the real-life implications are of this. How do we select the right candidates for psychotherapeutic training, how can we best train new psychotherapists, and how do we make sure that psychotherapeutic practice is consistently informed by the most updated knowledge? What should we focus on to secure evidence that our psychotherapists provide the best possible treatment? So far, the prevailing view has been that if only practitioners were trained to apply certain evidence-based therapeutic techniques, we would have the key factors in place to ensure an optimal treatment outcome for our patients. Experience shows that this assumption is far from accurate.

The specific treatment method and the therapist's technical interventions, as they are described in various treatment manuals, only make up one among multiple factors affecting the course and outcome of psychotherapy, and hardly the most important one. Factors pertaining to the individual therapist and patient and their mutual interaction are of far greater importance—although in practice, of course, it may be difficult to draw a clear-cut distinction between these elements of psychotherapy. Instead of striving to provide an evidence base for specific methods for the treatment of specific disorders, we should instead—or also—focus on securing an 'evidence base' for the individual psychotherapist's work, perhaps focused on their work with patients with certain specific issues.

Similarly, it is hardly helpful if our efforts to improve the practice of psychotherapy in the healthcare sector are focused exclusively on implementing what is identified as evidence-based specific treatment methods without paying sufficient attention to common therapeutic factors and the necessary conditions of psychotherapeutic work, including making sure that the individual psychotherapists has the necessary time, trust and professional latitude as well as access to continuous supervision. A wise man once said to me, 'Management loves techniques and standardized methods, it gives them a sense of being in control. But they don't get what it's really about. What the competent professional masters is something other and much more complicated, something that goes far beyond what can be captured by specific techniques and standardizations.' A one-sided focus on teaching practitioners to apply standardized treatment methods contains a risk that psychotherapists fail to sufficiently develop their clinical sensitivity, responsiveness, judgement, ability to listen, relational skills and ability to establish a viable therapeutic relationship with a wide range of different patients. If all you have is a big hammer, you may well tend to see nothing but nails. Practitioners with a narrow training focus may tend to think that a given symptom 'carries the same meaning' and should be handled the same way every time, in all patients; that the same specific interventions should be used with all patients. This reflects a failure to cultivate the ability to see what is unique in the patient and match one's treatment strategy to the given patient (Blatt 2001).

The effort to make psychotherapy evidence-based and standardized is driven, in part, by the essentially laudable ambition of providing the best possible treatment to as many patients as possible. The prevailing view of how best to achieve this ambition is to draw up guidelines detailing how to treat patients with a given disorder. In principle, this ought to increase the likelihood that patients receive fairly uniform, high-quality treatment across settings and geographic locations—including patients who are not treated in the most prestigious clinics or by high-profile therapists. All things being equal, this will serve to minimize the differences between the specific techniques used by different therapists, especially if the individual therapists are systematically trained to adhere to these guidelines or manualized treatment methods.

Further, one may imagine that the development of standardized treatment methods, which, typically, are brief treatment formats, will in some cases make psychotherapeutic treatment more efficient, so that more patients will be able to receive treatment in a system with limited treatment resources.

Treatment manuals and clinical guidelines may indisputably be helpful in training new therapists to apply certain treatment methods, just as standardized methods can support therapists, especially less experienced therapists, in their work. Besides, many practitioners will be able to draw inspiration from manuals for the treatment of specific disorders, if they are going to work with a patient who presents issues that they have little or no experience with (see Chap. 5, on the use of manuals). On the other hand, the spread of standardized treatment packages and the mandatory use of certain treatment methods in the healthcare sector appears to be a symptom of the growing lack of confidence in public-sector employees that permeates the introduction of public management methods with its associated regimen of standardization, documentation and evaluation across public institutions in recent decades. Turning this trend, which is so destructive in many regards, around will require renewed trust, including trust in the individual therapist's professional competence and judgement.

The prevailing approach to psychotherapy is rooted in medical science and the somatic treatment system, where the attempt is to develop specific techniques for the treatment of specific disorders and to secure evidence for these via randomized controlled trials (RCTs). Thus, the development of psychotherapeutic treatments has largely been driven by a predominantly medical understanding of psychotherapy, which in many regards is out of step with key elements in what might be called the classic psychotherapeutic culture, which has its roots in a predominantly humanistic approach to individuals and to psychotherapy. Moreover, and even more importantly, this approach to psychotherapy, as mentioned earlier, is not based on what empirical studies tell us about the effect of various forms of psychotherapy and what is effective in psychotherapy, in the sense that there is no indication that specific therapeutic techniques or treatment models are significantly more effective than other approved methods in the treatment of specific disorders (see Chap. 5).

Thus, we need to focus much more on something other and more than specific techniques for the treatment of patients with specific diagnoses. The prevailing strategy of optimizing psychotherapeutic treatment in the healthcare sector by means of a fairly one-sided implementation of so-called evidence-based treatment methods is misguided. We should instead—or, perhaps, also—apply a much broader strategy that focuses on individual therapists' personal qualities and relational skills: the therapist's ability to meet his or her patients with a fundamental psychotherapeutic stance and work with the diverse dynamics that play out in the therapeutic space. These dynamics are far from predictable and cannot be captured by a manageable number of categories—preconditions for formulating standardized guidelines for how they should be handled by the therapist, given the inherent logic of the medical model of therapy.

The Crucial Role of the Therapist's Personal Qualities

As early as 1936, the American psychologist Saul Rosenzweig poses the interesting question whether the factors that are claimed to be effective in a given therapeutic model or method are in fact the ones that determine the treatment effect, or whether psychotherapy outcomes might in fact be determined by other factors that are perhaps equally or even more important; factors that are common to the various treatment models. He addresses the question of how we can explain the fact that apparently dissimilar treatment methods—or 'psychotherapeutic ideologies', as he aptly calls them—have more or less similar effects in patients with the same disorder. A question that can only be said to have gained relevance since Rosenzweig first raised it. Rosenzweig recommends that we turn our attention to the individual therapist's personality and the good therapist's personal qualities, if we wish to uncover what determines the efficacy of psychotherapy, rather than focusing exclusively on possible differences in the efficacy of specific models for the treatment of specific disorders, as in, 'is cognitive behavioural therapy or psychodynamic therapy more effective in treating depression,' or 'is mentalization-based therapy more or less effective than dialectic behavioural therapy in treating personality disorders?'

As mentioned earlier, most outcome studies and meta-analyses indicate fairly clearly that there are no major differences in the outcomes of widely recognized psychotherapeutic methods, provided they are carried out by properly trained therapists and in an institutional setting with adequate resources. As will be discussed in more detail later (see Chap. 6) it seems increasingly likely that factors pertaining to the individual therapist are at least as important—in some cases probably much more important—for treatment outcomes than whether the therapist uses or adheres to one or the other psychotherapeutic method. Arguably, we should therefore stop devoting so many resources to comparing and expanding the evidence base of recognized treatment methods. Instead, we should consider how we can best ensure that individual psychotherapists are adequately or optimally prepared to work with their patients. This would include making sure that only people with the requisite personal qualities practise psychotherapy. This is especially important for psychotherapy with patients who have severe psychological disorders, where the effect of what happens in the therapeutic relationship can be particularly potent, in both a positive and a negative sense—and not all patients have the same capacity to handle or stand up to incompetent practitioners. In fact, several studies have found that there may be considerable differences between the average treatment outcomes for different practitioners, even when they claim to apply the same more or less manualized method to treat patients with the same disorder (diagnosis). This seems to be especially true when the patients have more severe psychological disorders (see Chap. 6).

Factors pertaining to the individual therapist's personal qualities, way of meeting and relating to the patient and ability to continually match his or her interventions to the patient's unique needs—aspects that are largely or completely ignored in the development of standardized treatment methods—thus seem to have considerable impact on the treatment process and its outcome. 'The psychotherapist matters,' as

Lester Luborsky, one of the 'grand old men' of psychotherapy research, wrote in an article on the topic quite a few years ago (Luborsky et al. 1997). Unfortunately, his observation has done little to draw attention away from the one-sided focus on specific and, in practice, verging on decontextualized treatment techniques. This focus implies that therapists must use particular interventions for the treatment of patients with a particular diagnosis, completely lacking the necessary awareness of the major differences one might see between people with the same diagnosis and, thus, differences in what the patient may need at different stages of the treatment. These are differences that the individual therapist must be able to notice and meet with an appropriate response by matching the treatment to the patient's current state and needs.

Although there is, thus, scant evidence of any close link between psychotherapy outcomes and the specific choice of treatment methods, the existence of such a link still dominates the prevailing view in most psychotherapeutic literature. Consequently, specific treatment methods are the primary focus of both empirical psychotherapy research and psychotherapy training, although there has in recent years been a certain softening in the very narrow focus on specific therapeutic techniques, including attempts to include some of the common therapeutic factors and maximize their impact by means of certain techniques (Safran and Muran 2000; Safran et al. 2011; Jørgensen 2009; Norcross 2011).

Matching the Method to the Individual Patient

The field of psychotherapy spans a range of fundamentally different perceptions of the nature of psychotherapy and what constitutes the core of good psychotherapy; perceptions that are rooted in very different views of human nature. The medical model of psychotherapy is thus far from the only one, despite its growing prevalence and dominance in recent decades. It is also important to remember that psychotherapy may de facto mean many different things and be used to address widely different issues. This makes it difficult to speak of psychotherapy as a uniform, homogenous concept. Among other things, this means that although the present book argues that the therapeutic relationship and the therapist's personal qualities—therapist factors—are absolutely crucial for the course of psychotherapy—the psychotherapeutic process—and its results—treatment outcome—there are forms of psychotherapy and individual psychological disorders where the use of a specific method is of crucial importance, while the therapist's personal qualities and the therapeutic relationship are of relatively limited importance. This is especially true of brief treatments of less severe disorders, including Internet-based 'therapy' and certain types of very focused cognitive treatment of less complex anxiety disorders.

Further, the book in no way argues that therapeutic technique is insignificant, only that in many cases it matters less whether the therapist chooses one or the other recognized psychotherapeutic methods, provided he or she is trained in one of these and has a reasonable mastery of it. Instead, we should be focusing much more on other factors besides the narrowly technical elements of psychotherapy. In practice, of course, it is no easy task to distinguish between the therapist's technique and the other elements of therapy, since the application of a particular technique with its underlying, scientifically informed understanding of psychopathology is a precondition for anything to unfold in the therapeutic space that warrants the term 'psychotherapy'. Moreover, technique is part of the foundation of the therapeutic relationship and for the therapist's ability to maintain a stable therapeutic stance and to intervene in ways that are meaningfully connected to what forms the core of the patient's difficulties.

In practical terms, this means, for example, that it is rarely a good idea to apply a method, with its associated perception of pathology, developed for brief cognitive therapy for less severe anxiety disorders if one is working with a patient with a severe depression or personality disorder. On the other hand, it will often be less important whether one chooses a cognitive, an interpersonal or a psychodynamic method developed for the treatment of depression, if the patient's main problems seem to conform to a diagnosis of depression. Or whether one draws one's main specific interventions from mentalization-based therapy, dialectic behavioural therapy or psychoanalytic therapy in working with a patient with a borderline personality disorder (BPD), even if the psychoanalytic treatment method in its more advanced versions does prepare the therapist much better for handling those aspects of the therapeutic relationships that appear to be key in working, for example, with BPD. Further, it will of course often be helpful if the therapist has received specialized training in working with a specific patient group—such as patients with severe personality disorders, eating disorders or chronic depression—if he or she is going to work with this patient group; training that is not focused on specific interventions or techniques.

The Therapist's Judgement

It is essential for a therapist to be able to judge what is the core element of the symptoms and challenges the patient presents. Based on a qualified diagnostic assessment—which does not necessarily require the use of authorized diagnostic systems but rather a systematic, qualified and scientifically informed assessment of the patient, including the patient's current level of functioning, personality organization and treatment needs—the therapist chooses a therapeutic strategy and method that is meaningfully related to this assessment. Among other factors, this requires empathy, a capacity for psychological thinking, extensive knowledge about a wide range of psychopathologies, good judgement and a reasonable sense of the limits of one's own ability and the need to seek advice from colleagues—all skills that do not readily lend themselves to being standardized and manualized.

Unlike many 'novices', experienced psychotherapy experts rarely base their work on a rigid application of guidelines and manualized treatment methods. They are much more likely to improvise, follow their intuition and match their strategy to the patient's present state. An experienced psychotherapist will often deem the rigid adherence to standardized guidelines for 'good psychotherapy' an obstacle to optimal treatment, which instead involves deviating from the standard treatment when it is called for. The seasoned therapist's ability to trust his or her intuition and engage in qualified improvisation stems from having completed extensive theoretical and practical training in the fundamental elements underlying good psychotherapy—and developing a sensitive psychotherapeutic stance, where tiny nuances in the patient's appearance, the therapist's own reactions in the therapeutic space (countertransference) and what happens in the therapeutic relationship continually shape the therapist's understanding of the patient, the specific choice of interventions and the continual revision of the therapeutic strategy. Often, this happens largely outside the therapist's conscious awareness.

To be able to relate to the patient in a way that is spontaneous, creative and professional the therapist must first internalize a fundamental therapeutic stance and the core therapeutic skills. To deviate from the standardized methods in a qualified way, the therapist must first know the approved methods or, ideally, internalize them until they become second nature and unfold naturally in the moment. This lets the therapist draw on these core methods without necessarily being aware of it consciously. In a sense, the psychotherapeutic stance and method gradually transform into a repertoire of procedural skills (and, to some extent, tacit knowledge) in the experienced and competent clinician (Pflichthofer 2012:31). On the other hand, deviating from the standardized methods without proper knowledge of them will, at best, be a sign of amateurism and a lack of professionalism. Any deviation from the standardized methods must occur within the basic framework of professional therapeutic practice, including the premise that the therapeutic process solely serves the patient's, not the therapist's, needs; that the therapist cannot violate the patient's personal boundaries and integrity; that the therapist is bound by confidentiality concerning what the patient says in the therapeutic space and so on.

In recent years, it has become increasingly obvious that factors pertaining to the individual therapist have a crucial impact on the outcome of psychotherapy, an impact that in many cases clearly outweighs the impact of specific treatment techniques. Moreover, the classic RCT approach that has dominated empirical therapy research is not without its problems, and we should therefore be to conclude too much from the findings of individual RCTs. We have to be critical—and aware—of the obvious shortcomings of the approach to psychotherapy and psychotherapy research that underlies RCTs, without rejecting the findings of these studies as irrelevant, which they are clearly not. However, in reading and interpreting them, we need to consider the context in which they were carried out. Generally, there is good reason to take a closer look at what might be the specifics of the so-called therapist factors: the non-technical elements of psychotherapy that do not readily lend themselves to being manualized and standardized, and which refer to the therapist's personal qualities and relational skills, the therapeutic relationship and the therapist's way of meeting the patient: in short, the psychotherapeutic stance. One of the key elements in the psychotherapeutic stance is that the therapist's approach to the patient and choice of treatment strategy should be matched to the individual patient. That is precisely what makes it so difficult to specify in exact terms what generally characterizes an optimal way of meeting and relating to a patient, which is an important aspect of the psychotherapeutic stance. Nevertheless, the present book attempts to do that, to the extent it is possible.

The dynamic-relational psychotherapeutic stance, as it is outlined in Part II of the book, is especially relevant in long-term individual psychotherapy and in work with patients with personality disorders of varying severity. The individual aspects of the psychotherapeutic stance, however, are clearly helpful and have the potential to enrich practitioners' work with all types of psychological disorders where it is relevant to apply a psychotherapeutic understanding of the issues the patient presents with. Thus, all types of therapeutic work with people who have psychological disorders call for the clinician to apply a qualified professional gaze to his or her patients' challenges, to understand and use his or her own reactions in the treatment process and to relate to the patients in a way that maximizes the chances of a positive treatment outcome. All elements that are addressed in the present attempt at understanding the psychotherapeutic stance. The book's intention is pragmatic in the sense that it attempts to define and understand the psychotherapeutic stance without explicitly addressing the many similarities and differences among the psychoanalytic, cognitive, interpersonal and other psychotherapeutic models with their related (often very vaguely phrased) ideas about what characterizes the psychotherapeutic stance. Although the more theoretical discussion about what separates and unites the great treatment traditions is interesting, it would inevitably become too far-reaching, too complex and not sufficiently relevant for most psychotherapists to fall within the scope of the present book.

The Structure of the Book

Part I takes a critical look at the medical model of psychotherapy and at the struggle between this view and what Bruce Wampold called a contextual model of psychotherapy, which the present text reinterprets, qualifies and instead refers to as the dynamic-relational model of psychotherapy. One could speak of an ongoing culture war in the field of psychotherapy, where some would argue that we are allocating too many resources to securing an evidence base for treatment models that we already know have more or less similar outcomes. Meanwhile, we do not devote nearly enough attention to the impact of the therapist's personal qualities, especially his or her relational skills and stance, on the course and outcome of psychotherapy. Part I outlines the therapist factors that seem to be important in individual psychotherapy with adults—factors that should have a central place in our understanding of psychotherapy, in the selection of therapists and in the training of new psychotherapists. Even if the more common practice today of training therapists to apply specific therapeutic techniques may seem less complicated than teaching therapists how to manage a therapeutic relationship, decode what the patient needs in the present moment and match his or her interventions and ways of being with the patient to this perception. Although the book does not claim that proper psychotherapy training programmes ignore the importance of the therapeutic relationship, the key question is to what extent the focus is on teaching specific techniques versus the somewhat more complicated development of personal qualities and the cultivation of a psychotherapeutic stance.

However, there is no way around it. Our understanding of psychotherapy and the training of new practitioners must reflect the actual complexity of psychotherapeutic practice, if we wish to optimize our psychotherapeutic treatment services. Although it may of course be tempting to look for shortcuts, such shortcuts are unlikely to exist. Practising psychotherapy is a complex, demanding but also tremendously interesting and rewarding endeavour. The medical model of therapy assumes that therapeutic techniques are key to treatment outcomes, and that the key goal for the individual therapist should be to learn to be as precise, competent and neutral as possible in implementing a specific technique. Thus, in principle, it should not matter who the therapist is that delivers the treatment. The therapist's subjectivity and personal qualities are viewed as potential source of errors or obstacles to the optimal implementation of the standardized treatment. At best, these factors are seen to be of secondary importance for the treatment outcome.

Part II is an attempt to unfold what characterizes the psychotherapeutic stance, how a psychotherapist should meet his or her patients, think about the challenges presented by his or her patients and handle what plays out in the therapeutic space. All things being equal, these aspects contain important information about and actualize what is at the core of the patient's difficulties. Part II is largely based on modern psychoanalytic theory, in part because psychoanalysis clearly offers the most nuanced insight into the phenomenology of psychopathology and psychotherapeutic skills, and in part because it is mainly psychoanalysts who have explored how we should interpret what happens in the therapeutic relationship and how to develop a psychotherapeutic stance to be able to handle it and use it therapeutically. While Part I is based mostly on knowledge from empirical studies, Part II may be criticized for not being similarly underpinned by empirical studies. This should be seen in light of the lack of empirical data on what defines the optimal therapeutic stance, and how the therapeutic stance should be varied depending on the patient's pathology (diagnosis). Part II may also be seen as an attempt to specify a possible set of common therapeutic factors, where the therapist's personal background, capacity for self-regulation, ability to be present in the therapeutic space—where the emotional intensity may at times run high—and strong relational skills become important aspects of developing as a psychotherapist.

The book should not be seen as yet another general psychotherapy textbook. There are already many such textbooks, of varying quality, including some excellent ones (see, e.g., Gullestad and Killingmo 2013; McWilliams 2004; Strupp and Binder 1984). The focus of this book is far more specific and aimed at what characterizes the psychotherapeutic stance or how a therapist should meet his or her patients across specific treatment models. The book is thus not intended as a collection of specific interventions or a 'new' treatment method; instead, its aim is to apply a sort of meta-perspective to psychotherapeutic practice. Thus, although I draw heavily on modern psychoanalytic thinking and literature—and incorporate modern psychoanalytic methods into my own psychotherapeutic practice (Jørgensen 2009)—I deliberately avoid associating the book with a particular treatment model, such as psychoanalytic psychotherapy, mentalization-based therapy, schema therapy or cognitive behavioural therapy, although that would undoubtedly be a wise strategic move in the sense that some of the practitioners who identify with the method in question would then probably be more likely to read and use the book.

Thus, it is one of the points of the book that these treatment models often develop into more or less entrenched positions in the psychotherapeutic culture, where they also—despite their often indisputable qualities—reflect one of the biggest problems in the psychotherapeutic culture: that people who develop new, promising treatment models gradually acquire a celebrity status, touring the world—in some cases almost as gurus or star therapists—'enlightening' the hungry practitioners with their treatment models and standardized guidelines for therapeutic practice. Guidelines and models which some therapists then subsequently tend to embrace too closely, assuming that they can practise without having acquired the necessary basic therapeutic skills and the fundamental therapeutic stance that are preconditions of all good psychotherapy. And without sufficient awareness that no specific treatment method is equally well suited for all patients and psychological challenges, not even for all patients with a given formal diagnosis. Just as most therapists have a greater talent for applying—and, for various (including personal) reasons, will find it easier to identify with—certain treatment methods rather than others.

The Need for a Scientifically Based Treatment Theory

There can be many good reasons for a psychotherapist to need a good theory and specific guidelines for 'what to do' in the therapeutic space, especially when working with patients with very severe disorders. In the therapeutic space, one may be confronted by powerful, painful and, to varying degrees, almost unbearable emotions and other mental states. That can lead to a need for 'something to lean on' and specific guidelines for 'what to do' from appointed authority figures—regardless whether these 'authority figures' themselves lay claim to this status or have simply been assigned this elevated status by the individual therapist using their method. Any practising psychotherapists will inevitably at times find it chaotic and difficult to grasp everything that happens in the therapeutic space. The therapist may feel powerless, experience shame over his or her (inner or, to varying degrees, expressed) reactions to the patient and be in doubt about what to do or whether he or she is even capable of helping the patient. At least, this is the case, if the psychotherapist has preserved the absolutely essential vulnerability, sensitivity and capacity for self-criticism. When this happens, treatment guidelines and directions about 'what to do' can reduce the therapist's sense of uncertainty and help him or her regain a sense of control and thus make it easier to remain present in the therapeutic space. In that sense, it can be quite helpful to rely on a treatment model. Subscribing to a specific treatment model can, however, become problematic if the therapist identifies so strongly with the model that it becomes an obstacle to alternative ways of thinking and understanding the therapeutic process. This can cause the therapist to become too focused on specific technical interventions and determining which technical intervention is prescribed by the model or its leading proponents—at the cost of his or her ability to listen, be present here and now, maintain a fundamental therapeutic stance and interact optimally with the patient in the present moment.

Scientific knowledge about human psychology, including developmental psychology, personality psychology, cognition psychology and social psychology, is an indispensable foundation for psychotherapeutic practice. It is supplemented by knowledge about psychopathology, psychotherapy and therapeutic change processes. Empirical knowledge and sound theories can help the therapist navigate in and make sense of complex processes and what may initially seem like 'incomprehensible' experiences in the therapeutic space, provided they do not become dogmatic and block the therapist's crucially important curiosity, openness and ability to be surprised by what is happening right now in the interaction with this (unique) patient. Good theory can support the therapist's capacity for nuanced and psychological thinking and his or her ability to contain and be present in the contact with the patient and to offer a balanced response in emotionally challenging situations in the therapeutic space. Similarly, knowledge of developmental psychology, personality psychology, affect regulation, psychopathology, factors affecting therapeutic efficacy and so on will improve the therapist's ability to act empathically in the meeting with a diverse range of patients.

However, theoretical knowledge and awareness of recent empirical research are not in themselves a sufficient basis for becoming a competent psychotherapist. Thus, there is reason to ask whether psychotherapy training sufficiently catalyses the development of the qualities in the therapist that seem to be crucial for good treatment. Questions may also be raised about the need for a systematic way to select and, perhaps, test individuals seeking psychotherapeutic training and authorization to practise psychotherapy, especially when it comes to severe psychological disorders. To the extent that clinical teachers in universities and continuing psychotherapeutic training programmes serve as role models for future generations of psychotherapists—and students, to varying degrees, internalize the stance these teachers model both explicitly and, not least, implicitly in their appearance and their expressed understanding of their patients, themselves and psychotherapy—it also becomes relevant to consider how best to select the people who train prospective psychotherapists. Moreover, the individuals who are going to train new psychotherapists should themselves practise psychotherapy in order to maintain and continue to develop their psychotherapeutic expertise and their sense of the complexity of the therapeutic process (Skovholt et al. 1997:367).

With Cushman (2013), it may be argued that a given historical period can be understood in the context of, among other things, the prevailing view of human psychology, psychological disorders and their treatment and the view of human nature that it reflects. From this perspective, it is worth noting how the currently prevailing focus on manualized treatment tends to reduce psychotherapy to an instrumental activity and the therapist to a technician charged with implementing standardized methods, in part in order to eliminate obstacles to adapting to the prevailing cultural logic and meeting the prevailing demands for optimal functioning (cf. Cushman and Gilford 2000) (see later) that we are subjected to in the competition state (Pedersen 2011).

1.1 Evidence-Based Clinical Practice

As mentioned earlier, few practitioners would disagree that psychotherapeutic practice should be evidence-based and informed by the best available recent research. The problem is, however, that the actual implications of this are far from clear. This ambiguity has led to intense conflict among different professional positions, just as the concept of evidence has been subjected to, at times, strong criticism, especially from scientists with a humanistic orientation, who see the concept as a seductive weapon of the social sciences against the humanities (Bollas 2013:115). The disagreement concerns both what can be considered (best) research evidence (APA 2006:274) and which specific treatment consequences could or should follow from available research findings. In 2005, the American Psychological Association (APA) adopted a policy for evidence-based clinical practice, defining evidence-based practice in psychology as 'the integration of the best available research with clinical expertise in the context of patient characteristics, culture, and preferences' (www.apa.org). Subsequently, a number of professionals have argued that the main emphasis should be on the clinician's use of the best available research, which typically implies that the clinician should use the specific treatment methods that have achieved the highest possible degree of evidence in empirical RCTs. In relation to this point of view, some have voiced a somewhat rigid and poorly documented criticism of practitioners who have not unquestioningly embraced the idea that the use of a specific evidence-based method is the most important factor in psychotherapy (Lilienfeld et al. 2013). Others have argued that it is downright unethical not to choose treatment techniques that have documented efficacy in RCTs (Chambless and Crits-Christoph 2006:193).

Other professionals have argued that the practitioner's clinical expertise is absolutely crucial, both with regard to decisions about what treatment to offer individual clients and about the subsequent practical implementation of the treatment. This viewpoint acknowledges that there is stronger evidence for the effect of some treatment methods compared to others, but it also views the choice of treatment method as one among many, equally important factors influencing treatment outcome. Thus, it warns against attributing too much importance to the choice of treatment method under the notion of evidence-based clinical practice at the cost of other aspects of therapy. Moreover, it argues that factors pertaining to the therapeutic relationship and the individual therapist are not given sufficient weight in most of the many treatment manuals and clinical guidelines that have been developed in recent decades, which typically describe how a practitioner, who is seen as a non-subject, should implement standardized methods for the treatment of specific disorders (Norcross and Lambert 2011:7). This view tends towards reducing the therapist to a neutral observer, an essentially replaceable professional technician or 'machine' delivering a standardized treatment (Nissen-Lie et al. 2013:484).

The professional dispute, or culture war, in the field of psychotherapy largely boils down to what is the key factor in psychotherapy: is it about specific treatment techniques curing specific disorders, or is it about therapeutic relationships and individuals healing human beings? (Norcross and Lambert 2011:3). A question that is closely related to the dispute between the medical and the contextual models of psychotherapy (see Chap. 3). Naturally, this question represents a simplification, as treatment technique, therapeutic relationship and the therapist's personal qualities are intimately interlinked and interdependent. Nevertheless, a polarization has occurred within the field that is counterproductive in many regards, where so far, the medical model of psychotherapy and its focus on the use of specific treatment techniques has a far stronger standing in large swathes of the research community, at the cost of the further development of our knowledge about some of the core elements of psychotherapy pertaining to the therapeutic relationship and the therapist's personal qualities and relational skills. It is rarely helpful when a single professional perspective gains near hegemonic status, and legitimate calls for evidence-based clinical practice should not be allowed to develop into a one-sided requirement for practitioners to be trained in and applying certain mandatory standardized methods.

Evidence-based practice is something other and far more than that, including bringing a qualified approach to clinical decision-making processes and therapeutic practice in general, underpinned by empirical research. Roughly speaking, the efforts to identify evidence-based treatment methods take their point of departure in a—typically relatively simple, brief, manualized—treatment method and queries whether RCTs show this method to be effective in the treatment of a given disorder. Evidence-based clinical practice, on the other hand, takes its point of departure in the patient, asking what research findings—including findings from RCTs—can help the therapist achieve the best possible treatment outcomes (APA 2006:273). Here it is important to note that with the increasingly intensive focus on certain types of evidence-basing (mainly RCTs), and especially on evidence-based treatment techniques, the latitude for practitioners in clinical practice may de facto become restricted. That is the case, for example, if insurers and public health services only fund or approve treatments that use certain methods in the treatment of certain diagnoses, with reference to the evidence for the efficacy of these (and only these) methods. Here too, the key problem is that it is based on the erroneous assumption that the applied treatment technique is what determines the treatment outcome, while all other factors—which, so far, have proved more difficult to document—are ignored, to varying degrees.

Clinical Expertise

Professional organizations and psychotherapeutic cultures try to maintain a focus on a broader range of factors in the understanding of psychotherapy. The APA has established two working groups that monitor the evidence for specific treatment methods and the interdependency of factors in the therapeutic relationship and treatment outcomes. Among other outcomes, work in the two groups has led to the publication of two influential anthologies, which have since been published in several editions: 'A guide to treatments that work' (Nathan and Gurman 2015) and 'Psychotherapy relationships that work' (Norcross 2011). Roughly speaking, the former focuses mainly on the issue of *what* the therapist should do—which technique/method the therapist should choose for the treatment of a patient with a given diagnosis—while the latter seeks to address the far more complex, but in many regards much more important, question of *how* the therapist should 'be' and work with the patient, including the possible implementation of a specific method with this particular patient, based on empirical research. The therapist not only needs to know what disorder (diagnosis) the person has but also what person has the disorder and address this in the treatment (APA 2006:279). This brings us closer to what the psychotherapeutic stance involves and to the specific content in one of the main elements in the APA's definition of evidence-based clinical practice: clinical expertise.

In an attempt at specifying what is included in the concept of clinical expertise, the APA points out that the psychotherapist must have highly developed competences within the following eight main areas, all of which promote good treatment outcomes (www.apa.org):

(1) Conducting assessments and developing diagnostic judgments, systematic case formulations, and treatment plans.
(2) Making clinical decisions, implementing treatments, and monitoring patient progress.
(3) Possessing and using interpersonal expertise, including the formation of therapeutic alliances.
(4) Continuing to self-reflect and acquire professional skills.
(5) Evaluating and using research evidence in both basic and applied psychological science.
(6) Understanding the influence of individual, cultural, and contextual differences on treatment.
(7) Seeking available resources (e.g., consultation, adjunctive or alternative services) as needed.
(8) Having a cogent rationale for clinical strategies. Expertise develops from clinical and scientific training, theoretical understanding, experience, self-reflection, knowledge of current research, and continuing education and training.

These elements all appear to be essential for qualified psychotherapeutic practice, and to varying degrees they form part of the basis for the psychotherapeutic stance that the therapist should adopt towards his or her patients. However, point 3 and, to some extent, points 2, 6 and 8—which concern the therapist's relational skills, judgement and ability to match his or her strategy to the patient's unique characteristics and needs—are especially relevant for the psychotherapeutic stance. APA (www.apa.org) adds that psychological treatments are most effective if they are matched to the patient's specific problems, resources, personality, sociocultural context and preferences, just as certain patient characteristics, such as functioning level, readiness for change and social network, should be expected to influence the treatment outcome. It is emphasized that in the effort to establish and maintain the therapeutic relationship and in the implementation of specific interventions, one should consider a number of factors, including individual differences in the specific manifestations of the disorder (specific symptoms and behaviours) and its aetiology, the patient's age and psychological development level, history, gender and gender identity, ethnicity, religion, social class, sexual orientation and factors in the patient's surroundings, including current stressors, for example due to unemployment, homelessness and critical life events, negative (traumatic) as well as positive.

It is difficult to disagree that the elements listed by the APA as key aspects of clinical expertise are desirable qualities in someone practising psychotherapy. We should strive to see these skills developed in new therapists by incorporating them, in various ways, in therapeutic training. Naturally, that is already happening, albeit to varying degrees. Still, the somewhat one-sided claim has been made that the use of particular manualized treatment method is all we can really train in a therapist (Chambles and Crits-Christoph 2006:199). Unfortunately, it is somewhat more difficult to operationalize, assess and document that these skills have actually been developed in persons seeking authorization to practise psychotherapy (Tracey et al. 2014). Indisputably, it is far from sufficient for a person to receive a certain amount of teaching and supervision, study specific literature and perhaps complete one or more written assignments—all factors that are relatively simple to quantify and assess, but which in isolation hardly say anything essential about a given therapist's actual clinical competence. If we want to treat this issue seriously, there seems to be no alternative to introducing some form of test and/or assessment of personal qualities in the individual therapist. Moreover, it seems clear that the development of relational skills, clinical judgement and the capacity for psychological thinking and for adopting a psychotherapeutic stance deserves a more central place in the training of psychotherapists.

1.2 The Psychotherapeutic Culture and Cultural Critique

As mentioned earlier, it is somewhat problematic to speak of the 'psychotherapeutic culture' as a well-defined and clear-cut phenomenon. However, there is some basis for saying that most properly trained psychotherapists represent and are tasked with defending certain fundamental human values, which are under pressure in late modern Western culture, and in that sense they counterbalance prevailing developments in contemporary culture. Some might even claim that the psychotherapeutic culture contains subversive elements in relation to some parts of our late modern society. Moreover, psychotherapists offer certain things that people living in the late modern Western culture appear to have a strong need for.

In a late modern culture characterized by the relentless quest for self-optimization, efficiency measures, pronounced individualization, competition, self-evaluation and quantification, only the things that can be quantified, measured and economized 'exist' or matter. That may cause people to develop a cynical and instrumental stance towards themselves and others, to their own body and mind—which have to remain functional, so they can get on with their self-optimization projects. In this cultural context, the classic psychotherapeutic culture and its perception of human beings as vulnerable, social and psychological beings, may seem controversial and anachronistic, with its insistent focus on our inner subjective life and very different values than the ones driving the late modern competition state (Pedersen 2011) and neoliberal ideas of the good society with its focus on economic rationales and its tendency to reject all other notions of the good life and the good society that go beyond an individual focus. The late modern competition state is driven by a fundamental fear of falling behind in overvalued ideas about competition with other states (which are similarly worried about falling behind). Thus, the focus is shifted from individual well-being to the competitiveness of replaceable individuals and their contribution to the human capital of the competition state, including a perceived and constant need to produce ever more in ever shorter time. Here we are dealing with a societal logic that is apparently so compelling that we lose sight of the original goal of our strivings for efficiency and optimization: maximizing human happiness and well-being. The relentless drive for efficiency and optimization has become a goal in itself, perhaps supplemented by the maximization of material wealth at the cost of mental balance and well-being.

Due to this relentless (societal) compulsion and (individual) urge for self-optimization it is difficult to accept and make room for the slow pace of psychological development processes. Similarly, psychological difficulties and disorders are seen as irksome obstacles that need to be cleared away as quickly as possible with various types of quick fixes in the form of psychoactive drugs or focused and action-oriented brief therapeutic treatments; both of them treatment forms that are well aligned with a Zeitgeist that calls for maximum efficiency and the development of technical solutions to virtually any emerging problem. From a psychotherapeutic point of view, it can be quite problematic if the measures taken in an attempt to treat psychological difficulties in their basic structure reproduce part of the condition that led to these difficulties in the first place: the instrumental perception of the self and the relentless quest for increased efficiency. As psychotherapists, we need to represent and stand up for values and perceptions of our patients and human psychology that act as a counterbalance, rather than reproducing those elements in contemporary culture and the patient's life that, to varying degrees, have led to the psychological difficulties that caused the patient to seek treatment.

The psychotherapist's task is not to provide simple answers or short-term quick fixes of complex problems, let alone to 'eliminate' irrational or socially undesirable behaviour, including contributing to the patient's unreflective adjustment to a given social reality. Although, naturally, it should never become a goal in itself for psychotherapeutic treatment to be long-term, a psychotherapist must insist that it is often a lengthy and in-depth process to help patients with more complicated psychological difficulties improve their life. We need the psychotherapist's qualified professional stance as a counterpoint to prevailing untenable ambitions of developing standardized quick fixes for severe emotional issues (Ogden and Gabbard 2010). There are limits to how much more we can accelerate basic psychological development processes without derailing the effort and arriving at a point where we are no longer promoting development but instead risk repeating harmful elements from the patient's life in the form of an impatient, inattentive, instrumental and excessively action-oriented approach to the patient's self. In psychotherapy, the patient is invited to linger in and explore his or her painful experiences and difficulties instead of following his or her potential urge to *act* as a means of escaping as quickly as possible or 'getting rid of' whatever it is that causes pain and difficulty and stands in the way of the idea of the optimal self—probably the patient's customary but not particularly successful strategy.

The psychotherapist catalyses the patient's ability to think about his or her difficulties and about how perceived problems, symptoms and dysfunctional behaviour can be understood and related to the patient's history, current life situation and way of living rather than simply looking for quick 'solutions' through concrete action. In keeping with the tradition in the psychotherapeutic culture, therapists must resist pressures that seek to reduce them to technicians who are supposed to 'fix' well-defined problems and eliminate symptoms and undesirable behaviour in the quickest, most pain-free and cheapest manner possible, including encouraging the patient to adjust, without reflection, to prevailing middle-class norms and ideas about 'the good life'. Instead, psychotherapists should draw attention to the possible link between psychological disorders and developments in contemporary culture, especially when we see major shifts in the share of the population seeking psychotherapeutic treatment and in the symptoms the patients present. Meanwhile, of course, the main task always remains helping the patient, as much as possible, to deal with painful emotional difficulties and symptoms and improving the patient's well-being and self-expression.

The psychotherapeutic process is structured around a number of elements that are in short supply and high demand in our late modern society, including undivided attention of the individual person's self, subjective experiences, emotions and well-being and a space with time for immersion and reflection, unconditional acceptance, confidentiality and clear boundaries, where the patient can feel confident that when he or she opens up to the therapist, sharing painful or shameful experiences, this is not going to be shared with a wider audience on various platforms and in the social media, let alone used against the patient in a potential later conflict or competitive situation. It stays in the therapeutic space and becomes part of the shared experience and story that the patient and the therapist co-create. Some of the key aspects of the psychotherapeutic space and the psychotherapeutic stance, characterized by a slow pace, patience and the therapist's calm 'presence' and readiness to listen (Strupp and Binder 1984:41), clash with—or stand in opposition to—a Zeitgeist and a culture characterized by restlessness and impatience, the relentless quest for quick fixes and shortcuts to optimization. Agendas that revolve around mutual competition, 'what's in it for me' and clamouring for attention are suspended in the therapeutic space.

A Humanistic Worldview

The psychotherapeutic culture is framed by a worldview and certain fundamental humanistic values that are arguably threatened, to varying degrees, in a late modern culture characterized by fairly different, if not actually anti-humanistic, values in the perception of, especially, fragile and socially marginalized individuals who do not live up to prevailing ideas about the optimal and, from society's point of view, productive individual. These humanistic values include respect for the patient as a subject with a meaningful and important inner life and personal autonomy—in contrast to meeting others as objects (inanimate things, functions) or instruments to one's own needs satisfaction—and an emphasis on the following aspects, among others:

- The individual's self-understanding, capacity for psychological thinking and for understanding psychological processes in him/herself, other individuals and groups.

- Accepting one's own vulnerability, painful aspects of reality, (mature) dependence on others and perceived powerlessness and helplessness in encountering inescapable aspects of life, such as loss, ageing, disease and the borderlands of human existence (overwhelming anxiety, psychosis, depression, traumatic experiences, 'the alien' in oneself or in others and so on).
- Developing trust and confidence in interpersonal relationships—beginning with the therapeutic relationship, where enhancing the patient's sense of security and fundamental trust in the therapist is sometimes the pivotal treatment focus.
- Striving for an appropriate balance between the basic human need for self-boundaries and the establishment of a unique identity (autonomy) versus the need to be a part of and contributing in a positive way to social communities (attachment) (Blatt 2008).
- Defending and contributing to the development of the (potential) human capacity for love, 'play', containing differences and different but equal perceptions of reality and acting in an age-appropriate manner.

Psychotherapeutic culture represents a non-instrumental approach to human beings and contributes to the critical thinking about developments in contemporary culture that may contribute to psychological overload in late modern individuals. Moreover, it helps put fragile people's experiences and situation into words and to defend people from psychological overload. Practising psychotherapy offers unique insights into the possible experiences of people living in socially marginalized environments and into the conditions underlying a wide range of human behaviour—insights that can be used as a basis for developing a more nuanced and qualified psychological understanding of people in contrast to prevailing tendencies to demonize, devalue and exclude socially at-risk and marginalized groups, including people who are unemployed, immigrants, people who have received psychiatric care and people who fail to live up to prevailing ideas about 'normal' heterosexual sexuality (LGBTQ persons and others); insights that are important to bring into the public debate.

In extension of this, psychotherapists should be reflective in the way they use concepts such as psychological disorder and avoid contributing to a further pathologization of the patients' experiences and psychological functioning, which may lead to an unhelpful distance to the patients. This also requires the therapist to be conscious of his or her own potential need to create such a distance to frightening irrationality, loss of control and unbearable mental states in the patients, precisely by pathologizing them. Without in any way romanticizing or trivializing the patients' sometimes severe challenges, the therapist should remain conscious that the line between normal and abnormal (psychological pathology) is often vague, a matter of degrees of 'disorder' or'dysfunction' that most of us will have some experience with and may have confronted in our own lives, if we dare. This approach can enhance the therapist's empathy for his or her patients and help normalize the patients' difficulties by varying degrees, something that may in turn help the patient feel less alone, alienated, 'different' and marginalized due to his or her perceived problems.

References

APA presidential task force on evidence-based practice. (2006). Evidence-based practice in psychology. *American Psychologist, 61,* 271–285.

Blatt, S. J. (2001). The effort to identify empirically supported psychological treatments and its implications for clinical research, practice and training. *Psychoanalytic Dialogues, 11,* 635–646.

Blatt, S. J. (2008). *Polarities of experience: Relatedness and self-definition in personality development, psychopathology, and the therapeutic process.* Washington, DC: American Psychological Association.

Bollas, C. (2013). *Catch them before they fall. The psychoanalysis of breakdown.* London, England: Routledge.

Chambless, D. L., & Crits-Christoph, P. (2006). The treatment method. In J. C. Norcross, L. E. Beutler, & R. F. Levant (Eds.), *Evidence-based practices in mental health* (pp. 191–200). Washington, DC: American Psychological Association.

Cushman, P. (2013). Because the rock will not read the article: A discussion of Jeremy Safran's critique of Irwin Hoffman's 'doublethinking our way to scientific legitimacy'. *Psychoanalytic Dialogues, 23,* 211–224.

Cushman, P., & Gilford, P. (2000). Will managed care change our way of being? *American Psychologist, 55,* 985–996.

Gullestad, S. E., & Killingmo, B. (2013). *Underteksten. Psykoanalytisk terapi i praksis* [Subtext. Psychoanalytic therapy in practice] (2nd ed.). Oslo, Norway: Universitetsforlaget.

Jørgensen, C. R. (2009). *Personlighedsforstyrrelser. Moderne relationel forståelse og behandling af borderlinelidelse* [Personality disorders. Modern relational understanding and treatment of borderline disorder] (2nd ed.). Copenhagen, Denmark: Hans Reitzels Forlag.

Lambert, M. J. (2007). Presidential address: What have we learned from a decade of research aimed at improving psychotherapy in routine care. *Psychotherapy Research, 17*(1), 1–14.

Lambert, M. J. (2013a). Introduction and historical overview. In M. J. Lambert (Ed.), *Bergin and Garfield's handbook of psychotherapy and behavior change* (6th ed., pp. 3–21). New York, NY: Wiley.

Lambert, M. J. (2013b). The efficacy and effectiveness of psychotherapy. In M. J. Lambert (Ed.), *Bergin and Garfield's handbook of psychotherapy and behavior change* (6th ed., pp. 169–219). New York, NY: Wiley.

Lilienfeld, S. O., Ritschel, L. A., Lynn, S. J., Cautin, R. L., & Latzman, R. D. (2013). Why many clinical psychologists are resistant to evidence-based practice: Root causes and constructive remedies. *Clinical Psychology Review, 33,* 883–900.

Luborsky, L., McLellan, A. T., Diguer, L., Woody, G., & Seligman, D. A. (1997). The psychotherapist matters: Comparison of outcomes across twenty-two therapists and seven patient samples. *Clinical Psychology: Science and Practice, 4,* 53–65.

McWilliams, N. (2004). *Psychodynamic psychotherapy: A practitioner's guide.* New York, NY: Guilford.

Nathan, P. E., & Gorman, J. M. (Eds.). (2015). *A guide to treatments that work* (4th ed.). New York, NY: Oxford University Press.

Nissen-Lie, H. A., Havik, O. D., Høglend, P. A., Monsen, J. T., & Rønnestad, M. H. (2013). The contribution of the quality of therapists personal lives to the development of the working alliance. *Journal of Counseling Psychology, 60,* 483–495.

Norcross, J. C. (Ed.). (2011). *Psychotherapy relationships that work: Evidence-based responsiveness* (2nd ed.). New York, NY: Oxford University Press.

Norcross, J. C., & Lambert, M. J. (2011). Evidence-based psychotherapy relationships. In J. C. Norcross (Ed.) *Psychotherapy relationships that work: Evidence-based responsiveness* (2nd ed., pp. 3–24). New York, NY: Oxford University Press.

Norcross, J. C., & Wampold, B. E. (2011). Evidence-based therapy relationships: Research conclusions and clinical practice. In J. C. Norcross (Ed.) *Psychotherapy relationships that work. Evidence-based responsiveness* (2nd ed., pp. 423–430). New York, NY: Oxford University Press.

Ogden, T. H., & Gabbard, G. O. (2010). The lure of the symptom in psychoanalytic treatment. *Journal of the American Psychoanalytic Association, 58,* 533–544.
Pedersen, O. K. (2011). *Konkurrencestaten* [The competition state]. Copenhagen, Denmark: Hans Reitzels Forlag.
Pflichthofer, D. (2012). *Spielregeln der Psychoanalyse* [Ground rules of psychoanalysis]. Gießen, Germany: Psychosozial-Verlag.
Safran, J. D., & Muran, J. C. (2000). *Negotiating the therapeutic alliance: A relational treatment guide*. New York, NY: Guilford.
Safran, J. D., Muran, J. C., & Eubanks-Carter, C. (2011). Repairing alliance ruptures. *Psychotherapy, 48,* 80–87.
Skovholt, T. M., Rønnestad, M. H., & Jennings, L. (1997). Searching for expertise in counseling, psychotherapy, and professional psychology. *Educational Psychology Review, 9,* 361–369.
Strupp, H.H., & Binder, J.L. (1984). *Psychotherapy in a new key*. New York: Basic books
Tracey, T. J. G., Wampold, B. E., Lichtenberg, J. W., & Goodyear, R. K. (2014). Expertise in psychotherapy. An elusive goal? *American Psychologist, 69,* 218–229.
Wampold, B. E. (2013). The good, the bad, and the ugly: A 50-year perspective on the outcome problem. *Psychotherapy, 50,* 16–24.
Wampold, B. E., & Imel, Z.-E. (2015). *The great psychotherapy debate: The evidence for what makes psychotherapy work* (2nd ed.). London, England: Routledge.

Part I
What Can We Learn From Psychotherapy Research?

Chapter 2
Psychotherapy as Sociocultural Practice

Psychotherapy has become a widespread practice in modern Western societies, and most modern people have at least an intuitive sense of what it is about. However, few consider the fact that the very fact that we use psychotherapy to treat mental disorders is rooted in a number of assumptions about human psychology, normality and psychopathology. Similarly, any attempt at defining psychotherapy implies certain ideas about human beings as psychological beings. The present text is based on an underlying understanding of human beings as inherently social beings who continuously attempt to understand themselves, others and their world in general, which includes levels of psychological thinking—or mentalizing—that attributes both oneself and others with an inner mental life, intentions and other mental states that serve as the basis of reactions and behaviour.

As meaning-seeking beings, we interpret and strive to understand events and subjective experiences, in part by attributing them causality and constructing meaningful narratives. In this endeavour, we are, to varying degrees, determined by our history and past experiences, particularly our interactions with those closest to us. On the other hand, we are also autonomous beings who, to varying degrees, make free choices and are rarely close to being fully determined by our history, brain processes or psychological processes. This may seem quite different from the impression one gets from reading certain types of literature about modern neuroscience, which come close to denying human subjectivity any basis in reality (or any impact on human behaviour), and where human experiences and behaviour are, somewhat one-dimensionally, explained by biochemical brain processes. As a rational being, the individual is free, but as a natural being, the individual is causally determined, and thus, severe psychopathology can shift the balance and reduce our space and capacity for exercising this freedom. Finally, among other processes, we use verbal language to categorize and understand the world, shape the aforementioned meaning-making narratives, communicate and convey information to others, influence others and build social communities.

In natural extension of this view of humanity, psychopathology will often be associated with disorders in several of these areas, including distorted, negative, profoundly simplified or one-dimensional notions of self and others—which may

C. R. Jørgensen, *The Psychotherapeutic Stance*,
https://doi.org/10.1007/978-3-030-20437-2_2

also be described as impaired or fragile mentalizing capacity (Bateman and Fonagy 2006) and identity disorders (Jørgensen 2008)—severe difficulties in perceiving or making sense of and understanding the basis of one's own and others' acts and a compromised capacity to make independent choices. It implies that human behaviour may be controlled by immediate and rapidly changing action urges, characterized by impulsiveness and associated with a sense of being unable to control one's own reactions and acts—whether this is driven by anxiety, inner psychological processes, brain processer or other features outside the person's control. In severe psychological disorders, the verbal language may 'fall apart' in various ways, and it may be difficult for others to understand exactly what the person is trying to communicate. Alternatively, the verbal language may not be used primarily to communicate content but as a form of action, a way of acting out or the evacuation of a subjectively perceived psychological reality. Psychopathology will typically be associated with what Jerome Frank (Frank and Frank 1993) has called demoralization, lack of faith in oneself, the world and the future, hopelessness, helplessness, confusion ('what's wrong with me?'), difficulty in making sense of one's own acts (symptoms) and a sense of alienation. This alienation is a kind of isolation or marginalization in relation to social communities that may occur because a person with a psychological disorder feels 'different', in a negative sense, inadequate, 'defective' and unable to live up to their own and others' expectations and ideals.

Individual psychotherapy can be defined as a predominantly interpersonal treatment based on psychological principles, revolving around verbal communication and the interaction between patient and therapist in the here-and-now. Psychotherapy involves a trained psychotherapist and a patient who is seeking help for psychological difficulties that have a predominantly psychological aetiology. From the outset, the patient has to have a minimum of trust and confidence in the therapist, in the psychotherapeutic process and thus in the therapist's competence and treatment approach. All forms of psychotherapy rest on a set of underlying principles and rules, including ethical guidelines for psychotherapeutic practice; one such principle is that the therapist and patient are, to varying degrees, restricted to specific roles as, respectively, the patient seeking help and the therapist providing help (see, e.g., *Etiske Principper for Nordiske Psykologer*, www.dp.dk, and *Ethical Principles of Psychologists and Code of Conduct*, www.apa.org/ethics/code/). This frames their interaction as a formalized, professional relationship that can be said to contain certain internal contradictions or even paradoxes, which the therapist may need to address explicitly. Moreover, psychotherapy can be viewed as a fundamentally ethical profession requiring highly developed ethics and ethical awareness from the therapist.

The relationship between patient and therapist is often (particularly in long-term therapy) characterized by a degree of trust, emotional closeness, confidence and attachment that is otherwise only—if at all—found in very close personal relationships. Nevertheless, the therapeutic relationship must never develop into a personal relationship, just as there are clear boundaries for the degree and expression of intimacy within the therapeutic relationship. It is always the therapist's responsibility to ensure that these boundaries are not violated, that the relationship does not develop into an intimate private one, and that the therapist's contribution to the therapeutic relationship remains strictly professional. Everything that happens in the therapeutic space must be solely directed at the patient's recovery and needs, not at the therapist's personal needs. The therapist has to create a space where the patient can reveal who she is (in the transference) and where she is seen, without the therapist filling the therapeutic space with his own needs, agendas, personal norms and prejudice about the patient. The therapist must under no circumstances abuse this 'power and position to take advantage of the client's dependence and trust' and must avoid all types of 'non-professional relations with a client that may reduce the professional distance and lead to conflicts of interest or exploitation' (*Etiske Principper for Nordiske Psykologer*). In that sense, the therapeutic relationship is asymmetrical, even though it is, at its core, a relationship between two equal human beings. The responsibility for maintaining these boundaries rests squarely with the therapist, who must also ensure that everything that takes place in the therapeutic space is driven by the purpose of meeting the patient's need for help. Hence, the therapist must remain conscious of the possibility that at some points during the course of the therapy, the patient may—as a result of her pathology and/or the unique nature of the psychotherapeutic space—wish to turn the therapeutic relationship into a private intimate relationship. The therapist must also remain conscious of the absolute need not to give into that wish and of the potential benefit of articulating and seeking to understand the background for it.

As a subject and as a human being, the therapist may become quite involved in the work with the patient, including in the interactions with the patient in the therapeutic space. Meanwhile, the therapist must establish and maintain a psychotherapeutic stance and thus an analytical psychotherapeutic perspective on what unfolds within the patient, the therapeutic space, the therapeutic relationship and the therapist himself. The psychotherapeutic relationship can also be described as paradoxical in another sense (Birksted-Breen 2016): on the one hand, it is a part of real life, with two persons interacting, and on the other hand, it takes place within the therapeutic space, which is, decidedly, not part of real life but some form of socially neutral situation, where it is possible say anything, analyse anything and seek to understand anything, but which also has very specific restrictions on what sort of action is allowed. In that sense, psychotherapy operates and exists in a space in between fantasy and reality, between an internal psychological reality and the concrete external reality, between the present moment and another place (commonly in the past). It represents a unique form of reality, where certain social conventions have been suspended, and where the patient can speak about experiences, act and 'use' the other (the therapist) in ways that are not possible in any other context.

The psychotherapeutic space represents a unique reality, where anything can be said and become the object of shared psychotherapeutic reflection without tangible consequences in the real world outside the therapeutic space (with few exceptions; for example if a patient describes issues or conditions that put herself or others at risk). If the relationship deteriorates into simply being a part of 'real life between you and me', without reference to some form of otherness, a space where the parties merely experience and interact (act out) with no analysis, the psychotherapeutic space—which is a condition for any lasting treatment effect beyond the possible beneficial effects of immediate gratification—has collapsed.

In that sense, psychotherapy and the psychotherapeutic stance are rooted in the concept of enlightenment—the notion that 'truth', understanding, nuanced thinking and insight enhance an individual's freedom and possibilities of self-expression.

The psychotherapist relies on a variety of interventions or techniques that, as much as possible, are individualized and applied in ways that match the patient's individual challenges and needs. The therapist's method and specific interventions help establish a structure for the scheduled meetings between patient and therapist while also bolstering the patient's confidence in the therapist's competence and her hope that the treatment will be effective. Any psychotherapy course involves elements of unlearning, new learning and revision of previous learning, as the patient makes new experiences in the interaction with the therapist and explores her perceptions of self, others and interpersonal interactions, including her thoughts about what happens when she makes emotional contact with herself and important others (Strupp 1986: 124).

Psychotherapy is not primarily aimed at treating psychological disorders where biological factors, including genetic dispositions, and brain processes outside the person's consciousness and control must be assumed to play a key role. This includes, for example, severe affective disorders, schizophrenia and certain types of autism. That is not to say that psychotherapy and others forms of talk therapy cannot in some cases make a highly meaningful contribution for persons with these disorders. That may include conversations where the patient is met as a human being and a subject, and where the focus might be on how he or she experiences the disorder and tries to make everyday life as manageable as possible—that is, conversations of a more supportive nature where the therapist does not necessarily adopt the same psychotherapeutic stance as in actual psychotherapy. Similarly, behavioural training, counselling, philosophical guidance, coaching, pastoring and classic behavioural therapy also do not constitute psychotherapy where the trainer, therapist, counsellor, coach or support person can be expected to adopt or have received training in establishing a psychotherapeutic stance.

References

Bateman, A., & Fonagy, P. (2006[2007]). *Mentaliseringsbaseretbehandling af borderline personlighedsforstyrrelse.* Copenhagen, Denmark: Akademisk Forlag.

Birksted-Breen, D. (2016). Bi-ocularity, the functioning mind of the psychoanalyst. *International Journal of Psychoanalysis, 97,* 25–40.

Frank, J. D., & Frank, J. B. (1993). *Persuasion & healing: A comparative study of psychotherapy.* Baltimore, MD: Johns Hopkins Press.

Jørgensen, C. R. (2008). *Identitet. Psykologiske og kulturanalytiske perspektiver* [Identity. Psychological and culture analysis perspectives]. Copenhagen, Denmark: Hans Reitzels Forlag.

Strupp, H. H. (1986). Psychotherapy: Research, practice, and public policy (how to avoid dead ends). *American Psychologist, 41,* 120–130.

Chapter 3
Medical Versus Dynamic-Relational Model of Psychotherapy

The American psychologist Bruce Wampold has been one of the leading critics of what he calls the medical model of psychotherapy, which has become increasingly dominant in psychiatry, clinical psychology and psychotherapy. Others have previously offered similar criticism, in part with reference to what has been called 'the drug metaphor' in psychotherapy research, arguing that psychotherapy research is misguided in examining the effect of psychotherapy in the same manner as we have traditionally examined the effect of drugs, through randomized controlled trials (RCTs) (Stiles and Shapiro 1989). In empirical psychotherapy research the growing dominance of the medical model of therapy has led to an overemphasis on examining the effect of specific technical aspects of psychotherapy—in an effort to find evidence for specific treatment methods—and a neglect of effective factors that are common to most forms of psychotherapy and of the inevitable interaction between treatment method, therapist, patient factors and treatment effect (Wampold and Budge 2012:602).

Wampold describes the main elements in the medical model, which has its origins in the health sciences (Wampold and Imel 2015:7ff). Based on the symptoms reported by the patient, observations of the patient's behaviour, clinical tests and examinations, the doctor makes a diagnosis. The diagnosis is assumed to be the result of specific disorders or dysfunctions, and in extension of this assumption, the doctor's primary task is to initiate a specific treatment directed at correcting these underlying disorders or dysfunctions. Roughly put, at the heart of the medical model lies a notion of specificity, where one specific treatment should be initiated to correct the specific disorders or dysfunctions that are assumed to be the origin of the specific diagnosed disorder. When this has been done, the diagnosed disorder is expected to be cured. This treatment specificity can be supported by documenting either that a specific treatment has greater effect than a placebo treatment in curing the specific disorder, or that the prescribed treatment actually works by correcting the disordered or dysfunctional processes that are assumed to lead to the specific diagnosed disorder. Within the medical model of therapy, the gold standard for evidence-based treatment is the randomized controlled experiment.

C. R. Jørgensen, *The Psychotherapeutic Stance*,
https://doi.org/10.1007/978-3-030-20437-2_3

Throughout the 20th century, the health sciences and their research designs and conceptual discourses have gained an ever stronger position within the scientific community. That is an important part of the explanation for the way in which large parts of the psychiatric field and clinical psychology have increasingly embraced key aspects of the medical research designs and ideas about what constitutes good, sound science. For psychiatry and psychotherapy to achieve any research-based legitimacy and thus have a chance of gaining a certain position in modern healthcare services, it was necessary, to some extent, to adapt to the medical research regimen. As a result, the aforementioned medical model of psychotherapy has now been embraced by many psychotherapy researchers and, not least, many academically trained psychotherapists, most of them physicians and psychologists trained in non-psychoanalytic forms of therapy, especially cognitive behavioural therapy. The discussion of a prototypical medical model of psychotherapy in no way implies that all medically trained therapists (psychiatrists) hold this view of psychotherapy, or that all psychologist or others with a non-medical background are necessarily operating from a dynamic-relational perspective. The two categories should be perceived as the prototypical opposite ends of a dimensional understanding that are not automatically associated with specific professions.

The core of the medical model of psychotherapy is that the treatment effect stems exclusively from the therapist's specific technical interventions, which, in principle, should be designed to treat specific disorders (diagnoses). This ignores the often very complex nature of psychopathology, where the individual patient's difficulties are rarely fully captured by the authorized diagnostic categories, and where comorbidity is widespread, which can make it difficult to determine which treatment to choose. The medical model does not attribute the therapeutic relationship any major independent impact on the treatment effect, and any effects associated with the individual therapist's personal qualities or the concrete implementation of the specific treatment are, in principle, viewed primarily as the result of errors in the therapists' application of the specific treatment method (which should be standardized and uniformly applied, regardless of individual temperaments and personalities). With a view to optimizing the individual therapist's technical skills and enabling randomized and controlled studies of the effect of specific treatment methods, it is thus necessary to develop detailed manuals describing the main techniques and principles in the specific treatment. Moreover, methods for assessing and controlling to what extent and how competently the individual therapist actually adheres to the guidelines for the specific treatment, as they are formulated in the treatment manual (the issues of adherence and specific competence are discussed later).

Examining the effect of specific manualized methods in the treatment of specific disorders further requires the development and application of a detailed and reliable diagnostic system for categorizing psychological disorders. That usually means relying on the American Psychiatric Association's authoritative diagnostic manual, the DSM-5. When we—psychotherapists and therapy researchers—thus strive to be accepted into 'good society' in the healthcare system and health sciences by leaning on or even embracing the medical model of psychotherapy, that may be a wise strategic choice. However, it may come at a high price if we lose sight of crucial core elements of psychotherapy—all the aspects that are not related to specific techniques, and which may be difficult to capture via predominantly quantitative methods.

The medical model of therapy has come under harsh criticism from many sides (Wampold and Imel 2015; Norcross 2011; Stiles and Shapiro 1989). The argument is, in part, that the medical model of therapy rests on the flawed notion that psychotherapy consists of a finite array of specific elements delivered more or less mechanically by a therapist—as prescribed by manualized procedures—to a largely passively receiving patient (Stiles and Shapiro 1989). This perception tends to reduce psychotherapy to a form of technology, where the crucial dialogic-interactional and meaning-making aspects are lost or, at least, slip out of focus in our understanding of psychotherapy as a cultural practice. The main issue is thus that psychotherapy cannot be reduced to an objective or neutral therapist's application of specific interventions, and that specifying the active ingredients of psychotherapy is far more complex than for a medical drug. In comparison to the dynamic model of therapy, which is rooted in classical humanities, the medical model of therapy reflects a reductionist and decontextualized view of psychotherapy that may in fact undermine the effect of psychotherapy by causing us systematically to focus on the 'wrong' aspects—standardized specific techniques—at the cost of focusing on the therapist's person and the patient-therapist interaction.

3.1 Psychiatric Culture War

As mentioned earlier, the growing spread of the medical model of psychotherapy has sparked what may be regarded as a sort of culture war in psychiatry and clinical psychology. This conflict is not just about which treatment approaches therapist ought to use; it is also about our more fundamental understanding of psychotherapy and of psychotherapeutic work. It is a struggle about whether psychotherapy consists primarily in implementing specific techniques in our work with patients with specific diagnoses, or whether contact, seeing the individual patient and using oneself in the treatment process are not at least as important. It is a struggle about what should be considered key measures of treatment effect, what meaning we attribute our patients' symptoms and what fundamental norms, values and ideals we, as psychotherapists, convey to our patients, often without being consciously aware of it. It is about norms, values and ideals that our patients, to varying degrees, internalize and make part of their self-understanding, and which may have a major impact on the way they perceive themselves and their psychological difficulties. Fundamentally, this culture war is also a struggle between different worldviews, just as it contains elements of a struggle between different scientific approaches, mainly the humanities and health or natural sciences. Similar to many of the world religions, our scientific paradigms contain strong monotheist tendencies, expressed in the idea that certain approaches and perceptions of the world are seen to represent the truth or the quest for truth (by means of certain specific methods), while alternative approaches, for one reason or another, should be excluded as less true or scientific (Dreher 2016:306f; Slife et al. 2005).

In empirical psychotherapy research, the effort to measure therapeutic effect and thus the goal of psychotherapy is dominated by the use of fairly simple questionnaires focusing on specific symptoms, perhaps supplement with assessments of the patient's behaviour. There is, however, reason to consider whether this focus on measureable symptoms and behaviours—which encourages a more short-term focus on immediate symptom relief, crisis management and improvements in the patient's adaptiveness—is always appropriate. Or whether we should perhaps focus more on changes in the patients' subjective experiences and ability to function as an autonomous subject, to experience meaning in their lives, intimacy, self-insight and a nuanced understanding of themselves and the world and to address the challenges that are part an parcel of the human condition in a more mature manner, including improving their ability to accept ambivalence, complexity and their own limitations.

Being a well-functioning human being, a subject, involves the ability to act with a fair degree of autonomy (not controlled by dysfunctional internal or external forces) and to experience or make meaning—a meaning that is sometimes only revealed or, rather, made in the psychotherapeutic process by examining the patient's history, recurring patterns in the patient's liv and the psychological functions that symptoms or 'disturbed' behaviour may serve (or have served) for the patient (avoiding anxiety, making contact, avoiding 'dangerous' emotional intimacy and so on). The psychotherapeutic stance that the present book seeks to examine and specify is rooted in these sorts of long-term goal and humanistically oriented norms and values—a humanistic worldview that the therapeutic work implicitly seeks to convey to the patient. In a culture with a strong emphasis on the immediately quantifiable (specific symptoms, specific behaviours) and with expectations of quick fixes to complex problems, a psychotherapeutic culture that seeks a deeper understanding of the individual person's uniqueness and subjective experience will invariably represent a contrasting world view and a critical humanistic opposition (Summers 2013:27f).

On reflection, it seems a somewhat peculiar—technically rationalist (Sassenfeld 2015:117)—assumption that we should be able to develop specific, universal prescriptions for the treatment of specific disorders, which we in principle assume can be applied more or less independently of the given context and the patient's general psychological (personality) function. That includes the idea that the application of standardized methods should be assumed to provide predictable and more or less uniform results, without any need for the individual therapist to reflect much or bring any creativity and judgment to the process. At least similarly remarkable seems the insistence that we should expect decisive differences in the effect of specific treatment methods, when the bulk of the available data suggests that this is rarely, if ever, the case—and that all we need to do is to develop better methods to capture these differences, which so far have largely appeared to be elements in certain researchers' and therapists' wishful thinking.

Subjectivity as a Source of Error

In the medical model of psychotherapy research (RCTs) the human (the therapist's) subjectivity is mainly seen as a source of error that should be minimized in order to achieve what is perceived as the best possible (standardized) implementation of a specific (manualized) treatment method, while the patient's and therapist's subjective experiences and being in in the therapeutic space are at best 'merely' considered to be subjective (not immediately quantifiable) and thus less important and valuable to our understanding and practice of psychotherapy. Moreover, we are currently seeing a tendency to apply causal logic to human subjectivity, which may reflect a tendency towards objectivism and naturalism with a considerable risk of reductionism, where subjectivity is de facto reduced to biochemical brain processes, interactions between entities described in cognitive psychology or other determinist frameworks, while human beings' free choice and more humanistically rooted approaches to human subjectivity are pushed out (Summers 2013:20ff). Throughout much of its history, psychiatry has existed in a span between approaches from the humanities and from the health/natural sciences, but especially in recent decades, certain variants of objectivizing neuroscience seem to have gained the upper hand at the cost of more subject-oriented, phenomenologically and hermeneutically informed approaches. Currently, humanistic values are under pressure in much of the world, just as the humanistic ethos is threatened, which has led some to ask whether 'humanistic perspectives are becoming anomalies in a new positivism' (Øyen et al. 2011:24).

Some studies suggest that a purely or predominantly biological understanding of psychological disorders is associated with less empathy for the patient, compared with a more psychosocial perspective (Lebowitz and Ahn 2014). Such a predominantly biological approach increases the risk of a mechanical dehumanization of the patient (Haslam 2006:258)—where the patient is no longer seen to be able to function as an autonomous individual (subjectivity) and is instead implicitly compared to a mechanical object controlled by biochemical brain processes—just as it also risks preparing the ground for an essentialist understanding of psychological disorders, where psychological states and processes are naturalized, the patient is perceived as qualitatively (categorically) different from other ('normal') people, and the patient's difficulties are largely attributed to genetic dispositions or biochemical brain processes that can be handled by more instrumental means (Werbik and Benetka 2016). Overall, such a strictly biological approach to the patient can hamper the development of a good therapeutic alliance and lead to a more emotionally detached and instrumental contact, although it is not, of course, in itself a problem that the therapist has a biological approach to the patient. The key point is how this is manifest in the therapist's fundamental understanding of the patient and his way of meeting her (as a subject rather than an object, with the purpose of identifying and correcting a mechanical or biochemical 'error'). Here, it is worth noting that a review of the existing empirical studies found that the study of medicine, with its largely biological orientation, leads to a significant decrease in the students' (self-reported) empathy (Neumann et al. 2011). That should be cause for concern and lends credence to the fear that a biological understanding of human beings in itself probably does not constitute a positive influence on the ability to work with psychotherapy, although the presented findings are, of course, open to different interpretations.

A Struggle for Legitimacy—And a Risk of Loss

There are many good arguments why it is essential for the legitimacy of clinical psychology and psychotherapy that we take part in the medically oriented game to provide scientific evidence. Similarly, there are certain conditions framing the use of psychotherapy in the healthcare services (such as budget restrictions that may make it necessary to offer certain patients short-term therapy and to deny treatment to others), which at present must be considered a fact of life that we simply have to deal with, in one way or another, for the time being. It is worth considering, however, whether the historical inferiority complexes of the more humanistically and philosophically based discipline of clinical psychology in relation to the natural sciences are now producing an urge to overcompensate in the form of an excessive focus on quantifiability (data-fetishism) and certain forms of evidence-based documentation (Werbik and Benetka 2016:94), while more complex dynamic-relational processes and aspects that do not readily lend themselves to being quantified are being pushed out of our shared attention.

In extension of this, it is worth noting that academic psychology and the understanding of psychology in most universities in the Western world are dominated by approaches based in health/natural sciences, just as researchers who embrace this paradigm stand to improve their career opportunities considerably, compared to those who are passionate about understanding practical clinical challenges from more qualitative and humanistically oriented perspectives (Buchholz and Gödde 2012). Currently, certain areas of psychology are being flooded with vast amounts of particularized data with nothing even close to an adequate effort to combine the data into a more coherent and meaningful understanding that also illustrates how these data may be of relevance to clinical practice. As the French mathematician Poincaré wrote more than a century ago, science is built of facts the way a house is built of bricks, but an accumulation of facts is no more science than a pile of bricks is a house (cf. Fonagy 2010:73). We clearly need works that seek to integrate the vast amounts of data and relate them to a more general understanding. Parts of the present book are intended as a humble attempt at contributing to this important task.

We also need to ask ourselves what the growing emphasis on quantification (management by objectives), specific treatment techniques, (a certain definition of) evidence and efficiency does to our own perception of ourselves as psychotherapists and to our perception of our patients. This includes considering whether the strong focus on specific techniques might also be driven by a desire to escape uncertainty by embracing the kind of certainty that comes from having clear guidelines for what to do in the encounter with the—anxiety-provoking to some—complexity of working with psychotherapy and with people with severe psychological disorders. Maybe we are not really ready or willing to acknowledge what the increasingly intense emphasis on evidence-based specific treatment techniques is doing to our understanding of psychotherapy and of ourselves as psychotherapists (Cushman

2013:222). Moreover, academic psychology is moving in a direction that might, over time, tip the balance, so that precise research methods and sophisticated statistical analyses come to be seen as being more valuable than the relevance of the content for psychological and psychotherapeutic practices (McWilliams 2013:920).

Even though it is, essentially, not quite meaningful to speak of psychotherapeutic culture as a clear-cut, well-defined phenomenon, in a sense psychotherapists and psychotherapy researchers are playing a sort of 'doublethinking' (cf. Hoffman 2009) with the goal of strengthening the legitimacy of psychotherapy: on the one hand, we play the scientific evidence game—striving for a specific kind of scientific legitimacy by conducting certain forms of efficacy studies (RCTs)—and on the other hand, we also maintain that key elements of the core of psychotherapy cannot be captured by this form of research, which means that the presented research findings have limited usefulness. The risk is that this strategy gradually gets out of hand, so that we increasingly identify with what Cushman (2013:213f) called the 'scientistic' understanding of psychotherapy, embedded in the medical model of psychotherapy.

To the extent that this has already occurred, it may in part explain why the traditional psychotherapeutic culture has had a remarkably difficult time resisting the colonization by administrative systems and their control regimens (Cushman 2012:264). The ability to conceive of and hold on to counter-images to the medical model of therapy is weakened, and strategies for monitoring and standardizing treatment, which form a natural extension of this understanding of psychotherapy, are increasingly accepted—with varying degrees of enthusiasm. Some may have more or less unquestioningly embraced the idea that this development represents progress, while others proceed with a mix of resignation, anger and frustration. On the other hand, categorically rejecting research and psychotherapeutic literature based on a medical model of therapy across the board would be uninformed; even though the medical model of therapy and research has certain obvious shortcomings and despite its problematic near-hegemonic position, it has obviously helped to qualify some aspects of our understanding of psychotherapy.

We need to strike an appropriate balance between boundless relativism on the one hand, where any therapeutic theory and method is considered just as good and 'scientifically' anchored as any other—which is obviously misguided—and, on the other hand, a regimen where therapists are required to apply certain specific methods for the treatment of specific disorders, based exclusively on individual randomized controlled efficacy studies. Similarly, we need a balanced approach to the use of categorical psychiatric diagnoses. On the one hand, we should not, out of hand, reject the use of diagnoses as a simplistic understanding of the patient, who cannot be adequately captured by rigid diagnostic categories. On the other hand, we should also avoid an unquestioning use of diagnoses, where a categorical diagnosis is viewed as capturing the patient's key difficulties and psychology and a satisfactory basis for initiating a standardized treatment with evidence for effect on the given diagnosis.

Moreover, we need to develop the psychotherapist's awareness that certain diagnoses—not least, significant changes in the prevalence of specific diagnoses—may be associated with a problematic individualization and psychologization (and, as a consequence, a decontextualization and depoliticization) of individual psychological manifestations of problematic trends in contemporary culture. This is seen, for example, in connection with the explosive growth in ADHD and depression diagnoses in recent decades, where the real problem is not the diagnoses as such, but the practice that has emerged in how these diagnoses are applied and the predominantly drugs-driven approach to helping the individuals who receive them (Jørgensen 2012, 2014).

Table 3.1 Key differences between the medical and dynamic-relational models of psychotherapy (cf. Wampold and Imel 2015:75)

Medical model	Dynamic-relational model
The therapeutic relationship is primarily a condition for the therapist's successful application of specific techniques. The cores of psychotherapy is a collection of specific techniques and procedures that have efficacy in themselves	The effort to establish and maintain a good therapeutic relationship is in itself a key part of the treatment. Psychotherapy is based on the contact and relationship between patient and therapist, where the therapist adopts a certain stance and implements techniques matching the individual patient
The therapist's primary task is to implement a specific treatment method, and in principle, the therapist is replaceable. The therapist's personal qualities are not seen as central	The therapist's more personal qualities are crucial for the treatment process and outcome, including for the optimal implementation of interventions
The therapist's specific technical competence is central to the treatment outcome	The therapist's relational skills, judgment and other more personal qualities are central to the development of the therapeutic alliance and outcome
Therapist effects are limited and should ideally be minimized by means of training in specific methods	Therapist effects are important—and often play a bigger role than specific methods—and should not be reduced through requirements to apply a standardized method
Specific efficacy factors are primary	Common efficacy factors are primary
The acquisition of specific evidence-based methods should be the key focus in the training of psychotherapists	Developing more personal qualities, such as ability to relate, good judgment, ability to contain intense mental states and ability to notice and repair ruptures in the therapeutic alliance, along with in-depth acquisition of a range of specific treatment techniques, should be the key focus in the training of psychotherapists
Precise categorical diagnostics is an important basis for the treatment work as a basis for choosing a specific treatment method with evidence for effect to the specific diagnosed disorder	Categorical diagnostics is less important than a nuanced psychological understanding and, perhaps, a case formulation of the individual patient's dynamics

Among others, Bruce Wampold has proposed an alternative, non-medical meta-understanding of psychotherapy. He calls his proposal a contextual model of psychotherapy, and it is introduced here as a basis for outlining what in my view should be called a dynamic-relational model of therapy (see Part 2). While the medical model of therapy assumes that factors related to the use of a specific treatment method are the only (or virtually the only) important and effective factors in psychotherapy, a dynamic-relational model of therapy has a far broader and more nuanced perspective, which considers both specific treatment techniques, elements in the therapeutic relationship, factors associated with the therapist's personal qualities, general therapeutic competence and ability to meet the patient with a responsive psychotherapeutic stance and the so-called common therapeutic factors as important for the psychotherapeutic treatment process and for the patient's benefit of the treatment. Although some disorders differ in this respect, the general picture is that *who* the therapist is carries far more weight than the specific method he or she applies (Rønnestad and Skovholt 2013:7). Empirical research thus suggests that in choosing a therapist, the patient is wise to consider the therapist's more personal qualities at least as much as specific treatment method he or she proclaims to use (Lambert 2013b:206) (Table 3.1).

This is not the place for an in-depth treatment of the history of psychotherapy (see, e.g., Ehrenwald 1976; Jackson 1999), but it should be mentioned that this somewhat categorical distinction between a medical and a dynamic-relational model of therapy fails to address the substantial disagreements that have historically existed between different representatives of the dynamic-relational model of psychotherapy (see, e.g., Wallerstein 1995; Makari 2008), including the transition from a classic one-person to a modern two-person model, and fundamentally different understandings of empirical research, for example what qualifies as valid empirical data, and how one can use empirical studies to understand and improve psychotherapeutic practice (see Chap. 8). The two approaches to psychotherapy outlined above are primarily intended as analytical categories, and it is debatable whether any specific, existing psychotherapeutic methods belongs squarely in either one of these categories, or whether most psychotherapists and psychotherapeutic treatment models to varying degrees contain elements from both. Nevertheless, it seems fairly obvious that some treatment models have a stronger element of assumptions from the medical model of therapy, while others align much more closely with the description of the dynamic-relational model of therapy.

References

Buchholz, M. B., & Gödde, G. (2012). Hexen und Besen und was sie fliegen macht. In G. Gödde & M. B. Buchholz (Eds.), *Der Besen, mit dem die Hexe fliegt. Wissenschaft und Therapeutik des Unbewußten. Bd. 1: Psychologie als Wissenschaft der Komplementarität* [The Broom with which the Witch flies. Science and Therapeutics of the Unconscious. Vol. 1: Psychology as a science of complementarity] (pp. 9–41). Gießen, Germany: Psychosozial-Verlag.

Cushman, P. (2012). Defenseless in the face of the status quo: Psychology without a critical humanities. *The Humanistic Psychologist, 40*(3), 262–269.

Cushman, P. (2013). Because the rock will not read the article: A discussion of Jeremy Safran's critique of Irwin Hoffman's 'doublethinking our way to scientific legitimacy'. *Psychoanalytic Dialogues, 23,* 211–224.
Dreher, A. U. (2016). In Babel. *Forum der Psychoanalyse, 32*(3), 299–316.
Ehrenwald, J. (Ed.). (1976). *The history of psychotherapy*. New York, NY: Jason Aronson.
Fonagy, P. (2010). Veränderungen der Klinischen Praxis: Wissenschaftlich oder pragmatisch begründet? [The changing shape of clinical practice: Driven by science or pragmatics?] In K. Münch, D. Munz, & A. Springer (Eds.), *Die Psychoanalyse im Pluralismus der Wissenschaften* (pp. 33–83). Gießen, Germany: Psychosozial-Verlag.
Haslam, N. (2006). Dehumanization: An integrative review. *Personality and Social Psychology Review, 10*(3), 252–264.
Hoffman, I. Z. (2009). Doublethinking our way to 'scientific' legitimacy: The desiccation of human experience. *Journal of the American Psychoanalytic Association, 57*(5), 1043–1069.
Jackson, S. W. (1999). *Care of the psyche: A history of psychological healing*. New Haven, CT: Yale University Press.
Jørgensen, C. R. (2012). *Danmark på briksen. Et psykologisk perspektiv på Danmark og danskerne i det senmoderne* [Denmark on the therapist's couch. A psychological perspective on Denmark and Danes in later modernity]. Copenhagen, Denmark: Hans Reitzels Forlag.
Jørgensen, C. R. (2014). *ADHD. Bidrag til en kritisk psykologisk forståelse* [ADHD. Contributions to a critical psychological understanding]. Copenhagen, Denmark: Hans Reitzels Forlag.
Lambert, M. J. (2013a). Introduction and historical overview. In M. J. Lambert (Ed.), *Bergin and Garfield's handbook of psychotherapy and behavior change* (6th ed., pp. 3–21). New York, NY: Wiley.
Lambert, M. J. (2013b). The efficacy and effectiveness of psychotherapy. In M. J. Lambert (Ed.), *Bergin and Garfield's handbook of psychotherapy and behavior change* (6th ed., pp. 169–219). New York, NY: Wiley.
Lebowitz, M. S., & Ahn, W.-K. (2014). Effects of biological explanations for mental disorders on clinicians' empathy. *PNAS, 111*(50), 17786–17790.
Makari, G. (2008). *Revolution in mind: The creation of psychoanalysis*. New York, NY: Harper Collins.
McWilliams, N. (2013). Psychoanalysis and research: Some reflections and opinions. *Psychoanalytic Review, 100*(6), 919–945.
Neumann, M., Edelhäuser, F., Tauschel, D., Fischer, M. R., Wirtz, M., Woopen, C., et al. (2011). Empathy decline and its reasons: A systematic review of studies with medical students and residents. *Academic Medicine, 86*(8), 996–1009.
Norcross, J. C. (Ed.). (2011). *Psychotherapy relationships that work: Evidence-based responsiveness* (2nd ed.). New York, NY: Oxford University Press.
Øyen, S. A., Müftüoglu, I. B., & Birkeland, F. I. (2011). De unyttige. Fortolkningsvitenskapenes fremtid i det nye akademia [The unproductive. The future of the interpretive sciences in the new academy]. In S. A. Øyen, I. B. Müftüoglu, & F. I. Birkeland (Eds.), *Humanioras fremtid. Kampen om forståelsen av menneske og samfunn* (pp. 9–27). Oslo, Norway: Cappelen Damm Akademisk.
Rønnestad, M. H., & Skovholt, T. M. (2013). *The developing practitioner: Growth and stagnation of therapists and counselors*. London, England: Routledge.
Sassenfeld, A. (2015). *Relationale Psychotherapie. Grundlagen und klinische Prinzipien* [Relational psychotherapy. Basics and clinical principles]. Gießen. Germany: Psychosozial-Verlag.
Slife, B. D., Wiggins, B. J., & Graham, J. T. (2005). Avoiding an EST monopoly: Toward a pluralism of philosophies and methods. *Journal of Contemporary Psychotherapy, 35,* 83–97.
Stiles, W. B., & Shapiro, D. A. (1989). Abuse of the drug metaphor in psychotherapy process-outcome research. *Clinical Psychology Research, 9,* 521–543.
Summers, F. (2013). *The psychoanalytic vision*. New York, NY: Routledge.

Wallerstein, R. S. (1995). *The talking cures: The psychoanalyses and the psychotherapies*. New Haven, CT: Yale University Press.

Wampold, B. E., & Budge, S. L. (2012). The 2011 Leona Tyler award address: The relationship—And its relationship to the common and specific factors of psychotherapy. *The Counseling Psychologist, 40*(4), 601–623.

Wampold, B. E., & Imel, Z.-E. (2015). *The great psychotherapy debate: The evidence for what makes psychotherapy work* (2nd ed.). London, England: Routledge.

Werbik, H., & Benetka, G. (2016). *Kritik der Neuropsychologie. Eine Streitschrift*. GieBen: Psychosozial-Verlag.

Chapter 4
Common Therapeutic Factors

The dynamic-relational model of therapy is based on the so-called common therapeutic factors in combination with the modern psychoanalytic and psychodynamic understanding of therapy. Among others, the American psychiatrist Jerome Frank has made important contributions to the description of common therapeutic factors.

As mentioned earlier, empirical psychotherapy research has for decades sought to crystallize specific therapeutic methods that show markedly better effect than others in the treatment of specific disorders. Generally, this effort has not been successful. The widely approved psychotherapeutic methods show largely similar outcomes for most disorders, and the difference between individual therapists' outcomes within a given treatment model often exceeds the difference between the treatment models (Miller et al. 2013:89). The impact of therapist factors on treatment effect is equal to or larger than the impact of technical factors (see also Chap. 5). Moreover, the so-called component studies—which, roughly put, examine the impact on treatment effect of adding or removing a specific treatment element—generally find limited or no influence of adding or removing specific elements to/from established treatment methods (Wampold and Imel 2015:214ff; Bell et al. 2013). The idea that specific methods or specific technical interventions are crucial for the efficacy of psychotherapy is thus, at best, tenuous, and there is reason to assume that the factors that are common to most or virtually all types of psychotherapy play a greater role for its course and outcome. Based on findings from empirical psychotherapy research, Norcross and Lambert (2011:13) estimate that patients' benefit from psychotherapy can generally be attributed to four main factors with the following relative weights:

(1) Expectancy factors (15%): the patient's positive expectations of the therapist and the therapy.
(2) Technique factors (15%): treatment effect stemming from specific treatment techniques.
(3) Common therapeutic factors (30%): factors that are common to most or all treatment methods.

C. R. Jørgensen, *The Psychotherapeutic Stance*,
https://doi.org/10.1007/978-3-030-20437-2_4

(4) Extra-therapeutic change factors (40%): an unspecified residual category that may include, for example, that the patient expands his or her social network, finds a girl/boyfriend or finds work.

Based on a meta-analysis of various methods for the treatment of depression, Cuijpers et al. (2012:289) later estimated that as much as 50% of the effect of psychotherapeutic treatment can be attributed to common therapeutic factors, while a little over 15% stems from factors related to the specific treatment method. These very general estimates may of course be criticized on a number of counts, including that they do not account for any—probably substantial—differences between specific disorders. Also, it must be assumed that certain treatment methods contribute more to the treatment effect than others, including that treatment models designed specifically to maximize the effect of the common therapeutic factors can be said to challenge the distinction between technical and common therapeutic factors and must also be assumed to make a greater contribution to the treatment effect. It is important to note that the relatively large impact of the common therapeutic factors in no way implies that the psychotherapeutic method or the therapists' training in specific psychotherapeutic methods is irrelevant. On the contrary, a therapist must have solid basic training—for example in psychology or medicine—and be trained in one or more of the approved treatment methods; that is particularly crucial when it comes to dealing with the more severe psychological disorders.

The key point is that it is not essential which of these treatment methods the psychotherapist embraces, identifies with and primarily relies on in his therapeutic work, provided that the treatment planning and the choice of specific interventions are coherent and matched to the condition and needs of the individual patient. This ability to match the treatment to the individual patient requires certain non-technical skills from the therapist—skills that must be numbered among the common therapeutic factors. It is also worth noting that some therapists will pursue an eclectic approach, drawing their specific intervention methods from a variety of therapeutic traditions. Moreover, different treatment models appear to be growing increasingly similar, in the sense that therapists use closely related interventions, sometimes under different labels.

Further, to activate both the patient's positive expectations and the common therapeutic factors, the therapist must use a coherent method that the patient (and the therapist) perceives as meaningful, and which addresses the patient's central problems. In that sense, breaking the therapeutic efficacy factors into four separate and distinct elements is not quite viable—or a reflection of the real world. Any psychotherapeutic intervention is a relational act or event, a point that further underscores the impracticality of operating with a clear-cut distinction between the different therapeutic elements. Technical interventions always take place within and affect the therapeutic relationship, just as the quality of the therapeutic relationship affects the patient's responsiveness to the therapist's technical interventions. If the therapist's interventions make the patient feel seen and understood, that may improve the therapeutic relationship, in addition to possibly improving the patient's self-perception. Moreover, the therapist's empathic contact with the patient may change and improve the patient's self-perception while also serving as a necessary condition for well-timed and well-chosen interventions. Interventions may also be aimed at improving the therapeutic relationship, for example in the form of healing ruptures in the therapeutic alliance (see Chap. 11). Moreover, some of the change factors that are not directly linked to the therapy will often be indirectly related to it, in the sense that the patient may be able to find work or engage (differently) in a romantic relationship thanks to changes brought about by the therapy. The therapy may also give rise to positive synergy effects, where extra- and intra-therapeutic factors mutually intensify one another.

4.1 Corrective Emotional Experiences and Other Common Factors

As suggested earlier, a distinction is often drawn between specific and common efficacy factors or mechanisms of change in psychotherapy. The field suffers under a lack of consensus about exactly how to define and delimit the two concepts. There have also been tendencies to develop simplistic and tenuous dichotomies claiming, for example, that technical or common factors alone—or virtually alone—determine the treatment effect. Theoretically, the therapeutic efficacy factors can be defined as those elements of psychotherapy that explain the effect of psychotherapeutic treatment. In practice, however, it can be very difficult to define and study these factors empirically, since virtually all mechanisms of change in psychotherapy are interrelated and transactional. They do not lend themselves readily to observation, and they relate, to varying degrees, to the individual patient's subjective experience of what happens in the therapeutic space. Historically, a distinction has been drawn between specific and nonspecific efficacy factors:

- Specific therapeutic factors refer to a given treatment method's unique and theoretically founded techniques and mechanisms of change, possibly mechanisms targeted at specific disorders or problem areas. The specific therapeutic factors are often highlighted when prominent representatives of a treatment method seek to define what makes the method unique—what sets it apart from other methods—and explains its alleged ability to achieve particularly good effects in the treatment of specific disorders. The specific factors have a key position in the medical model of psychotherapy.
- Nonspecific therapeutic factors are efficacy mechanisms that are not theoretically founded in a specific treatment method or associated with effect in the treatment of specific disorders, but which are assumed to account for part of the effect of most or all treatment methods for most or all psychological disorders. The concept suffers under that fact that it is often confused with the placebo effect, which has a low status in parts of the health sciences as a kind of random or uncontrolled effect.

Even though it can be argued that the distinction between specific and nonspecific factors is interesting on a theoretical level, in practice it has proven difficult to specify the precise difference between the two categories of efficacy mechanisms. In part, this is because factors that are considered to be specific in one treatment method (such as exposure in cognitive behavioural therapy) are viewed as nonspecific or irrelevant in other treatment methods (such as psychoanalytic treatment), even if they appear to account for much of the efficacy of these methods, whether or not they apply specific techniques to activate or strengthen the efficacy factors in question. In part, it is because certain treatment methods more or less deliberately seek to develop more specific strategies and techniques to maximize the effect of the nonspecific factors, thus rendering the nonspecific factors specific. This applies in particular to more relationally oriented treatment methods, including modern relational psychoanalysis (Jørgensen 2009) and methods focused on repairing ruptures in the therapeutic alliance (Safran and Muran 2000; Muran and Barber 2010, see Chap. 11). As the field has sought to describe, specify and thus maximize the effect of what used to be called nonspecific factors, the concept has, to some extent, become obsolete, which makes it more meaningful to speak of common therapeutic factors.

- Common therapeutic factors are efficacy factors that are common to most or all psychotherapeutic methods, and which, to varying degrees, are part of the theoretical foundation of one or more treatment methods, just as they only have a limited association with the treatment of specific disorders or problem areas. Thus, the common therapeutic factors are not readily suited to highlighting what is unique about a given treatment method—branding it—which may be part of the reason why they have received considerably less attention in psychotherapy research. The common factors are central in the dynamic-relational model of psychotherapy and are far from arbitrary or theoretically unfounded—unlike placebo factors. On the other hand, however, they are also not linked to any specific treatment method.

Common Therapeutic Factors as Part of the Foundation for the Psychotherapeutic Stance

This is not the place for a comprehensive discussion of the common therapeutic factors, but in addition to the ones mentioned above, there are certain common factors that it is helpful to be aware of in the therapeutic work, and which may form part of the foundation for the psychotherapeutic stance (see Jørgensen 2004; Pfammatter and Tschacher 2012; Pfammatter et al. 2012; Pflichthofer 2012; Tschacher et al. 2014). Still, it should be noted that although we can point to many possible therapeutic efficacy factors, based on theory, clinical-psychological experiences and reflection, we have very limited empirically founded knowledge about exactly why (via what processes and mechanisms) psychotherapy works (see, e g., Kazdin 2009):

- *Corrective emotional experiences*. In the interaction with the therapist the patient gains important new corrective emotional experiences that help her revise her perception of self, others, interpersonal relations (inner object relations) and the world in general. Maladaptive interaction patterns or object relations from the patient's past life are actualized in the therapeutic relationship, where the patient unconsciously expects and invites the repetition of patterns that have dominated her relations until now. In a well-functioning treatment process, however, that does not happen, or only to a very limited extent, and if (when) it does happen, the therapist brings it into focus so they can work together to discover what is happening and why. The patient's more or less conscious expectations and fears that maladaptive patterns and experiences from interactions with others will be repeated in the relationship with the therapist are disproven. More or less unconsciously, the patient reacts to the therapist the same way she typically reacts to important others in her life, assigning the therapist a familiar role in the initial re-enactment of maladaptive interpersonal patterns from the patient's life. Guided by the psychotherapeutic stance, however, the therapist does not (or only to a limited extent) react the way the patient unconsciously expects and invites. By reacting differently, the therapist corrects the patient's established ides about herself, others and interpersonal interactions (Melcher 2013:99f; Alexander 1956; Alexander and French 1946). The therapist appears as a new object to the patient, and it is precisely thanks to the therapist's ability to appear as a real other, beyond the patient's projections and transference, that the patient is able to achieve corrective experiences in the therapeutic relationship (Pohl 1979:36f). The patient (re)experiences emotionally intense situations in the therapeutic space that remind her, in important ways, of similar situations earlier in her life. At the time she was unable to handle them, but because these situations now occur under other, more advantageous circumstances and have a different, more positive and less emotionally overwhelming outcome, they serve to correct the inner psychological consequences of the original experiences (Alexander and French 1946:66). This enables a revision of the patient's procedural memory and implicit relational knowledge, which have been dominated by unhelpful and, to varying degrees, distorted perceptions of self, others and interpersonal interactions. What the therapist *does*, the way he acts in the interaction with the patient, her intersubjective emotional contact with the therapist—not only what the therapist says, but who the therapist *is* (Nacht 1962:207)—thus contain essential efficacy factors. Another concept that is sometimes applied is moments (of meeting) or episodes in the therapeutic process characterized by intense intersubjective contact between patient and therapist (Stern et al. 1998) (see Chap. 11), just as corrective experiences also clearly contain elements of exposure (see below). The corrective emotional experience is not a specific technique or tied into the use of specific interventions but primarily concerns the therapist's way of meeting and relating to the patient, that is, the therapist's stance and the emotional climate in the therapeutic space (cf. Alexander 1956:78). This should not be taken to mean that the therapist acts inauthentically, taking on a false role, as some critical interpretations of the concept of corrective emotional experiences have claimed (Treurniet 1997:607). In extension of this, therapists must be driven by a genuine desire to help their patients, which includes examining himself and having an authentic presence that goes beyond a nine-to-five job—without going to the other extreme of boundless self-sacrifice.

- *A trusting relationship reduces isolation.* Patient and therapist develop a relationship built on mutual trust, appreciation and respectful cooperation that helps reduce the patient's perceived social isolation, loneliness and sense of being on her own as she struggles to overcome her problems.
- *Catharsis.* The patient has powerful emotional experiences in the therapeutic space, which also offer an opportunity to release pent-up emotions.
- *Dismantling avoidance strategies.* The patient is confronted with and gradually dismantles her maladaptive avoidance strategies, mainly because they gradually (initially in the therapeutic space, later outside it) prove superfluous and are replaced by more adaptive strategies for self-regulation. Maladaptive strategies for avoiding emotional contact, thematization of traumatic experiences or other situations that are anxiety-inducing for the patient, are dismantled.
- *Exposure.* Via therapeutic work with emotionally intense past experiences and the interactions that play out in the therapeutic space, the patient is exposed to powerful emotions and other mental states that gradually allow her to become desensitized and better able to contain and handle a wider range of diverse and intense mental states. The patient learns that intense emotions and other mental states are not dangerous and that they can be regulated, for example by articulating and reflecting on how they might be understood, and what they pertain to or communicate.
- *Constructing a new self-narrative.* In the therapeutic work, the patient's story is thematized, and new meaning-making connections are established between different elements of the patient's past, present and imagined future life. The patient's existing self-narrative is deconstructed, and a new, more positive, coherent and nuanced story about the patient's life and self is constructed with the therapist as a catalyst and co-author.
- *Appreciating the patient as an intentional subject.* In the way he meets and cooperates with the patient, the therapist signals an appreciation of her as an intentional and responsible person ('you have your reasons to act and perceive things the way you do; let's try to take a closer look at that together'), which promotes the patient's own experiences of agency and of being an intentional person. The patient 'finds' herself as a subject in the therapist's way of meeting and mirroring her as a subject. Thus, the psychotherapist creates a very different starting point than the behavioural therapist, who does not ask the patient why she (as an intentional subject) acts the way she does but mainly tells her that she (as a stimulus-response machine) should act differently.
- *From passive to active.* Because the therapist invites the patient into a partnership and an equal dialogue about how to solve the patient's perceived difficulties, where the patient is expected to contribute actively to the treatment effort, the patient becomes conscious of—and activates—her resources. Over time, the patient leaves the role of passive, paralysed and helpless victim of others' actions and circumstances that lie beyond her control behind in favour of a position as a competent actor in her own life, who, based on a realistic assessment of the circumstances, is capable of making her own choices.
- *Demonstrating self-regulation, inner integration and tolerance.* Through his behaviour in the interaction with the patient and his way of handling intense

mental states in the therapeutic space, the therapist demonstrates how powerful affects and other mental states can be regulated. These are strategies for self-regulation that the patient comes to internalize and gradually learns to use. The patient thus internalizes the therapist's ability to contain and tolerate the patient's emotions, other mental states and aspects of the patient's self. This improves the patient's ability to contain and tolerate aspects of herself as well as her ability to integrate different aspects of the self (and reclaim aspects of the self that had been evacuated and projected into the therapist, cf. projective identification, see Chap. 10). The therapist is the good and tolerant object that the patient can internalize and identify with, which over time can help change the patient's (typically negative) self-perception (Nacht 1962:210).

- *Secure base*. With his person and personal integrity the therapist provides stability, clear boundaries, security, emotional presence, tolerance and authentic attention. The therapist thus fulfils a number of parental functions (by providing a secure base), something that is often important to promote the patient's psychological development, including exploring her internal and external reality, developing her ability to set boundaries and developing her ability to function in social contexts (cf. that psychotherapy in some cases contains elements of socialization into contemporary culture, where the therapist represents norms and values that the patient can internalize). For some patients, the therapeutic relationship is the first stable relationship in their life, a novel meeting with another human being who is focused, authentically present and attentive to their needs rather than his own.
- *Mentalizing develops the patient's mentalizing capacity*. The persistent focus on psychological processes in the patient and in the therapeutic space develops the patient's ability to articulate and think nuanced thoughts (mentalize) about psychological processes in herself, others and interpersonal interactions. In the verbal conversation about the patient's inner life and her subjective experiences and difficulties, the therapist offers nuanced mental representations of the patient's subjective sensations, experiences, affects and other mental states, and these mental representations or verbalizations make the patient's inner life accessible to conscious reflection and more advanced mental processing. The patient improves her ability to understand herself and others, including the possible motivations for human behaviour. With Wilfred Bion we can say that the therapist contributes to the development of the patient's alpha function, that is, the patient's ability independently to create mental representations of experiences (raw, non-verbalized sensations) and mental states (raw affective states and so on), which is the condition for psychological thinking (the ability to build connections between internal and external life) and for understanding and perceiving, especially, emotional experiences as meaningful (Symington and Symington 1996:59ff).
- *Strengthening epistemic trust*. With the progression of the therapeutic work and the patient's positive experiences from the interaction with the therapist, the patient's epistemic trust in what happens in interactions with important others increases correspondingly. Gradually, the patient comes to trust that what the therapist and selected others communicate is credible, generalizable and relevant to her. This engages her capacity for new learning and for learning from experi-

ences in interactions with others (Fonagy and Allison 2014; Allison and Fonagy 2016). The patient's capacity to learn from social experiences is (re)activated. This enables the patient to let go of fixed perceptions of reality—perceptions that the patient has often needed to hold on to as a perceived bulwark against anxiety, chaos and a sense of the self as vulnerable and threatened by information that challenges the patient's established perception of reality—and to be open to new experiences in social interactions offering corrections to previously fixed working models for interactions with others, including rigid notions of self and others. This may counteract the epistemic mistrust, loneliness and blocked capacity to take in new experiences that often come with an insecure attachment pattern, where the patient mistrusts others' communication and intentions. In patients with a severe attachment disorder, the inability to profit from new experiences may be a core pathological aspect where epistemic mistrust prevents the patient from 'hearing', let alone taking in, what the therapist says and does. This underscores the crucial importance of the relational work. The epistemic trust can be strengthened in part by healing ruptures in the alliance and by not repeating maladaptive patterns from the patient's life in the therapeutic relationship but also through what may seem as minute aspects of the therapist's way of meeting the patient, including eye contact, using the patient's name, a certain tone of voice that signals emotional significance and continuous attunement in the therapeutic approach to the patient based on her state and needs in the moment (Allison and Fonagy 2016:289f).

- *Encountering different perspectives on reality*. In a safe setting, the patient is introduced to the existence of multiple possible perspectives on reality, which enhances her tolerance of ambiguity, complexity and the idea that different people can have different subjective perceptions of reality. This improves the patient's ability to contain and manage interpersonal conflicts, which often stem from the presence of different subjective perceptions of events (disagreement), the underlying intentions behind acts and so on. Mentalization-based therapy in particular emphasizes how important it is that the therapist insists on the existence of multiple equally valid perspectives on reality, offering a nuanced specification of these possible perspectives on a given incident and explicitly stating the differences between the patient's and others' perspectives, including the therapist's own (Bateman and Fonagy 2016:183). When the therapist introduces alternative perspectives on the patient's self and perceptions, the key is not the specific content or any notion that these alternative perspectives reflect some kind of 'truth', but rather the very point that the introduction of new perspectives on the patient's material opens new possibilities for self-understanding and new ways for the patient to understand her own history and experiences. That may help the patient gradually abandon previous rigid and fixed interpretations of reality.
- *Nuanced understanding promotes coping skills*. By working with current difficulties and their background in her inner life and history, the patient gains a new and deeper understanding of her challenges. She becomes aware of connections between past events and current difficulties and between inner psychological processes and perceived symptoms/behaviour. At the same time, her cognitive

coping skills improve, as she gets better at decoding the possible motives behind and the meaning of her own and others' behaviour as well as correction or reality-testing of distorted thought patterns.

Key Point: Corrective Emotional Experience

Overall, these common efficacy factors convey the point that a wide range of aspects in the therapeutic process and relationship can impact the patient's treatment outcome. Perhaps the most important common factor, and related to many of the others, is the patient's encounter with new experiences in an emotionally intense, significant and (largely) fundamentally secure context that may correct the patient's maladaptive ideas about herself, others, relationships and the world in general. These corrective emotional experiences form the basic structure, so to speak, of effective treatment. However, it is important to remain aware, especially when working with patients with severe attachment disorders, that a key focus area may be to establish the patient's fundamental sense of security and epistemic trust, which is such a crucial condition for acquiring corrective experiences within the therapeutic space. Generally, the organization of the therapeutic space, a stable framework (same time and place every time) and the therapist's personal credibility, tolerance and authentic interest in the patient can create a sense of calm, structure and tolerance ('holding'), which may in itself serve as a corrective for many patients whose life has been characterized by persistent and erratic changes, turmoil, lack of structure and an absence of any who has shown a genuine interest in their subjective experiences and inner life.

A young woman with a severe attachment disorder and a history of abandonment by key attachment figures has learned to protect herself from further disappointment by never allowing others to get too close and become emotionally significant to her. In that way she avoids the pain from being betrayed or abandoned (again) or, alternatively, from inadvertently causing the relationship to fall apart through her own actions. When she finds that another person is becoming too significant to her, she is overwhelmed by anxiety of being betrayed, taken advantage of and abandoned, which causes her to withdraw from the contact; she breaks off the relationship or looks for/finds flaws in the other to convince her that the person is not trustworthy and should be avoided. As a result, she feels lonely and has a large unmet need for emotional contact. This pattern is now played out in the therapeutic relationship, where the patient long keeps the therapist at arm's length without allowing him to become emotionally significant to her. He is merely a function, someone who happens to play the role of therapist; if he were to be replaced with someone else, (in her opinion) that would make no difference to her. She projects her experiences from past relationships into her relationship with the therapist, expecting and acting as if he is also, naturally, going to let her down and take advantage of her in order to serve his own needs (see also the section on transference in Chaps. 9 and 11). Over time, the patient finds over and over again that the therapist in fact does not let her down, does not try to take advantage of her and does not walk out on her; instead he contains and sticks with her, even in situations when she perceives herself as being most 'ugly', aggressive, repulsive and defective. The therapeutic relationship does not even fall apart even when she shows the therapist aspects of herself that she normally tries to hide from others because she thinks they are too shameful and 'toxic' for others to see.

After bringing these corrective experiences over a prolonged period in the therapeutic relationship, the therapist verbalizes his experience that she may be trying to keep him and their relationship from becoming important to her, perhaps because she perceives that as dangerous and as something that she needs to protect herself from, for a variety of reasons. Initially, this makes her very nervous, she is overwhelmed by anxiety, and she aggressively rejects his intervention: 'So you want me to sit here and praise you and tell you great you are, just so later you can use it against me?' Afterwards, however, she begins to reflect, as she begins to realize that she may not have the same 'good reasons' to keep the therapist (and certain others) from becoming significant to her. She sees that, objectively speaking, she may have no reason to be overwhelmed by anxiety at the thought that the therapist might become important to her, the way she did in earlier (traumatizing) attachment relationships, where she paid a high price for emotional contact with significant others. Precisely because the therapist does not act the way she has been used to from other important relationships, she gradually realizes that her behaviour in the interaction with the therapist—in the transference—is one-sided shadow boxing (Alexander 1956:67), and she gradually acknowledges that her emotional reactions to the therapist have been irrational, non-realistic and maladaptive. She begins to revise her basic perceptions of self and others and of how she can be in the contact with others. She begins to be able to be in emotional contact and to feel more secure in and enjoy the contact.

Existing treatment models can, to varying degrees, promote the activation of the common efficacy factors, and to some extent they draw explicitly on them in their attempt to explain the effect of specific interventions. There is reason to assume that therapists who are trained in different therapeutic methods disagree as to which of the common mechanisms of change are most important, and that they will differ in which common factors they highlight and, respectively, reject (cf. Tschacher et al. 2014:93).

Most proponents of a given treatment method will insist that specific interventions from their chosen treatment model are crucial for treatment effect, while common efficacy factors (which run across seemingly fundamentally different treatment methods) are assigned less importance or are ignored completely, in part because they do not readily lend themselves to arguing the benefits of a given treatment method. In a similar vein, there are countless examples that common efficacy factors are associated with more method-specific strategies, which on closer inspection are quite closely related with strategies from other treatment methods. For example, schema therapy (Young et al. 2003:182f) recommends 'reparenting', meaning that the therapist to some extent enters into parent mode in interactions with the patient, as a way of compensating for shortcomings in the way the patient's parents handled these functions during the patient's childhood and youth ('limited parenting'). This offers obvious possibilities for corrective emotional experiences in the therapeutic relationship to counterbalance previously established interaction patterns in the patient, as the therapist adopts a certain stance and relates to the patient in a particular manner.

More specifically, reparenting, is described as the therapist appearing honest and trustworthy, creating a warm, nurturing and empathic atmosphere, representing a source of stability in the patient's life, setting appropriate boundaries, being accepting and nonjudgmental towards the patient and adopting a tolerant and forgiving view of both his own and the patient's flaws and imperfections (Young et al. 2003:203ff). This also implies that the therapist in some situations need to adopt what Young et al. (2003:278) call 'healthy adult mode', setting boundaries, showing nurture and protecting the patient (who in this context is seen as the 'vulnerable' or 'angry child')—all of them elements that are associated with the common therapeutic factors, which may counterbalance traumatic experiences earlier in the patient's life (in the therapeutic relationship). Although the factors have a tenuous link to specific interventions, they are verbalized in a particular way with the aim of linking them with a specific treatment method.

That the common therapeutic factors have a crucial impact on the treatment effect does not imply that it one might simply develop an otherwise atheoretical—hyper-eclectic and pragmatic—treatment method with a view to using the same common factors with all patients, regardless of their more specific disorder or issues. Maximal activation of the common efficacy factors cannot be elevated into a particular therapeutic technique or method and a model of pathology (Lambert and Ogles 2014; Laska and Wampold 2014). As mentioned earlier, it is in itself an important common efficacy factor or condition for treatment effect that the therapist's work is based on a model of pathology that is focused on and relevant to the individual patient with her specific challenges, and that the therapist's work is rooted in a comprehensive and coherent understanding of psychopathology and psychotherapy. It matters less which of the widely approved treatment theories the therapist applies, provided it is attuned with the individual patient's primary difficulties.

References

Alexander, F. (1956). *Psychoanalysis and psychotherapy: Developments in theory, technique, and training*. New York, NY: Norton.

Alexander, F., & French, T. M. (1946). *Psychoanalytic therapy: Principles and application*. New York, NY: Ronald Press.

Allison, E., & Fonagy, P. (2016). When is truth relevant? *Psychoanalytic Quarterly, 85,* 275–303.

Bateman, A., & Fonagy, P. (2016). *Mentalization-based treatment for personality disorders: A practical guide*. Oxford, England: Oxford University Press.

Bell, E. C., Marcus, D. K., & Goodlad, J. K. (2013). Are the parts as good as the whole? A meta-analysis of component treatment studies. *Journal of Consulting and Clinical Psychology, 81*(4), 722–736.

Cuijpers, P., Driessen, E., Hollon, S. D., Oppen, P., Barth, J., & Andersson, G. (2012). The efficacy of non-directive supportive therapy for adult depression: A meta-analysis. *Clinical Psychology Review, 32,* 280–291.

Fonagy, P., & Allison, E. (2014). The role of mentalizing and epistemic trust in the therapeutic relationship. *Psychotherapy, 51,* 372–380.

Jørgensen, C. R. (2004). Active ingredients in individual psychotherapy: Searching for common factors. *Psychoanalytic Psychology, 21*(4), 516–541.

Jørgensen, C. R. (2009). *Personlighedsforstyrrelser. Moderne relationel forståelse og behandling af borderlinelidelse* [Personality disorders. Modern relational understanding and treatment of borderline disorder] (2nd ed.). Copenhagen, Denmark: Hans Reitzels Forlag.

Kazdin, A. E. (2009). Understanding how and why psychotherapy leads to change. *Psychotherapy Research, 19,* 418–428.

Lambert, M. J., & Ogles, B. M. (2014). Common factors: Post hoc explanation or empirically based therapy approach? *Psychotherapy, 51,* 500–504.

Laska, K. M., & Wampold, B. E. (2014). Ten things to remember about common factor theory. *Psychotherapy, 51,* 519–524.

Melcher, I. (2013). *Franz Alexander und die moderne Psychotherapie. Gießen.* Germany: Psychosozial-Verlag.

Miller, S. D., Hubble, M. A., Chow, D. L., & Seidel, J. A. (2013). The outcome of psychotherapy: Yesterday, today, and tomorrow. *Psychotherapy, 50,* 88–97.

Muran, J. C., & Barber, J. P. (Eds.). (2010). *The therapeutic alliance: An evidence-based guide to practice*. New York, NY: Guilford.

Nacht, S. (1962). The curative factors in psychoanalysis. *International Journal of Psychoanalysis, 43,* 206–211.

Norcross, J. C., & Lambert, M. J. (2011). Evidence-based psychotherapy relationships. In J. C. Norcross (Ed.), *Psychotherapy relationships that work: Evidence-based responsiveness* (2nd ed., pp. 3–24). New York, NY: Oxford University Press.

Pfammatter, M., & Tschacher, W. (2012). Wirkfaktoren der Psychotherapie – eine Übersicht und Standortsbestimmung [Efficacy factors of psychotherapy—An overview]. *Zeitschrift für Psychiatrie, Psychologie und Psychotherapie, 60,* 67–76.

Pfammatter, M., Junghan, U. M., & Tschacher, W. (2012). Allgemeine Wirkfaktoren der Psychotherapie: Konzepte, Widersprüche und eine Synthese [General efficacy factors of psychotherapy: Concepts, contradictions and a synthesis]. *Psychotherapie in Psychiatrie, Psychotherapeustischer Medizin, 17,* 17–31.

Pflichthofer, D. (2012). *Spielregeln der Psychoanalyse* [Ground rules of psychoanalysis]. Gießen, Germany: Psychosozial-Verlag.

Pohl, V. H. (1979). Psychoanalytische Haltung und Technik als Formen zwischenmenschlichen Umgangs [Psychoanalytic stance and technique and forms of interpersonal interactions]. *Zeitschrift für Psychosomatische Medizin und Psychoanalyse, 25,* 34–48.

Safran, J. D., & Muran, J. C. (2000). *Negotiating the therapeutic alliance: A relational treatment guide*. New York, NY: Guilford.

Stern, D. N., Sander, L. W., Nahum, J. P., Harrison, A. M., Lyons-Ruth, K., Morgan, A. C., et al. (1998). Non-interpretive mechanisms in psychoanalytic therapy: The something more than interpretation. *International Journal of Psychoanalysis, 79,* 903–921.

Symington, J., & Symington, N. (1996). *The clinical thinking of Wilfred Bion*. London, England: Routledge.

Treurniet, N. (1997). On an ethic of psychoanalytic technique. *Psychoanalytic Quarterly, 66,* 596–627.

Tschacher, W., Junghan, U. M., & Pfammatter, M. (2014). Towards a taxonomy of common factors in psychotherapy: Results of an expert survey. *Clinical Psychology and Psychotherapy, 21,* 82–96.

Wampold, B. E., & Imel, Z.-E. (2015). *The great psychotherapy debate: The evidence for what makes psychotherapy work* (2nd ed.). London, England: Routledge.

Young, J. E., Klosko, J. S., & Weishaar, M. E. (2003). *Schema therapy: A practitioner's guide*. New York, NY: Guilford.

Chapter 5
Randomized Controlled Trials

> Just as experimenters cannot afford the loss of statistical power that invariably follows from implementation of impure treatments, clinicians cannot afford the loss of therapeutic power that follows from implementation of pure treatments, particularly where common factors play a role in outcome (Westen et al. 2004:643).

In empirical psychotherapy research the randomized controlled trial (RCT) is considered the gold standard. Its fundamental rationale in connection with outcomes research is that studying the efficacy of a given treatment method requires a way to systematically compare the effect of this method with the effect of another—preferably approved—treatment, alternatively the treatment patients are normally offered ('treatment as usual', TAU), or (less optimally) with patients on a waiting list, including patients who are not receiving any other treatment. As it is not practically possible to construct a placebo psychotherapeutic treatment (cf. Wampold et al. 2016), this option is not used, although it would be the ideal approach as seen from the medical RCT logic. Outcome studies involve selecting a relatively large sample of patients with a specific diagnosis. In this selection it is important to ensure a systematic diagnostic assessment based on reliable diagnostic methods (structured diagnostic interviews, certified diagnostic systems and so on) and to ensure that any comorbidity is systematically diagnosed and described. Ideally, patients with severe comorbid disorders are excluded to ensure as 'pure' a patient group as possible. The included patients are randomly divided (randomized) into two or more groups.

In an exemplary RCT, the patients in each group are offered a specific manualized treatment by therapists who have received systematic training in the treatment method they are going to apply, and various types of controls are put in place to verify that they in fact apply it and to assess their competence in doing so. Based on video recordings of the therapy sessions, independent observers assess how closely the therapists adhere to the treatment manuals (adherence), and how competent they are (specific therapeutic competence). Treatment duration is determined ahead of time and is the same for all patients, regardless whether any of the involved patients might in fact benefit from different treatment durations. The patients' benefit from the treatment is assessed via different outcome measures, typically primarily based

C. R. Jørgensen, *The Psychotherapeutic Stance*,
https://doi.org/10.1007/978-3-030-20437-2_5

on questionnaires where each patient self-reports the severity and character of his or her difficulties before and after the treatment, possibly supplemented with effect measurements during the treatment and for a period after completion (follow-up). These effect measurements may be accompanied by various diagnostic assessments and assessments of the patient's symptomatology or functioning level by the therapist or other, more or less professional individuals (in some cases clinical trainees).

Within its own inherent logic the RCT has many important qualities. It aims to ensure that the patient group included in the study is relatively homogenous, in the sense that they all have a given diagnosis. There are controls to ensure that the therapists involved actually perform the therapeutic methods whose efficacy the study sets out to examine, and which are described in the treatment manuals that are used in the study. This includes verifying the integrity and differentiability of the treatments that are being compared (that is, that the treatments performed are in fact the ones the study aims to compare, and that they differ clearly in practice), just as a battery of widely approved effect measures are used to ensure that findings are reasonably comparable across different RCTs.

The basic assumption in the optimal RCT is that adherence to the RCT guidelines offers a fair degree of certainty that the primary factor distinguishing the outcome of the different patient groups is the treatment they were offered. Any other variables that influence treatment outcome are either controlled for or are so relatively insignificant and randomly distributed between the groups that their impact is eliminated or is evened out by the sheer number of patients and therapy courses in each of the groups. That assumption is an important one, and in a sense it is critical for the RCT, as it supports the assumption that any statistically significant differences in average treatment outcome between the groups can be largely attributed to the specific methods that were applied in the respective groups. If there are significant differences in the average patient outcomes between the groups, it is thus reasonable to conclude that there is a real difference in the efficacy of the specific methods or techniques in the treatment of patients with the specific diagnosis.

Fundamental Problems with RCTs

As mentioned earlier, many of the RCTs that have been published, especially in recent decades, have clearly contributed to our understanding of psychotherapy and, not least, to the scientific validation of the efficacy of psychotherapy. Nevertheless, RCTs are characterized by certain fundamental problems, which require us to be cautious to draw very far-reaching practical implications of RCT findings, particularly when it comes to individual studies (see the section on meta-analyses)—for example by concluding that patients with a certain diagnosis should always be offered a certain specific treatment, because an RCT 'indicated' that it produces significantly better outcomes than another widely approved treatment method. Moreover, the spread of and focus on RCTs has distorted the perception of what are the key elements of psychotherapy, for example that specific technical factors are supposed to be particularly important for the effect of psychotherapy, which is not the case, as mentioned earlier. The more extensive and fundamental discussion about RCTs lies outside the scope of the present text, but some of the main issues bear mentioning here (cf. Wampold and Imel 2015; Stiles 2013; Orlinsky 2008; Westen et al. 2004, 2005).

- *Overestimating the importance of specific methods*. RCTs are based on the somewhat problematic assumption that the specific psychotherapeutic method or technique is the decisive efficacy factor in psychotherapy and that the effect of a specific therapeutic method can thus be detached from other important (contextual) treatment factors, including aspects of the therapeutic relationship and factors pertaining to the individual therapist applying the method in question. Many of the studies are based on an implicit assumption that psychotherapy can be reduced to an assembly of methods or procedures that are efficacious in themselves. It should be remembered that manualized treatments may range from tightly structured prescriptions for standardized interventions to attempts at formulating more general treatment principles which it is more up to the individual therapist to translate into practice in his work with the individual patient.
- *Therapist effects*. Even the most stringently conducted studies have a considerable therapist effect (see Chap. 6), meaning that there is usually considerable variation in treatment outcomes between the therapists involved in the RCT. This indicates that the therapist's individual qualities have a significant impact on treatment effect that goes beyond the effect of treatment method itself. Moreover, the vast majority of RCT outcomes studies ignore the expectable variance in effect between the participating therapists, meaning that, all things being equal, the studies overestimate how big a share of any variance in treatment effect can actually be attributed to the treatment methods that are being compared (Kim et al. 2006:167).
- *Efficacy versus effectiveness*. Treatments in RCTs rarely match real life in the clinic, where the patient group is far more heterogeneous and is characterized by considerable comorbidity and other factors that make it difficult to generalize the findings of an RCT to real life in clinic. Although they are scientifically weaker, more naturalistic studies are closer to the daily work in the clinic. In psychotherapy research, this difference between RCTs and naturalist studies is often referred to as the difference between efficacy and effectiveness. Generally, RCTs are less problematic in relation to shorter treatments for less severe and clearly defined disorders without major comorbidity, including, in particular, symptom disorders with no accompanying disorders in the patients' personality function.
- *Weak control treatments*. Many RCTs, particularly the older ones, compare the effect of a specific treatment with an obviously weaker and imprecisely described TAU. Thus, in practice, what the finding usually indicates is that it is better to 'do something' for the patient than to do virtually nothing, which is in itself both highly predictable and of little interest.
- *Major structural differences between the treatments that are being compared*. Often, there are major structural differences between the compared treatments in the sense that one treatment method—typically the one that the RCT sets out to verify the efficacy of—has far more resources than the comparison treatment. These differences may pertain to therapist training, dedication, access to super-

vision and so on. Moreover, RCTs often use relatively inexperienced therapists, which means that it is uncertain whether the findings can be generalized to therapists with many years of experience. Thus, it can be argued that only RCTs that compare 'real' (bona fide) and actually comparable treatments should be taken seriously (Wampold and Imel 2015:266f).

- *Allegiance effects*. Both researchers and therapists typically have an affinity for a particular treatment method. Numerous studies have shown that this, to varying degrees, influences the way efficacy studies are designed and conducted, and that this may influence (bias) the presented findings. This is sometimes referred to as allegiance effects: varying degrees of connection between researchers' and clinicians' 'belief' in a specific treatment method and the tendency for the same researchers and clinicians to conclude that the method is more effective than others. In a review of this phenomenon from some years ago, Luborsky et al. (1999:101) found that researchers' allegiance explains up to 70% of the found variance in effect sizes in efficacy studies of various treatment methods. More recent meta-analyses of the phenomenon suggest that its impact has been decreasing over time with improvements in the applied research designs. A review of existing meta-analyses (Munder et al. 2013:508), however, has not found allegiance effects generally to be lower in more recent efficacy studies; there are signs that improved research designs are associated with smaller allegiance effects, but the effects are not quite eliminated (Munder et al. 2011).
- *Overestimating diagnostic precision*. Typically, it is assumed that any comorbid disorders are random and additive in relation to the selected primary disorder that is the focus of the RCT. From a dynamic clinical point of view, this assumption may be problematic, since different symptoms are often mutually connected and rooted in a common underlying dynamic or disorder. What we call comorbidity, based on a medical understanding and our authorized diagnostic systems, should thus in some cases be considered rather as complex symptomatologies stemming from a complex and multifactorial aetiology, not as two or more parallel and essentially distinct disorders that should be treated sequentially and with different 'evidence-based' methods. An overemphasis on sharply delimited and possibly comorbid disorders may shift the focus away from more fundamental psychological issues that run across specific diagnoses. Thus, symptoms and disturbed behaviour should far from always be understood and treated as separate from the patient's life and personality in general, just as it is often problematic to assume that the typical patient has just one, clearly delimited problem (captured by the specific diagnosis), or that the treatment may proceed as if that were the case (cf. Budd and Hughes 2009:514; Westen et al. 2004).
- *Problematic assumptions about psychotherapy*. Implicitly, RCTs are based on a perception of psychotherapy as a finite array of definable elements that individual therapists can learn, and which they will then implement in a fairly uniform manner. Another implicit assumption is that the therapist can perform the standardized treatment more or less independently of the patient, who is considered a largely passive recipient of the therapist's interventions. These assumptions are clearly problematic.

- *Mechanical experimental logic*. As suggested, RCTs are based on the experimental logic that if all significant variables, bar one (the independent variable, the treatment method), are kept constant or controlled for, any outcome differences that emerge (the dependent variable), can be attributed to the variable that was 'manipulated' (choice of treatment method). The problem is, however, that individual differences make it impossible, in practice, to treat even two people the same way in every regard (except for one—the applied treatment method). Similarly, two therapists will never conduct a given treatment in the same manner—and if they did, that would imply that they were reduced to technocrats without subjectivity, who would hardly be able to establish or maintain a therapeutic alliance, let alone be able to use the central therapeutic efficacy factors in the therapeutic relationship. On a more fundamental level, it could be argued that this experimental logic reflects a mechanistic and behaviourist understanding of psychotherapy where the patient is perceived as an object, the passive target or recipient of interventions from a technician-therapist.
- *Uniformity myths*. For decades, empirical psychotherapy research has been characterized by what Kiesler (1966) more than half a century ago labelled 'uniformity myths', for example the myth that all patients with a given diagnosis are fairly uniform on all the factors that are relevant for psychotherapeutic treatment, and that they thus require the same treatment. Another uniformity myth is that it is possible to control or eliminate the variability across the patients participating in an efficacy study by only including patients with a specific diagnosis (Beutler 1997), which in practice ignores the importance of individual differences between patients who happen to share the same diagnosis (Levitt et al. 2005:118). Another such myth is that psychotherapy is a static entity, meaning that all therapists who embrace and are trained in a specific method in practice can be assumed to apply this method uniformly, and that it is thus acceptable to ignore therapist factors, possibly supplemented with methods for controlling the participating therapists' adherence and specific competence. In light of recent meta-analyses of the substantial impact of therapist effects on outcome, this assumption must be rejected as clearly unfounded, even if training in a specific manualized treatment method does tend to reduce the effect of therapist factors (see Chap. 6).
- *Interaction between patient factors and therapist factors*. To the extent that more complex analyses seek to incorporate individual patient and therapist factors, they typically do so by means of relatively primitive but operationalizable variables (sex, age, experience). Moreover, patient and therapist are typically viewed as two distinct variables as opposed to interacting ones. In effect, this renders the study de facto unable to address how, for example, the patient's negative reactions to the therapist's invitation to contact or interventions might influence the therapist's subsequent behaviour in the therapeutic space. The therapist may, for example, become insecure, irritated or defensive and thus less effective in his role as a therapist, or, conversely, the therapist may seize upon and work with this response as one that reflects a rupture in the alliance and reveals the patient's relational difficulties.

- *Randomization and responsiveness*. The randomized distribution of patients to different treatment methods reflects a lack of responsiveness in matching patient, therapist and treatment that is normally avoided in clinical practice; this is a crucial condition for the research design, but it is therapeutically problematic. On the other hand, the individual therapists may compensate for it in practice by attuning his interventions to the individual patient. This requires certain personal qualities or general therapeutic competencies (common therapeutic factors) in the individual therapists. However, it undermines the inherent logic of the RCT because the therapists' responsiveness (see Chap. 10) may compromise the uniformity of the treatments offered to a given patient group. It is not, however, an either/or issue but a matter of degrees, which relates to the degree to which the examined treatment methods allow for or even require the therapists to be responsive in their implementation of a given treatment method.

Overall, these weaknesses in RCTs mean that we should give up our sometimes blind acceptance of this research design as the gold standard for psychotherapy research. It should be seen as one among several other, equally valid options for studying psychotherapy. Here, we should note that it may lead to considerable cognitive dissonance and, thus, resistance, especially for researchers who have invested much of their career and themselves in traditional outcome studies, to acknowledge that empirical effect research will probably never come close to satisfying the considerable expectations of developing standardized techniques for treating specific diagnoses with significantly better effect than existing treatment forms.

The scientific-evidence trend and the prevailing focus on RCTs may potentially decrease the quality of the therapeutic training provided to future therapists due to an excessive focus on manualized techniques aimed at rigid categories of 'disorders' (specific diagnoses) rather than on the individual, whole person (Henry 1998). On the other hand, it will likely be possible to improve the effect of our treatments considerably by allocating more resources to the field, improving the selection of people who are going to work with psychotherapy and improving their therapeutic training. The latter would include adopting a much broader focus than simply conveying a specific treatment method (although therapists naturally also need training in the application of various coherent treatment techniques, possibly aided by treatment manuals), including enhancing the new psychotherapists' relational competences and their ability to adopt and maintain a psychotherapeutic stance under pressure.

5.1 The Use of Treatment Manuals

> The extraordinary diversity of the psychological constellations concerned, the plasticity of all mental processes and the wealth of determining factors oppose any mechanization of the technique; and they bring it about that a course of action that is as a rule justified may at times prove ineffective, whilst one that is usually mistaken may once in a while lead to the desired end (Freud 1913:123).

One of the first to develop a manual for psychotherapeutic treatment was Aaron Beck, who during the 1970s presented a manual for the cognitive treatment of depression (Beck et al. 1979, however, see also Greenson 1967; Glover 1955). Since then it has become increasingly common to develop descriptive manuals of psychotherapeutic methods for the treatment of specific disorders. A manual describes the basic theory, concept of pathology and treatment principles of a specific treatment method and—in varying degrees of specificity—individual interventions, including when and how these interventions are to be used. This is all based on the implicit or explicit assumption that the described treatment principles and, not least, the specific interventions are central to the course and outcome of the treatment, and that the described interventions capture the psychotherapeutic treatment's active ingredients and key change mechanisms.

Both research-related and clinical arguments can be made in favour of developing and using treatment manuals. In the training of new therapists it may be helpful to have a manual that specifies the key elements of a treatment method, just as novice therapists in particular may, in some contexts, benefit from consulting a treatment manual in their search for answers to questions concerning 'what to do' in a given situation with a given patient. The questions is, of course, whether it is an illusion to think that a manual can in fact offer adequate and sufficiently nuanced answers to the often complex questions that come up during the course of psychotherapeutic work. The short answer is that, yes, it is an illusion, but there is no denying the degree of security and certainty a manual may offer to some therapists, in the sense that they now believe they know 'what to do'. Further, it could be argued that the standardization associated with the manualization of a treatment can in some regards ensure a certain uniformity and provide a professional foundation for the treatment patients are offered in different settings.

Novice therapists will often underestimate the complexity of the therapeutic work and only gradually develop the necessary grasp of timing and flexibility and the ability to attune their—perhaps manualized—interventions with the individual patient; skills that are absolutely central to the psychotherapeutic work and which cannot manualized (Castonguay et al. 1999). While novice therapists often, for example in an attempt at managing their anxiety and insecurity, stick fairly rigidly to the instructions from textbooks, manuals or supervisors, thus acting without the necessary responsiveness and sensitivity to the patient's needs, experienced and competent therapists will be far more flexible and likely to deviate from the standardized, manualized method when necessary. The experienced therapist is much more able to improvise, revise his understanding of the patient in light of new information and adapt his strategy to it in ways that cannot be formulated in a treatment manual (cf. Binder 2004:12). This ability to improvise, to handle the unexpected and to react in a balanced way in difficult situations (for example when a problem occurs in the therapeutic relationship) is particularly important when working with patients with more severe disorders (cf. Binder 1999:713).

In a high-quality manual and, not least, in the talented use of it, there is an awareness that the manual's instructions should always be implemented in ways that are attuned to the individual patient. The potential problem, however, is that if the purpose of developing and applying a manual is to achieve a certain degree of standardization and uniformity in the treatment of a specific disorder, that goal becomes increasingly difficult to realize with the growing awareness that the use of the manual requires many complex skills in the individual therapist, which cannot be manualized and, hence, not standardized. Moreover, the psychotherapeutic process and psychotherapy work are so complex that it could not possibly be standardized or manualized in detail.

Psychotherapy is not an applied science, and it cannot be reduced to the implementation of a science- or evidence-based (manualized) method; rather, it is a professional discipline (Buchholz 2006:435) whose practitioners are bound by scientific theory and knowledgeable about the most recent empirical knowledge. In extension of this, it should be considered whether professional psychotherapy should primarily be conducted by persons with—psychological or medical—professional training, particularly when it concerns severe psychological disorders. Any notion that psychotherapeutic treatments and psychotherapeutic work can be governed by empirical research and authoritative treatment manuals is, at best, naive and at worst destructive, if it is translated into a requirement for all therapists to adhere to a centrally determined framework and to document that they use a particular standardized method (Buchholz 2006:448). Here, it should be remembered that treatment methods based in psychoanalysis emerged mainly from clinical practice and experiences from psychotherapeutic work, which were subsequently expanded with the (largely inductive) development of scientific theories. Behavioural therapy, on the other hand, sprang mainly from an existing learning theory, that is, from academic psychology, which subsequently (in a largely deductive process) served as the basis for the development of a treatment method (Körner 2013a:242f). These differences in origins and methodological preferences continue to be evident in fundamentally different perceptions of the rationale and usefulness of treatment manuals.

From a research perspective it may be necessary to prepare a detailed manual for the principles and specific interventions of a treatment method in order to examine its effect in an RCT-design, which, as mentioned earlier, has become the gold standard for efficacy studies. The underlying logic is that in order to examine the efficacy of a given treatment, one has to be able to specify, in detail, what sort of treatment the study pertains to. Also—and even more importantly—one has to be able to document, to some extent, that when a group of therapists taking part in an efficacy study are tasked with performing a given treatment, they actually practise that method and not a different one. The treatment manual must therefore be supplemented with instruments that enable independent raters to assess the extent to which the individual therapist adheres to the treatment instructions and methods in the manual (adherence) as well as the competence of the practice (specific therapeutic competence).

The main purpose of using treatment manuals in efficacy research is thus to maximize the integrity and differentiability of the performed treatments, meaning that the therapists who are tasked with implementing a specific (manualized) treatment actually do just that, without veering too far into the territory of other treatment methods, and to minimize the variability between the therapists providing the manualized treatment. From an RCT perspective, the manual and the related instruments for rating adherence and competence should thus minimize or, ideally, eliminate the variability of the independent research variable, the psychotherapeutic treatment method. The manual represents an attempt at standardizing and controlling the treatment process. As mentioned earlier, individual studies have found that the variation in treatment effect across therapists is actually less in studies that rely on a treatment manual, just as the variation appears to be less among novice therapists (Crits-Christoph et al. 1991). However, it never quite goes away. Whatever we do, we must expect considerable variation between different therapists' actual treatment work and outcomes. In an imagined scenario where therapist effects are completely eliminated, it will not matter which therapist a patient is assigned to (cf. Barkham et al. 2017:14). A purist approach to the use of manuals, where one imagines that the core of psychotherapy can be formulated in a treatment manual that could, in principle, be implemented by a replaceable technician, inevitably comes up against the problem that psychotherapeutic work is always conducted in the meeting between at least two persons, both of whom—including the therapist—are influenced in their behaviour, to varying degrees, by unconscious processes and factors related to each individual's person and individuality (cf. Cremerius 1979:579).

Problems Related to the (Inappropriate) Use of Treatment Manuals

At least three key problems can be pointed out in the use of treatment manuals that are relevant in the present context, and which may potentially undermine the therapist's psychotherapeutic stance if the manuals are not used with sufficient judiciousness. The point is not that treatment manuals cannot be used in a clinically meaningful way. They can. But they must be used with flexibility and with respect for, especially, more experienced and competent therapists' professional judgment, not as a weapon in primitive arguments between different professions about what is the 'technically correct' way to treat patients with specific disorders. Treatment manuals should never be used as a weapon to mandate that therapists use a particular method for the treatment of all patients with a given diagnosis.

(1) *Failure to capture the core of psychotherapy*. From a dynamic-relational perspective, where the meeting between patient and therapist, the therapist's psychotherapeutic stance and what unfolds in the relationship between patient and therapist are considered the core of psychotherapy, the typical treatment manual does not capture the most important aspects of the psychotherapeutic work. Its primary focus is on the technical elements of the therapy that can be standardized, and although these may, at best, may make some contribution to the treatment, they are not nearly as important as the common therapeutic factors. It is an illusion to imagine that the use of a manual would offer decisive control over the core elements of psychotherapy, which are notoriously difficult to control, such as the individual therapist's ability to enter into a relationship with the patients and to notice important nuances in the interaction with the patient and offer an appropriate response to them—aspects that depend mainly on the therapist's more personal qualities (Strupp and Anderson 1997:78).

(2) *Prescriptive use*. Originally, the main intention with developing treatment manuals was to offer a descriptive presentation of the key ingredients of various

treatment methods. Increasingly, however, manuals are also being used prescriptively, to varying degrees, as a basis for authoritative clinical guidelines or even to mandate therapists to use and stick to certain specific treatment methods (for example as a condition for working in certain institutional settings or for patients to have access to funding for their treatment). That is problematic, as treatment manuals are not suited to be used as weapons in conflicts between different professions about which specific treatment methods are superior and recommended. Moreover, these conflicts may be further intensified and muddled by economic concerns, including demands for drastic efficiency increases in psychotherapeutic work, which may in practice compel therapists to offer short-term therapy, also in cases when that is far from optimal from a clinical point of view.

(3) *Reducing the therapist to a technician.* It is obviously uninformed to claim either that the use of treatment manuals should govern all clinical work, or that all manuals are inherently useless in any situation. As is the case with our diagnostic systems, it is not manualization as such that is the problem. However, to the extent that manuals are used rigidly—rather than as an open description of general treatment principles—and prescriptively, requiring therapists to apply methods they do not identify with professionally, that will in itself diminish the quality of their therapeutic work, their flexibility and creativity and, consequently, their treatment outcomes. An excessive focus on specific, behavioural 'how-to' guidelines promote a superficial instrumental thinking, where the therapist may be reduced to a kind of 'psychotechnician', charged with delivering a standard product to standard patients with a given diagnosis. Generally, the least knowledgeable and skilful therapists are the ones who stand to benefit most from manualized training (Beutler et al. 2004:246).

Studies in the Use of Treatment Manuals

A slightly older study among practising psychologist in the United States (Addis and Krasnow 2000) found considerable resistance to the use of manuals, especially among more dynamically oriented therapists, while cognitive therapists are somewhat more positive. Therapists who reject the use of manuals in their treatments say, among other things, that they find it reduces them to technicians, keeps them from using their intuition, forces patients into arbitrary categories and leads to an excessive focus on therapeutic techniques rather than the needs of the individual patient. They also comment that manuals are 'appropriate for research clients but not for "real-world" clients' (Addis and Krasnow 2000:335). By contrast, psychologists who are less critical of the use of manuals say that it helps them utilize only interventions that have been demonstrated to be effective, that manuals can keep therapists on track during therapy, and that they can help them improve their clinical skills.

These findings reflect the wide range of opinions of what psychotherapy is about, what is the core of psychotherapy (the use of specific evidence-based techniques or more complex relational processes) and the ability of empirical research to inform therapeutic work. The psychologists who participated in the study also stated that manuals are more appropriate for the treatment of certain disorders, including anxiety and depression, while it seems much less obvious to use manuals for personality disorders, among other diagnoses (Addis and Krasnow 2000:336). That is probably a very valid point, and it contributes to a more nuanced view on treatment manuals, including when we might want to use them and how, and when they unlikely to be helpful.

Implicitly or explicitly, the use of treatment manuals often, to varying degrees, requires that the therapist has established a good therapeutic alliance and continuously evaluates exactly when a given technical intervention should be applied for the manualized treatment method to be effective. The problem is, however, that these core aspects of psychotherapy, which depend on the therapist's judgment, relational skills and basis psychotherapeutic stance, cannot be readily manualized. To some extent, manuals have the wrong focus, as they deal with elements of psychotherapy that are relatively easy to operationalize and change in the individual therapist as part of basic and continuing training. Although these treatment aspects are naturally not without importance, they are secondary. To be effective, therapy must have a structure and contain elements that activate the patient and therapist in ways that are meaningfully related to the patient's perceived difficulties.

Just as diagnostic systems and instruments in themselves are fine and often necessary elements of clinical work, so long as they are not used rigidly and without reflection, treatment manuals in themselves are a fine tool for certain tasks, including training new therapists. What can be problematic, however, is the way these manuals are sometimes used. Treatment manuals rarely require the therapist to follow techniques as a ballistic action (see Chap. 10) but recommend that the therapist uses his judgment to determine when and exactly how the specified techniques should come into play; thus, the therapist has to be responsive in his use of the manual. This reflects the implicit awareness that this crucial treatment element cannot be manualized (Stiles et al. 1998:446). Hence, any discussion of the pros and cons of manualization should distinguish between different types of manuals – from manuals that provide detailed guidelines for what should be addressed in the individual sessions, and how, to (more intelligent) manuals that focus on more general treatment principles, incorporating the therapist's flexibility and ability to match his interventions to the given patient and situation and accompanied with guidelines for rating adherence and competence (see, e.g., Karterud and Bateman 2010:64f).

William Henry's classic study of how intensive manualized training (cf. Strupp and Binder 1984) alters therapists' work, including the way they interact with their patients, illustrates the complexity of training psychotherapists and some of the potential challenges in using treatment manuals (Henry et al. 1993a, b). The study includes 16 therapists who undergo one-year training in time-limited dynamic psychotherapy and examines how the therapists' interpersonal style and technical interventions changes after the training programme. Generally, the participating therapists' work moves closer to the manualized prescriptions—their technical adherence increases. The therapists also become much more active in the therapy, which may be excellent in some cases (but far from all). The problem is that for some therapists, the training has a negative effect on certain aspects of the therapeutic relationship; this appears to be associated with personality features in the individual therapists that are unaffected by the training. Also, the therapists generally do not improve their ability to deal with negative countertransference (see Chap. 7) and keep it from being acted out in the interaction with the patient.

Therapists with self-hostile, self-controlling and self-indicting introjects, that is, therapists who place very high demands on themselves to do things correctly, and who struggle to forgive themselves when they fail, are the ones who achieve the highest technical adherence. Therapists with these introjects (possibly related to more compulsive personality features and issues with juggling multiple perspectives on reality)—which, as mentioned, are not altered through training—also show the poorest treatment outcomes (Strupp and Anderson 1997:77; Henry et al. 1993b). Thus, there are indications that for therapists with this type of negative introject, the training actually increases the introjects' negative contribution to their interpersonal interaction with the patients. Moreover, these therapists are also more likely to engage in countertherapeutic interpersonal processes with their patients after training (Henry et al. 1993b:446). Taken together, these findings suggest that a high degree of technical adherence may be associated with poorer treatment outcomes, and that manualized training does not necessarily change the therapist's more personal qualities, which may constitute the most crucial aspects of the treatment.

evidence thatThe individual therapist's person and subjectivity will always have a—presumably decisive—influence on the therapeutic work and process and thus on treatment outcomes. Therapists' ability to handle those aspects of the therapy that have the greatest impact on the treatment process and on the patient's treatment outcome is not necessarily improved through traditional therapeutic training with a focus on learning the application of a specific treatment method—not even when the treatment method in question, as in this case, is aimed at addressing patients' interpersonal challenges. Henry and colleagues find no indication that therapists' treatment outcomes have improved after the one-year training course in manualized time-limited dynamic therapy (Bein et al. 2000). Generally speaking, there is thus little evidence that manualization in itself has a positive influence on treatment outcome (Beutler et al. 2004:246).

It should also be noted that it was subsequently found that only a minority of the participating therapists actually implemented the manualized treatment at a competent level, and that more than one in four (28%) was not found to apply the manualized method with at least a minimal level of skill in the treatment courses included in the study (Bein et al. 2000:128). Careful analysis thus suggests that even after completing the one-year training course, the participating therapists perform manualized interventions without the necessary sense of timing and attunement with the patient; this includes asking patients about the therapeutic relationship 'out of the blue' and focusing on the patient's possible transference in ways that appear to confuse the patients and heighten their anxiety (Bein et al. 2000:129). In any circumstance, that is a strategy that may be best suited for therapy with patients with varying degrees of personality pathology, not as a general treatment strategy applied to all groups of patients and psychopathology (cf. Binder and Henry 2010:295).

5.2 The Therapist's Adherence and Competence

Generally, there does not seem to be any connection between the therapist's adherence to technical prescriptions in a treatment manual and treatment effect. Similarly, there does not seem to be any major connection between the therapist's specific technical competence—in applying specific manualized treatment techniques—and treatment outcome. A meta-analysis based on 32 studies of adherence and 17 studies of specific technical competence found an effect size for the link between adherence score and treatment outcome that was be close to none (0.02) (Webb et al. 2010:203). The similar effect size for the link between the therapist's specific technical competence and treatment outcome was found to be 0.07, signifying that the link has no real-life impact (ibid.).

For both links, there is a certain variation in effect size across the existing studies, but overall, there does not seem to be any meaningful connection. This finding could be argued to seriously challenge the traditional notion that therapists' application of a specific treatment technique has a real impact on outcome—a core assumption in the medical model of therapy. Similarly, these findings support the notion that common efficacy factors (and therapist factors) have a greater impact on outcome than factors associated with specific interventions, and that we should strive to maximize common factors in psychotherapy, rather than only increasing therapists' adherence to—and specific technical competence in—manualized treatment methods (Webb et al. 2010:207), which is an effort that involves specifying and training in the psychotherapeutic stance.

There is, however, reason to consider whether the adherence-outcome link might be slightly more complicated, and perhaps it is still too early to draw any final conclusions (Baldwin and Imel 2013:283). Individual studies have thus found that therapists' adherence can vary considerably from session to session (Tschushke et al. 2015:427) and across a single therapist's treatment courses (Boswell et al. 2013). Further, therapists' adherence and, in part, their demonstrated technical competence must be considered interactional in nature, in the sense that patients with more severe disorders—including patients with an interpersonal style that may be difficult for many therapists to handle, for example because they show aggression towards the therapist or withdraw from contact—may make it harder for the therapist to stick to a treatment strategy and adhere to technical prescriptions (Wampold and Imel 2015:237). This may be because such prescriptions rarely specify exactly what to do when in relation to particularly challenging patients, and because any prescriptions typically do not match the specific patient and problematic situation in the given treatment course—they simply fail to capture real-life complexity.

Patients with an aggressive, hostile, dismissive interpersonal style often 'invite' complementary reactions from therapists, in a sense calling for responses that are similarly aggressive and hostile and thus therapeutically inappropriate (Kiesler 1996). Patients with severe attachment disorders and externalizing behaviour may put the therapist under pressure, which may lead to a poorer performance and cause him to deviate significantly from his normal treatment method and strategy (lower adherence). That may be helpful in many cases, provided the therapist acts competently, maintaining the psychotherapeutic stance ('let's try and understand what's happening here') instead of resorting to defending himself against perceived attacks or criticism from the patient, alternatively meeting the patient's 'attacks' with 'deskilled' counterattacks or various forms of 'punishment' or acting out the role as the 'disappointed' or 'hurt' victim of the patient's 'unfair' attack or criticism (cf. Boswell et al. 2013).

There is reason to consider whether both very low and very high technical adherence may reflect therapist difficulties on a more personal level, leading to 'deskilled' or incompetent therapist behaviour and thus lower outcome effect. Very high adherence may, as mentioned earlier, reflect rigidity and a lack of flexibility and responsiveness in the therapist's work; alternatively, especially novice therapists may adhere very closely to a manualized method when they find that their patients do not profit from the treatment, thus, high adherence and low treatment outcome interact (Webb et al. 2010:207). Very low adherence may in some cases reflect the therapist's inability to implement a therapeutic method consistently and coherently (cf. Barber et al. 2006), or it may capture the incompetent therapist's tendency to vacillate between fundamentally different treatment models and strategies in response to perceived difficulties in the treatment process. Novice or insufficiently skilled therapists who struggle to contain and regulate their own inner conflicts, maladaptive action urges or mental states (see projective identification in Chap. 11) may try to handle them by adhering closely to a standardized method. A novice therapist may seek to stabilize a still-fragile professional identity as psychotherapist through overidentification with a particular treatment method (cf. Wirth 2012:307), clinging rigidly to a particular (seemingly easy-to-grasp) technique (Zwiebel 2007:210).

Similarly, the inexperienced or professionally insecure therapist may try to manage perceived anxiety by adhering rigidly to specific guidelines and a manualized method that does not match the patient's needs here and now or reflect what it takes to handle problems that arise in the therapeutic relationship. In some contexts these processes may lead to very high adherence, which may superficially give the impression that the person is a skilled therapist, but which may in fact be quite problematic for the therapeutic process and, not least, for the patient. All of this should, of course, be viewed in relation to exactly how the individual study and the individual treatment model rates therapist adherence, including whether and to what extent the assessment includes considerations about the therapist's flexibility and responsiveness (for example of more nuanced and intelligent instruments for assessing therapist adherence, see Karterud and Bateman 2010; Karterud 2012).

Moderate adherence is probably optimal, if we believe that the therapist's application of a coherent and approved treatment method has some impact on treatment outcome—a moderate level of adherence that is informed and guided by the therapist's ongoing evaluation of the patient's state and needs, the therapist's attunement of interventions in light of this evaluation and the maintenance of a psychotherapeutic stance. Thus, some studies have found that variability in the therapist's adherence or technical flexibility during a treatment course is associated with better outcome (Owen and Hilsenroth 2014:284). Such variability may reflect an appropriate flexibility in the therapist's work, although in theory, of course, it may also reflect less desirable characteristics, including an inability to apply a treatment method coherently (incompetence and arbitrariness), just as it may also be a product of variation in the patient's treatment motivation, resistance (hostility towards the therapist, withdrawal from contact with the therapist and so on) and responsiveness to the therapist's interventions (ibid.), which the therapist seeks to address by altering the treatment strategy.

Finally, there is reason to consider the impact of the person who rates adherence and competence. Based on the assumption that the therapist's responsiveness, that is, his ability to attune his interventions to the patient's needs (see Chap. 10), is crucial for the treatment course and outcome, and that the optimal application of a given intervention (frequency and specific delivery) depends on individual patient factors, it is far from simple to rate adherence and competence in a qualified way. It requires a well-developed ability to assess the individual therapist's work in light of the patient's current state and needs, which in itself is not readily standardized, and that may complicate the likelihood of achieving sufficient reliability of these ratings. What may at first glance appear to be a reflection of low adherence and poor therapeutic competence may in fact reflect very competent work, if it is seen and understood in a larger context than the one that is normally formulated by a given rating scale.

It is generally problematic when adherence and competence ratings are carried out without sufficient concern for the actual treatment context in which a given technique or method is applied, since psychotherapeutic competence is context-specific and includes the therapist's ability to use a given method in a manner that is attuned with the given patient and situation (Zilcha-Mano and Barber 2014:70). Psychotherapeutic competence can thus not be reduced to the therapist's ability to implement a standardized method but has to be understood more broadly and include the therapist's sense of the patient and context and his ability to attune his interventions accordingly. One may choose to distinguish between (method-) specific and general competence. In that light, adherence and competence ratings should be carried out by experiences psychotherapists, not by novice therapists or therapeutic trainees, as is often the case in RCTs.

References

Addis, M. E., & Krasnow, A. D. (2000). A national survey of practicing psychologists' attitudes toward psychotherapy treatment manuals. *Journal of Consulting and Clinical Psychology, 68,* 331–339.

Baldwin, S. A., & Imel, Z. E. (2013). Therapist effects: Findings and methods. In M. J. Lambert (Ed.), *Bergin and Garfield's handbook of psychotherapy and behavior change* (6th ed., pp. 258–298). New York, NY: Wiley.

Barber, J. P., Gallop, R., Crits-Christoph, P., Frank, A., Thase, M. E., Weiss, R. D., et al. (2006). The role of therapist adherence, therapist competence, and alliance in predicting outcome of individual drug counseling: Results from the national institute drug abuse collaborative cocaine treatment study. *Psychotherapy Research, 16,* 229–240.

Barkham, M., Lutz, W., Lambert, M. J., & Saxon, D. (2017). Therapist effects, effective therapists, and the law of variability. In L. G. Castonguay & C. E. Hill (Eds.), *How and why are some therapists better than others?* (pp. 13–36). Washington, DC: American Psychological Association.
Beck, A. T., Rush, J. J., Shaw, B. F., & Emery, G. (1979). *Cognitive therapy for depression*. New York, NY: Guilford.
Bein, E., Anderson, T., Strupp, H. H., Henry, W. P., Schacht, T. E., Binder, J. L., et al. (2000). The effects of training in time-limited dynamic psychotherapy: Changes in therapeutic outcome. *Psychotherapy Research, 10,* 119–132.
Beutler, L. (1997). The psychotherapist as a neglected variable in psychotherapy: An illustration by reference to the role of therapist experience and training. *Clinical Psychology: Science and Practice, 4,* 44–52.
Beutler, L. E., Malik, M., Alimohamed, S., Harwood, T. M., Talebi, H., Noble, S., et al. (2004). Therapist variables. In M. J. Lambert (Ed.), *Bergin and Garfield's handbook of psychotherapy and behavior change* (5th ed., pp. 227–306). New York, NY: Wiley.
Binder, J. L. (1999). Issues in teaching and learning time-limited psychodynamic psychotherapy. *Clinical Psychology Review, 19,* 705–719.
Binder, J. L. (2004). *Key competencies in brief dynamic psychotherapy: Clinical practice beyond the manual*. New York, NY: Guilford.
Binder, J. L., & Henry, W. P. (2010). Developing skills in managing negative process. In J. C. Muran & J. P. Barber (Eds.), *The therapeutic alliance: An evidence-based guide to practice* (pp. 285–304). New York, NY: Guilford.
Boswell, J. F., Gallagher, M. W., Sauer-Zavala, S. E., Bullis, J., Gorman, J. M., Shear, M. K., et al. (2013). Patient characteristics and variability in adherence and competence in cognitive-behavioral therapy for panic disorder. *Journal of Consulting and Clinical Psychology, 81,* 443–454.
Buchholz, M. B. (2006). Profession und empirische Forschung in der Psychoanalyse – ihre souveränität und Integration [Profession and empirical research in psychoanalysis—Sovereignty and integration]. *Psyche, 60,* 426–454.
Budd, R., & Hughes, I. (2009). The dodo bird verdict—controversial, inevitable and important: A commentary on 30 years of meta-analyses. *Clinical Psychology and Psychotherapy, 16*(5), 510–522.
Castonguay, L. G., Schut, A. J., Constantino, M. J., & Halperin, G. S. (1999). Assessing the role of treatment manuals: Have they become necessary but nonsufficient ingredients of change? *Clinical Psychology: Science and Practice, 6,* 449–455.
Cremerius, J. (1979). Gibt es zwei psychoanalytische Techniken? [Are there two psychoanalytic techniques?] *Psyche*, *33*, 577–599.
Crits-Cristoph, P., Baranackien, J.S., Kurcias, J.S., Beck, A.T., Carroll, K., Perry, K., Luborsky, L., McLellan, A.T., Woody, G.E., Thompson, L., Gallagher, D. & Zitrin, C. (1991). Meta-analysis of therapist effects in psychotherapy outcome studies. *Psychotherapy reseach, 1*(2), 81–91
Freud, S. (1913). Om indledningen af behandlingen. In: Freud, S. (1992). *Afhandlinger om behandlingsteknik*. København: Hans Reitzels forlag, 123–43
Glover, E. (1955). *The technique of psychoanalysis*. New York, NY: International University Press.
Greenson, R. R. (1967). *The technique and practice of psychoanalysis*. London, England: Hogarth Press.
Henry, W. P. (1998). Science, politics, and the politics of science: The use and misuse of empirically validated treatment research. *Psychotherapy Research, 8,* 126–140.
Henry, W. P., Strupp, H. H., Butler, S. F., Schacht, T. E., & Binder, J. L. (1993a). Effects of training in time-limited dynamic psychotherapy: Changes in therapist behavior. *Journal of Consulting and Clinical Psychology, 61*, 434–440.
Henry, W. P., Schacht, T. E., Strupp, H. H., Butler, S. F., & Binder, J. L. (1993b). Effects of training in time-limited dynamic psychotherapy: Mediators of therapists' responses to training. *Journal of Consulting and Clinical Psychology, 61*, 441–447.

Karterud, S. (2012). *Manual for mentaliseringsbasert gruppeterapi (MBT-G)* [Manual for mentalization-based group therapy]. Oslo, Norway: Gyldendal Akademisk.

Karterud, S., & Bateman, A. (2010). *Manual for mentaliseringsbasert terapi (MBT) og MBT vurderingsskala. Versjon individualterapi* [Manual for mentalization-based therapy (MBT) and MBT assessment scale. Version individual therapy]. Oslo, Norway: Gyldendal Akademisk.

Kiesler, D. J. (1966). Some myths of psychotherapy research and the search for a paradigm. *Psychological Bulletin, 65,* 110–136.

Kiesler, D. J. (1996). *Contemporary interpersonal theory & research: Personality, psychopathology, and psychotherapy.* New York, NY: Wiley.

Kim, D.-M., Wampold, B. E., & Bolt, D. M. (2006). Therapist effects in psychotherapy: A random-effects modeling of the national institute of mental health treatment of depression collaborative research program data. *Psychotherapy Research, 16,* 161–172.

Körner, J. (2013a). Plädoyer für eine Direktausbildung zum Psychotherapeuten. Entwurf eines Studiengangs "von der Profession her" [Plea for direct training of psychotherapists. Draft of a profession-based study curriculum]. *Forum Psychoanalyse, 29*(2), 235–257.

Levitt, H. M., Neimeyer, R. A., & Williams, D. C. (2005). Rules versus principles in psychotherapy: Implications for the quest for universal guidelines in the movement for empirically supported treatments. *Journal of Contemporary Psychotherapy, 35,* 117–129.

Luborsky, L., Diguer, L., Seligman, D. A., Rosenthal, R., Krause, E. D., Johnson, S., et al. (1999). The researchers' own therapy allegiances: A 'wild card' in comparisons of treatment efficacy. *Clinical Psychology: Science and Practice, 6,* 95–106.

Munder, T., Gerger, H., Trelle, S., & Barth, J. (2011). Testing the allegiance bias hypothesis: A meta-analysis. *Psychotherapy Research, 21,* 670–684.

Munder, T., Brütsch, O., Leonhart, R., Gerger, H., & Barth, J. (2013). Researcher allegiance in psychotherapy outcome research: An overview of reviews. *Clinical Psychology Review, 33,* 501–511.

Orlinsky, D. E. (2008). Die nächsten 10 Jahre Psychotherapieforschung. Eine Kritik des herrschenden Forschungsparadigmas mit Korrekturvorschlägen [The next 10 years. A critique of the prevailing research paradigms with suggestions for adjustments]. *Psychotherapie, Psychotherapeutische Medizin, 58,* 345–354.

Owen, J., & Hilsenroth, M. J. (2014). Treatment adherence: The importance of therapist flexibility in relation to therapy outcomes. *Journal of Counseling Psychology, 61,* 280–288.

Stiles, W. B. (2013). The variables problem and progress in psychotherapy research. *Psychotherapy, 50,* 33–41.

Stiles, W. B., Honos-Webb, L., & Surko, M. (1998). Responsiveness in psychotherapy. *Clinical Psychology: Science and Practice, 5,* 439–458.

Strupp, H. H., & Anderson, T. (1997). On the limitations of therapy manuals. *Clinical Psychology: Science and Practice, 4,* 76–82.

Strupp, H. H., & Binder, J. L. (1984). *Psychotherapy in a new key: A guide to time-limited dynamic psychotherapy*. New York, NY: Basic Books.

Tschuschke, V., Crameri, A., Koehler, M., Berglar, J., Muth, K., Staczan, P., Wyl, A. V., Schulthess, P., & Koemeda-Lutz, M. (2015). The role of therapists' treatment adherence, professional experience, therapeutic alliance, and clients' severity of psychological problems: Prediction of treatment outcome in eight different psychotherapy approaches. Preliminary results of a naturalistic study. *Psychotherapy Research, 25*(4), 420–434.

Wampold, B. E., & Imel, Z.-E. (2015). *The great psychotherapy debate: The evidence for what makes psychotherapy work* (2nd ed.). London, England: Routledge.

Wampold, B. E., Frost, N. D., & Yulish, N. E. (2016). Placebo effects in psychotherapy: A flawed concept and a contorted history. *Psychology of consciousness: Theory, Research and Practice, 3,* 108–120.

Webb, C. A., DeRubeis, R. J., & Barber, J. P. (2010). Therapist adherence/competence and treatment outcome: A meta-analytic review. *Journal of Consulting and Clinical Psychology, 78,* 200–211.

Westen, D., Novotny, C. M., & Thompson-Brenner, H. (2004). The empirical status of empirically supported psychotherapies: Assumptions, findings, and reporting on controlled clinical trial. *Psychological Bulletin, 130,* 631–663.
Westen, D., Novotny, C. M., & Thompson-Brenner, H. (2005). EBP- EST. Reply to Crits-Christoph et al. (2005) and Weisz et al. (2005). *Psychological Bulletin, 131*(3), 427–433.
Wirth, H-J. (2012). Zur latenten Anthropologie der Therapeuten im Kontext unterschiedlicher psychoanalytischer Therapierichtungen [On the latent anthropology of therapists in the context of different psychoanalytic therapy forms]. In G. Gödde & M. B. Buchholz (Eds.), *Der Besen, mit dem die Hexe fliegt. Wissenschaft und Therapeutik des Unbewußten* (pp. 279–317). *Bd.2.* Gießen, Germany: Psychosozial-Verlag.
Zilcha-Mano, S., & Barber, J. (2014). Learning from well-trained and experienced dynamic psychotherapists: Research on the efficacy of dynamic psychotherapy and its mechanisms of change. *Contemporary Psychoanalysis, 50,* 58–88.
Zwiebel, R. (2007). *Von der Angst Psychoanalytiker zu sein* [On the fear of being a psychoanalyst]. Stuttgart, Germany: Klett-Cotta Verlag.

Chapter 6
The Efficacy of Specific Treatment Methods

A large number of studies have been published on the efficacy of various treatment methods for a wide range of psychological disorders, albeit with a clear emphasis on studies of variations on the use of cognitive and behavioural treatments to treat mild and moderate depression and anxiety disorders (generalized anxiety, obsessive-compulsive disorder, various types of post-traumatic stress disorder (PTSD) and so on). Recent years have also seen a fair number of studies of psychodynamic therapy and of treatments for certain personality disorders (particularly borderline).

As anyone who has been involved in efficacy studies will know, they are inevitably based on a large number of compromises and tough choices; the perfect efficacy study is an illusion. They all contain inherent methodological issues and compromises, which make it important to be cautious in generalizing the findings, although, on the other hand, one should not conclude that efficacy research is inherently irrelevant to clinical practice. Because of the large number of studies that have been published, it is far from simple to achieve an overview, and the best and simplest approach is to turn to the growing number of meta-analyses of efficacy studies. The use of meta-analyses, however, comes with its own methodological challenges, including that they (1) to varying degrees collate studies of disorders and treatment methods that are not really the same, (2) fail to adequately consider the indisputable interaction between patient factors and treatment methods, which may obscure actual differences in effect, (3) may show publication bias because studies which find no discernible differences in treatment effect are much less likely to be published, just as they (4) typically include studies of very varying quality in order to maximize the empirical basis and, thus, the statistical power. Moreover, meta-analyses are often based on a very large (but also problematically heterogeneous) data set, which means that in some cases researchers may find (and be tempted to overstate) statistically significant differences between treatment methods that, from a clinical vantage point, are so small as to be of no practical relevance (Wampold et al. 2017).

Meta-analyses have also been criticized for overstating the effect of specific treatment methods—at the cost of common factors—because they hardly every randomize the assignment of therapists to specific treatment methods. Hence they fail to attribute enough weight to therapist effects (see later)—a problem that has

C. R. Jørgensen, *The Psychotherapeutic Stance*,
https://doi.org/10.1007/978-3-030-20437-2_6

the estimated potential to reduce found differences between treatment methods by anything from 20 to 80% (Owen et al. 2015). Issues concerning the content and methodology of the many efficacy studies and meta-analyses will not be discussed further in the present context. The following briefly outlines what the existing meta-analyses tell us about the efficacy of psychotherapy and specific therapeutic methods. For a more extensive treatment of these issues, the reader may turn to the following books, among others: *Bergin and Garfield's Handbook of Psychotherapy and Behavior Change* (Lambert 2013a, b), *What Works for Whom?* (Roth and Fonagy 2006) and *A Guide to Treatments that Work* (Nathan and Gorman 2015).

As mentioned earlier, research studies provide a firm basis for claiming that psychotherapy generally has a substantial effect in the treatment of most predominantly psychogenic psychological disorders, although there is some variation across specific disorders, just as a not insignificant share of patients in psychotherapy fail to achieve any real effect or may even be worse off at the (often premature) completion of treatment than they were when the treatment began. It is far from simple, however, to estimate how big a share of patients fail to benefit or may even have a negative outcome of psychotherapy, as there is reason to assume that this depends in part on the pre-treatment severity of the patient's disorder, treatment duration, drop-out rates (where the patient might have benefited from the treatment if it had not been prematurely terminated) and the individual therapist's competence. Further, as a general point, there is little or no substantial difference in the effect of well-reputable treatment methods for psychological disorders, including, especially, cognitive behavioural therapy, interpersonal therapy, psychodynamic therapy and humanistic psychotherapy (Lambert 2013b:194).

Symptom Disorders

Looking more specifically at the treatment of, for example, mild or moderate depression, the effect of psychotherapy is generally quite good and at least on par with or superior to medical treatment; there are some indications that a combination of psychotherapy and medicine is often the most effective approach (Lambert 2013b:172f). As for severe and chronic depression, including dysthymia, and bipolar disorders, the empirical basis is somewhat weaker, but it does appear that in this area medical treatment has slightly or somewhat better effect than psychotherapy (ibid.). Finally, relapse rates for affective disorders are generally somewhat smaller for psychotherapy than for medical treatment (Lambert 2013b:173). With regard to the effect of various psychotherapeutic methods there are a number of meta-analyses, which arrive at slightly different conclusions. Cuijpers et al. (2008) compared the effect of seven different methods for treating mild to moderate depression in adults—based on 53 studies with about 2800 patients—and found that no treatment method shows substantially better effect than any other, although interpersonal therapy does seem to have slightly better effect (effect size approximately 0.2), while unspecified supportive therapy has slightly lower effect (effect size about –0.2) compared with other treatment methods. Drop-out rates are significantly higher for cognitive behavioural therapy (Cuijpers et al. 2008:917).

On the other hand, Tolin (2010) presented a meta-analysis comparing the outcomes of cognitive behavioural therapy (CBT) with what he classifies as other bona fide methods for the treatment of a wide range of psychological disorders, including depression and anxiety. This analysis was based on 26 studies published until 2007 with a total of 1900 patients. It finds that CBT has better outcomes for anxiety and depression than psychodynamic—but not interpersonal or supportive—psychotherapy when measured post-treatment and at the one-year follow-up (Tolin 2010:715). The differences are relatively small, however (effect sizes of 0.2–0.5), and when publication bias, the findings are no longer significant (Tolin 2010:714f). Similarly, a smaller meta-analysis comparing short-term psychodynamic psychotherapy for mild to moderate depression with a range of other treatments found that the outcome of short-term psychodynamic psychotherapy is significantly poorer at post-treatment, while there is no significant difference at the 3–12-month follow-up (Driessen et al. 2010). However, some of the studies included in this meta-analysis have serious methodological problems, including insufficient sample sizes and diagnostic procedures for the involved patients, lack of randomization and a lack of distinction between individual therapy and group therapy.

Tolin's meta-analysis came under heavy criticism (Baardseth et al. 2013; Wampold et al. 2017:15f), in part because the analysis of the effect of anxiety treatment is based on only four studies, two of which are more than 40 years old, while other relevant outcome studies were excluded, for reasons that were not apparent. A new and expanded meta-analysis of the studies included in Tolin's study (supplemented with additional ones) found that CBT is slightly more effective for depression if the focus is solely on disorder-specific effect (effect size only 0.2), while no different is found for non-disorder-specific effect size (Baardseth et al. 2013:398). No difference was found in the effect of various bona fide methods for the treatment of anxiety disorders (Baardseth et al. 2013:401f), and it is concluded that there is no evidence that CBT is a more effective treatment for anxiety disorders than other bona fide methods (Baardseth et al. 2013:402).

Anxiety disorders—like affective disorders—cover a wide and diverse spectrum ranging from mild and generalized anxiety to severe and complex PTSD disorders and obsessive-compulsive disorders (OCD), where anxiety symptoms are combined with severe behavioural dysfunction. Generally, prognosis, treatment duration and treatment effect differ a great deal across these disorders. The field is dominated by studies of cognitive behavioural therapy, which generally has good effect—typically substantially better compared with patients on a waiting list or in various forms of unstructured control treatments, particularly for patients with generalized anxiety, less complex PTSD and OCD (Lambert 2013b:173f). However, it is also a field with certain methodological issues, including too many studies where the effect of a specific treatment is compared with patients on a waiting list or patients who are offered an obviously poorer treatment and, not least, an insufficient number of systematic comparisons of bona fide treatments. Among others, Wampold and Imel (2015:149) therefore conclude that there is no evidence for substantial differences in the effectiveness of bona fide treatments for anxiety. Similarly, there is no basis for claiming that any specific method for the treatment of depression has significantly better effect than any other, including CBT (Baardseth et al. 2013:402; Wampold and Imel 2015:135ff; Normann et al. 2014). For similar findings concerning the treatment of symptom disorders in young people, see Weisz et al. (2017:94).

Personality Disorders

A meta-analysis examined the effectiveness of various treatments for personality disorders (Budge et al. 2013). The first part of this analysis includes 30 studies characterized by a high degree of heterogeneity with regard to treatments, patients and the quality of the research methods. The conclusion is that the effect of what is somewhat vaguely referred to as evidence-based treatment methods (in formal terms, the participating therapists apply a treatment method with previously documented outcome effect) is significantly better than the effect of a somewhat vaguely defined category of 'treatment as usual' (TAU) (Budge et al. 2013:1061). If we leave out the studies where it is unclear whether the applied TAU can even be characterized as actual psychotherapy, we arrive at a moderate effect size (0.37) in favour of the evidence-based treatment methods. It is worth noting, however, that in the authors' own assessment, almost three-quarters of the included studies apply a TAU of no or poor quality (Budge et al. 2013:1062). Further, they find that the effect of the evidence-based treatment methods is generally greater in patients with a borderline personality disorder than in patients with other types of personality disorders. The explanation may be that the borderline patient group often has quite severe symptoms pre-treatment, and that what may be the most successful methods for the treatment of personality disorders—mentalization-based psychotherapy and dialectic behavioural therapy—were initially developed specifically for borderline disorders. A more recent and somewhat more narrowly focused meta-analysis, which only deals with the treatment of borderline personality disorders, similarly finds that dialectical behaviour therapy and psychodynamic therapy (but not cognitive behavioural therapy) are slightly more effective (respective effect sizes of 0.34 and 0.41) than nonspecific methods in the treatment of borderline disorders (Cristea et al. 2017).

The second part of the meta-analysis only includes efficacy studies that compare two or more bona fide methods for the treatment of personality disorders (Budge et al. 2013). Hence, this part of the meta-analysis includes only 12 studies, again of varying quality and focused on different personality disorders. Here, the finding is a significant difference in the respective effectiveness of the included bona fide treatment methods. On closer analysis, however, most of the difference is seen to stem from just two studies, which found, respectively, that mentalization-based psychotherapy has a clearly better effect than structured clinical management for borderline personality disorder (Bateman and Fonagy 2009), and that schema-focused therapy is a more effective treatment for borderline disorders than transference-focused psychotherapy (GieBen-Bloo et al. 2006)—the latter a study that later received some criticism for methodological weaknesses (Yeomans 2007; Grenyer 2007). If these two studies are excluded from the meta-analysis, there is no significant difference in the effect of the compared bona fide methods for the treatment of personality disorders (Budge et al. 2013:1063, Jørgensen et al. 2013, 2014). Finally, there is reason to consider whether allegiance effects should be addressed in the interpretation of the study which found that mentalization-based therapy is significantly more effective, as that study was conducted by Bateman and Fonagy, who developed the method (Jørgensen et al. 2013, 2014).

In summary, although the quality of published outcome studies has clearly improved over time, the field continues to be marred by certain methodological problems, including, not least, that too many studies are based on comparing treatments that really are not comparable (new and well-structured treatments compared with 'intended-to-fail' treatments) rather than bona fide treatments, just as we generally do not know enough about the long-term effect of psychotherapy, the extent to which the results of RCTs can be transferred to clinical practice (the relationship between efficacy and effectiveness) (Wampold et al. 2011), and how more complex elements in the therapeutic process interact with treatment effect.

Overall, there is no evidence that any given method is significantly more effective in the treatment of specific disorders, although one might get that impression from individual outcome studies that find a significant advantage for a specific method used to treat a specific disorder compared to TAU or an alternative treatment that, to some extent, appears to meet the criteria for being classified as a bona fide treatment. In particular, more psychoanalytically oriented researchers and therapists may—as the author of the present book—be tempted to argue that more 'in-depth' treatment methods cause more structural changes in the patient, which in some cases take longer to manifest in the symptom measures that are typically applied in classic efficacy studies, and that psychoanalytic treatment should therefore be expected to have a better effect in the long term. A meta-analysis of existing follow-up studies, however, does not lend support to that proposition but finds that the long-term outcome more or less matches that of other approved treatment methods (Kivlighan et al. 2015). Generally, however, there is a need for substantial studies of this interesting issue.

6.1 Therapist Effects—The Impact of Therapist Factors on Treatment Outcome

> Amongst the factors which influence the prospects of an analysis (…), we must reckon not only the structure of the patient's own ego but the personal characteristics of the analyst. (…) So there is some reason in the demand for a high degree of psychic normality and correct adjustment in the analyst as evidence of his qualifications for his work (Freud 1937:377).

Naturally, the typical finding of no or very limited differences in the effect of generally approved treatment methods has caused some researchers to ponder what might explain why the choice of specific therapeutic methods at best have limited impact on treatment outcome. In addition to the possibility that different therapeutic methods may of course represent different and fairly similarly effective paths leading to the same goal, other factors under consideration include whether differences between the therapists taking part in the efficacy studies may help explain the remarkably small differences in effect size between very different standardized treatment methods.

Efficacy researchers speak of *therapist effects* or *therapist factors* influencing the effect of the treatment methods that have been examined.

Definitions of therapist factors vary slightly, but generally, the term refers to the effect that a given therapist has on outcome compared to other therapists or to those elements of a documented variance in treatment effect that in various statistical analyses appear to stem from factors pertaining to the individual therapists rather than to characteristics of patients and treatment methods. It refers to the finding that certain therapists have much better average treatment outcomes than others, independently of patient characteristics and the specific treatment method applied (Wampold and Imel 2015:78; Baldwin and Imel 2013:259f). The term thus refers to a phenomenon that points in a somewhat different direction than what has for decades been the dominant focus of psychotherapy research and of the medical model of therapy, which is to determine which specific treatment method is most effective. Generally, the emphasis on the efficacy of specific treatment methods has left little room for attending to, let alone securing research funding for studying, therapist effects. In the fifth edition of the authoritative handbook on empirical psychotherapy research *Bergin and Garfield's Handbook of Psychotherapy and Behavior Change*, Beutler et al. (2004:289f) thus conclude that research attention on elements of psychotherapy that are unrelated to outcome measures of specific treatment methods has been steadily decreasing. That applies especially to therapist variables, although several factors have emerged as promising predictors of treatment outcome in earlier studies (ibid.). In recent years in particular we have, however, begun to see renewed interest in the empirical study of therapist factors (cf. Baldwin et al. 2017:39f).

Apart from certain important studies from the early 1990s, generally speaking, empirical studies of this important field are few and far between. In the latest edition of *Bergin and Garfield's Handbook of Psychotherapy and Behavior Change* (2013) it is pointed out that we still lack research in this area; that, for several reasons, we need to pay more attention to the impact of therapist variables on outcome; and that we may find substantial differences between different therapists' outcomes—so substantial that this aspect should attract far greater attention in clinical practice (Baldwin and Imel 2013:290f).

As early as the 1960s, progressive researchers (Kiesler 1966) criticized the psychotherapy profession for ignoring important differences between therapists and for acting as if these differences between therapists is of no importance for the treatment process and outcome. Similarly, certain individual researchers at an early stage pointed out the—one would think, obvious—fact that some psychotherapists are much more successful than others (Ricks 1974). Another topic of debate is one of the aforementioned 'uniformity myths' in psychotherapy research: the usually unstated assumption that psychotherapists who take part in efficacy studies are more alike than different (Kiesler 1966:112) (see Chap. 5 concerning problematic aspects of the RCT format). During the 1980s, Lester Luborsky published the first small and, by today's standards, fairly primitive studies on the individual therapist's impact on treatment effect, and in 1991 Paul Crits-Christoph, one of Lester Luborsky's followers, presented the first meta-analysis of the impact of therapist factors on treatment effect in classic efficacy studies. From around 2005, bigger studies begin to appear on differences between individual psychotherapists' outcomes (Okiishi et al. 2003, 2006), which may shed some light on the role of therapist factors in determining the course and outcome of psychotherapy.

Underestimating Therapist Factors in Efficacy Studies

The vast majority of efficacy studies are not designed to address the role of therapist effects, and hence these are typically assessed using various forms of explorative post hoc meta-analyses of studies that were originally designed to compare the outcomes of specific treatment methods. In recent years, a number of post hoc meta-analyses of efficacy studies have set out to examine the impact of therapist factors on treatment effect. Generally, 3–9% of the variation in treatment effect is attributed to therapist factors (Wampold and Imel 2015:176; Baldwin and Imel 2013; Crits-Christoph et al. 1991), in some studies as much as 17% or more (Lutz et al. 2007; Huppert et al. 2001; Erickson et al. 2012), depending, in part, on the choice of effect measure, research design (RCT or naturalistic study), who the raters of treatment effect are, and which methods for statistical analysis are applied. Although some might find 3–9% a relatively low share, it should be noted that the impact of therapist factors often clearly exceeds the impact of differences between the compared treatment methods, which typically account for 0–1% of the outcome variation (Wampold and Imel 2015:176), again, somewhat dependent on the chosen method of statistical analysis and effect measures.

There is a clear risk of underestimating the role of therapist factors in these post hoc meta-analyses of efficacy studies, which were not designed to address therapist factors in the first place, in part because patient factors, all things being equal, will interact with therapist factors, and thus, any therapist factors might disappear in a meta-analysis. For example, more dysfunctional patients often have a poorer treatment prognosis, and their behaviour in the therapeutic space may requires greater skill from the therapist if the treatment is to have any effect. Thus, therapists who treat patients who on average are more severely disturbed pre-treatment—despite having the same formal diagnosis as other therapists' patients—but achieve fairly similar average treatment outcomes as other therapists who treated patients who initially did better have in fact solved a more demanding task. This is not captured in the published meta-analyses or in traditional outcome studies. Again, we are confronted with the fact that the psychotherapeutic process is inherently too complex to readily lend itself to traditional (quantitative) empirical studies; hence, researchers try to isolate and quantify individual key factors, which in real-life therapy interact continuously throughout the process.

To examine the impact of therapist factors, researchers should therefore ensure that the participating therapists have patients with fairly similar functioning levels (and that the heterogeneity of the patient group assigned to each therapist is limited), or they should attempt to control for the variation in their analyses, which is rarely done in traditional efficacy studies (Baldwin and Imel 2013:260). Further, it should be ensured that each therapist has a fairly large case load (to ensure sufficient statistical power), just as the assignment of patients to therapists should in principle be randomized. The latter is never the case in traditional randomized controlled efficacy studies, where the randomization pertains to the assignment of patients to treatment methods, because variations in the efficacy of specific treatment methods is the primary focus. On the other hand, one might argue that such a randomization would reflect a problematic lack of responsiveness in the coupling of patients and therapists; indeed, it is completely incompatible with normal clinical practice, where the match of patient and therapist, to varying degrees, is based on—partially conscious and explicit—'knowledge' about which therapists are more successful with certain types of patients and psychological issues.

Some Crits-Christoph and Gallop (2006) argue that because we lack a sufficient number of studies designed specifically to explore the role of therapist factors, and because it is generally assumed that any negative findings concerning therapist effects are unlikely to be published, we need to be very cautious in drawing conclusions on this topic, since we still lack sufficiently valid information about the impact of therapist factors on treatment effect. However, the real problem seems to be that we have not long since concluded that we need to devote far fewer resources to traditional efficacy studies and instead direct our limited research resources at investigating how the therapist influences the course and outcome of psychotherapy, even if we still lack reliable information about the precise effect size of therapist factors. There are indications that therapist factors have at least as much, and in some cases substantially greater, impact on treatment outcome than the choice of specific therapeutic method when it comes to psychotherapeutic treatment for most psychological disorders.

Meta-Analyses of Therapist Factors

The published meta-analyses show a tendency for therapist factors to carry more weight in older and more naturalistic studies compared with RCTs. This is hardly surprising, since more recent RCTs aim deliberately to minimize or eliminate therapist effects by selecting, training and supervising the participating therapists to ensure that they adhere as closely as possible to a standardized and manualized treatment method. All things being equal, such a strategy will reduce the differences between the participating therapists' work and thus any differences in outcome. As mentioned earlier, the strategy also has the potential to reduce the quality and success rate of some therapists' work, because expectations or mandates to adhere to a particular standardized treatment method may diminish the competent therapist's flexibility and creative latitude. It is worth noting that even these studies, which aim to minimize therapist factors, nevertheless often find that therapist factors account for a greater share of outcome variance than the specific treatment methods, which underscores that our exclusive focus on the effect of treatment techniques is misguided. We are similarly out of touch with reality if we consider the therapist a neutral, subjectless provider of certain treatment methods; the therapist is an important independent factor in psychotherapy (Luborsky et al. 1985:609).

As mentioned earlier, the impact of therapist factors on outcome may depend on the chosen outcome measures, including who assesses the effectiveness (patient, therapist, independent rater), and how (questionnaires, interviews or other methods). Thus, the effect size for therapist factors has been found to vary from 0 to 28%, depending on the outcome measure applied by the individual study and whether the rating was done by the patient or the therapist (Huppert et al. 2001; Nissen-Lie et al. 2013). Further, some studies have found the impact of therapist factors to be related to the severity of the patients' condition, where factors in the individual therapist seem to carry more weight in the treatment of more severely disturbed patients (Saxon and Barkham 2012). One of the most important studies of this phenomenon found that therapist factors may explain as little as 1% of outcome variance for the patients with the least severe conditions, compared to 10% for the most severely disturbed (Saxon and Barkham 2012:539). Other studies too have found a greater impact of therapist factors on outcome for patients with more severe pathology pre-treatment (Kim et al. 2006:168). One study found that as much as 17% of the difference in treatment effect can be attributed to therapist factors in the patients with the highest severity scores pre-treatment (Von Wyl et al. 2016:145; Barkham et al. 2017:25f, 33). Saxon and Barkham (2012) find indications that therapists who generally have poorer outcomes are negatively affected by increases in patient severity at intake. Thus, it appears that the more severe the patient's condition is pre-treatment, the more essential it is which therapist the patient is assigned to, regardless of treatment method.

Generally, the patient's severity rating is very important for the treatment outcome and general prognosis, but this seems to be less pronounced if more severely affected patients are assigned to the therapists who generally have the best outcomes. From a clinical point of view, that makes sense, since working with severely disturbed patients, including patients with severe personality disorders, often places greater demands on the therapist's general therapeutic competence, personal qualities (ability to contain intense affects, conflicts in the therapeutic relationship and so on) and ability to maintain a psychotherapeutic stance. Here, it is worth noting that Saxon and Barkham's aforementioned study is based on patients with depression and anxiety in brief time-limited treatment (6–7 sessions), who had not been assessed for other psychiatric pathologies—a clear limitation of the study—but who did not show obvious signs of suffering from very severe personality pathology. Had the latter been the case, there is reason to assume it would have further increased the difference in the impact of therapist effects, depending on the severity of the pathology.

That therapist factors account for such a relatively large share of treatment effect—typically accounting for more than the specific treatment method—is important for at least two reasons. First, it points to serious problems with the traditional efficacy study, where the main focus is on the link between treatment techniques and outcome, while therapist factors are typically either ignored or considered a source of error or 'noise' that the research design seeks to minimize (Beutler et al. 2004:227). Since the focus is not on the most important aspects of psychotherapy, there is a risk of overestimating the impact that the specific treatment techniques has on outcome. Second, it underscores the need for studies that focus more on differences in individual therapists' treatment outcomes and—as the next step—on uncovering what sets therapists with excellent outcomes apart from therapists who are less successful in helping their patients achieve a satisfactory outcome. In particular, we should be interested in what characterizes therapists who achieve superior outcomes with high-severity patients. Finally, of course, it may also have implications for clinical practice in the sense that we should look more at individual therapists' outcomes rather than which treatment methods they identify with, regardless whether they claim to rely on 'evidence-based' methods. Moreover, we should address the issue of therapists who systematically have poorer treatment outcomes than should be expected—either by making sure they receive additional training or by arranging for them to take on other tasks, although the latter may obviously be controversial.

The discussion about the relative contribution—or lack of contribution—of therapist factors and specific treatment methods to outcome strikes at the core of certain therapists' and psychotherapy researchers' professional identity. Essentially, it raises the question of what psychotherapy is really about—what is the core of psychotherapy and thus determines its efficacy, and what we should focus on in the training and evaluation of psychotherapists. A similar point pertains to the professional disagreements about whether the medical or the psychodynamic concept of therapy is more appropriate. The sometimes intense professional debate about the role of therapist factors for outcome has been manifest, in part, in discussions about how to interpret the results of the large NIMH outcome study of methods for the treatment of depression—in many regards, an excellent study that was conducted on behalf of the American National Institute of Mental Health (Elkin 1994). This RCT was originally designed to compare the efficacy of medical and various psychotherapeutic treatments of patients with varying degrees of depression, but it is based on such a large high-quality data set that it can also be used to shed light on other interesting questions.

Several years after the completion of the original study, new teams of researchers thus re-analysed the data. One team concludes that 8% of the outcome variance between the different treatments in the study can be attributed to therapist factors, while the specific treatment methods do not seem to play any role (0% of the treatment effect is attributable to the specific treatment method), after these therapist factors have been factored in (Kim et al. 2006). Other analyses, on the other hand, find no impact of therapist factors on treatment outcome once individual therapists with especially good or poor outcomes (outliers) have been eliminated from the data set—even though the analysis still finds substantial differences between the individual therapists' drop-out rates (0–75%) and the share of patients (0–63%) who 'recovered' (patients who no longer meet pre-determined criteria for depression post-treatment) (Elkin et al. 2006). On that basis, this research team concludes that the role of therapist factors has been overstated (Elkin et al. 2006:154).

Subsequently, it has been pointed out that the widely different conclusions to these two analyses of the same data set emerge because the two teams use different statistical analyses and focus on different outcome measures (Soldz 2006). Among other points, it may seem problematic that one research team (Elkin et al. 2006) eliminates those therapists from the data set who have outlier outcomes before it goes on to analyse the contribution of therapist factors to treatment effect (Wampold and Bolt 2006). It has also been argued that the design of the NIMH study does not generate data that is suited for estimating the effect size of therapist factors (Lutz et al. 2007). Overall, there is no easy path to consensus on exactly how to estimate the role of therapist factors in traditional efficacy studies, just as the relative impact of therapist factors, for a number of reasons, remains a controversial issue in psychotherapy research. For an overview of studies that can help elucidate the role of therapist factors, see, e.g., Baldwin and Imel (2013:264–275).

Significant Differences in Treatment Outcomes

There are, however, a number of studies that look at average outcome differences across a large number of therapists. These studies consistently suggest that there may be quite substantial differences in the average benefit for patients from treatment provided by different therapists. Thus, we need to distinguish between good and less successful therapists, although it is rarely the case that any therapist is successful with all his patients, let alone that any one therapist systematically has sub-par outcomes for all his patients.

One of the first studies in this field was conducted by Lester Luborsky (Luborsky et al. 1985). He compares the outcomes of nine therapists' treatment of a total of 110 patients—all male drug-dependent veterans—in fairly brief treatment courses (up to 24 sessions). The patients were randomly assigned to different therapists, and no meaningfully significant differences were found between the nine therapists' assigned groups of patients pre-treatment. Luborsky finds substantial differences in average effect size between the nine therapists, varying from 0.13 (very low, bordering on no average effect) to 0.74 (quite a large treatment effect) (Luborsky et al. 1985:604). In a later, slightly larger but related study Luborsky not only finds considerable differences between the individual therapists' average effects—from therapists whose patients on average have deteriorated slightly post-treatment to therapists who see 80% of their patients improve—but also an indication that the most successful therapists have the lowest drop-out rates as well and thus must be assumed to be better at retaining patients and at securing a good outcome for most of them (Luborsky et al. 1997). None of the participating therapists have convincing outcomes for all their patients.

Okiishi has presented one of the first large-scale studies of differences in therapists' average treatment outcomes. The study is based on 1780 college students receiving treatment for mild or moderate disorders (fewer than 2% of the patients have a personality disorder) from 56 therapists. The treatment is largely brief time-limited therapy (with an average of about five sessions), and there is no difference in the average degree of pre-treatment severity between the individual therapists' patient groups. This study, too, finds large differences in the participating therapists' average treatment outcomes. Patients who received treatment from the least successful therapists on average deteriorate slightly during the course of the treatment, while patients working with the most successful therapist achieve an average improvement that is ten times the average rate of change for all the therapists in the study (Okiishi et al. 2003:366). The therapists with the best average outcomes also saw clients for a shorter time (ibid.:368).

Roughly put, the patients who receive treatment from the most successful therapists on average see greater improvement faster. None of the findings can be explained with reference to the type or extent of the therapists' training (theoretical orientation or duration), which underscores the importance of the therapist's more personal qualities for the course and outcome of therapy. It is unclear, however, whether these findings can be generalized, for example to longer-term treatment of more severe psychological disorders. The study also has a number of fairly serious methodological limitations, including that it uses only one, relatively simple, outcome measure, that many of the patients are only mildly disturbed, and that patients are not assigned to therapists in a randomized process.

Several more recent studies, involving hundreds of therapists, who together have treated thousands of patients, add to the general picture of quite substantial differences between individual psychotherapists' average treatment outcomes (Brown et al. 2005; Okiishi et al. 2006; Kraus et al. 2011; Saxon and Berkham 2012; Berglar et al. 2016) and drop-out rates (Berglar et al. 2016), including that a small subset of therapists appear to have negative treatment outcomes in some areas (Kraus et al. 2011). These are mainly naturalistic studies based on patients with mild, and in some cases moderate, pathology—typically, anxiety or affective disorders—for fairly short treatments (typically 5–10 sessions), where the severity of the patients' pre-treatment disorders does not explain the outcome differences between individual therapists. Okiishi et al. (2006:1167) find a 22% recovery rate for the patients who receive (short-term) treatment from the most successful among a large group of therapists (in the course of nine sessions on average), while only 5% deteriorate during the treatment. By comparison, there is only a 11% recovery rate among the patients who receive treatment from the therapists with the worst treatment outcomes, while 10% deteriorate. Generally, the findings suggest that we can identify 10–20% of therapists who are characterized by having significantly poorer or better treatment outcomes than a larger middle group (about 60%) of therapists who do not show any substantial variation in treatment outcomes, and who generally are fine, effective therapists (cf. Barkham et al. 2017:26f).

Kraus et al. (2011) have presented material suggesting that therapists are often better at treating certain disorders or dysfunctions within certain domains than within others, while some therapists (as many as 16% of the nearly 700 therapists who take part in their study) appear to have a harmful effect on dysfunctions in certain areas, particularly abuse and violent behaviour. This might suggest that therapist effectiveness is not a general feature but varies across problem areas, just as virtually all the therapists in the study have positive effects in at least a few areas, and none have positive outcomes in all problem areas. That matches the typical clinical experience: that most therapists are better at working with and helping some types of patients than others, and that therapist competence and effectiveness are, to some degree, domain-specific.

On the other hand, other studies (Nissen-Lie et al. 2016) have found that therapists who achieve good (or poor) treatment outcomes in one area often do so in other areas too; this might be seen as an indication that therapist competence and effectiveness constitute a more general individual characteristic, which cannot be reduced to specific skills in treating patients with a certain disorder or certain types of difficulties (Green et al. 2014). Finally, Saxon and Barkham (2012:542) have found that therapists who have many patients with a high score for self-reported risk behaviour (risk-to-self or risk-to-others), have a poorer average treatment outcome, possibly because they feel under greater pressure, which may negatively affect their performance or, certainly, their outcomes. In extension of this, one might imagine that the individual therapist's ability to contain and respond effectively to more dysfunctional and challenging patients (maintaining the psychotherapeutic stance and avoiding acting out countertransference) is an important part of the explanation for the documented differences in therapist effectiveness or average treatment outcomes (Lambert 2013a, b:198).

Overall, it appears that characteristics in the individual therapist have a significant impact on treatment outcome, and that there may be substantial differences in the therapists' average outcomes. In extension of this point, there is reason to query what sets the effective (and perhaps the exceptional) therapists apart from the less competent ones. Empirical psychotherapy research cannot tell us a great deal about this, but it does offer some insights. Generally, variability in treatment effect between therapists seems to be primarily associated with differences in interpersonal skills (Barkham et al. 2017:31).

Apart from obvious and trivial points, for example that a good psychotherapist has to have a good capacity for empathizing and for conveying this quality to the patient, there are no simple answers as to what generally characterizes the good therapist. This is in part because patient factors play such a large role, and because different patients need very different things from the therapist; for example, patients with a deactivating attachment style need a therapist with a different relational style than patients with a hyperactivating attachment style (Tyrrell et al. 1999). In these scenarios, the key therapeutic competence is centred on the therapist's ability to read what the individual patient needs, continually, and adapt his response accordingly (therapeutic responsiveness, see Chap. 10). This includes the ability to maintain a psychotherapeutic stance and to regulate the acting out of countertransference, also in situations where emotions run high, or when there is a high level of conflict in the therapeutic space. On the other hand, it does not appear that therapist factors that are fairly simple to operationalize and verify (sex, age and so on) have any impact on outcome; nor can they help us define what characterizes the good therapist. Things are more complicated than that, which reflects the complexity of the psychotherapeutic process.

References

Baardseth, T. P., Goldberg, S. B., Pace, B. T., Wislocki, A. P., Frost, N. D., Siddiqui, J. R., et al. (2013). Cognitive-behavioral therapy versus other therapies: Redux. *Clinical Psychology Review, 33,* 395–405.

Baldwin, S. A., & Imel, Z. E. (2013). Therapist effects: Findings and methods. In M. J. Lambert (Ed.), *Bergin and Garfield's handbook of psychotherapy and behavior change* (6th ed., pp. 258–298). New York, NY: Wiley.

Baldwin, S. A., Wampold, B. E., & Imel, Z. E. (2007). Untangling the alliance-outcome correlation: Exploring the relative importance of therapist and patient variability in the alliance. *Journal of Consulting and Clinical Psychology, 75,* 842–852.

Barkham, M., Lutz, W., Lambert, M. J., & Saxon, D. (2017). Therapist effects, effective therapists, and the law of variability. In L. G. Castonguay & C. E. Hill (Eds.), *How and why are some therapists better than others?* (pp. 13–36). Washington, DC: American Psychological Association.
Bateman, A., & Fonagy, P. (2009). Randomized controlled trial of outpatient mentalization-based treatment versus structured clinical management for borderline personality disorder. *American Journal of Psychiatry, 166*(12), 1355–1364.
Berglar, J., Crameri, A., Von Wyl, A., Koemeda-Lutz, M., Köhler, M., Staczan, P., et al. (2016). Therapist effects on treatment outcome in psychotherapy: A multilevel modelling analysis. *International Journal of Psychotherapy, 20,* 61–80.
Beutler, L. E., Malik, M., Alimohamed, S., Harwood, T. M., Talebi, H., Noble, S., et al. (2004). Therapist variables. In M. J. Lambert (Ed.), *Bergin and Garfield's handbook of psychotherapy and behavior change* (5th ed., pp. 227–306). New York, NY: Wiley.
Brown, G. S., Lambert, M. J., Jones, E. R., & Minami, T. (2005). Identifying highly effective psychotherapists in a managed care environment. *American Journal of Managed Care, 11,* 513–520.
Budge, S. L., Moore, J. T., Del Re, A. C., Wampold, B. E., Baardseth, T. P., & Nienhuis, J. B. (2013). The effectiveness of evidence-based treatment for personality disorders when comparing treatment-as-usual and bona fide treatments. *Clinical Psychology Review, 33,* 1057–1066.
Cristea, I. A., Gentili, C., Cotet, C. D., Palomba, D., Barbui, C., & Cuijpers, P. (2017). Efficacy of psychotherapies for borderline personality disorder: A systematic review and meta-analysis. *JAMA Psychiatry*, *74*(4), 319–328.
Crits-Christoph, P., & Gallop, R. (2006). Therapist effects in The National Institute of Mental Health treatment of depression collaborative research program and other psychotherapy studies. *Psychotherapy Research, 16*(2), 178–181.
Crits-Christoph, P., Baranackie, K., Kurcias, J.S., Beck, A.T., Carroll, K., Perry, K., Luborsky, L., McLellan, A.T., Woody, G.E., Thompson, L., Gallagher, D. & Zitrin, C. (1991). Meta-analysis of therapist effects in psychotherapy outcome studies. *Psychotherapy Research, 1*(2), 81–91
Cuijpers, P., Straten, A., Anderson, G., & Oppen, P. (2008). Psychotherapy for depression in adults: A meta-analysis of comparative outcome studies. *Journal of Consulting and Clinical Psychology, 76,* 909–922.
Driessen, E., Cuijpers, P., de Maat, S. C. M., Abbass, A. A., de Jonghe, F., & Dekker, J. J. M. (2010). The efficacy of short-term psychodynamic psychotherapy for depression: A meta-analysis. *Clinical Psychology Review, 30,* 25–36.
Elkin, I. (1994). The NIMH treatment of depression collaborative research program: Where we began and where we are. In A. E. Bergin & S. L. Garfield (Eds.), *Handbook of psychotherapy and behavior change* (4th ed., pp. 114–142). New York, NY: Wiley.
Elkin, I., Falconnier, L., Martinovich, Z., & Mahoney, C. (2006). Therapist effects in the National Institute of Mental Health treatment of depression collaborative research program. *Psychotherapy Research, 16*(2), 144–160.
Erickson, S. J., Tonigan, S., & Winhusen, T. (2012). Therapist effects in a NIDA CTN intervention trial with pregnant substance abusing women: Findings form a RCT with MET and TAU conditions. *Alcoholism Treatment Quarterly, 30,* 224–237.
Freud, S. (1937). Analysis terminable and interminable. *The International Journal of Psychoanalysis, 18,* 373–405.
GieBen-Bloo, J., van Dyck, R., Spinhoven, P., van Tilburg, W., & Dirksen, C. (2006). Outpatient psychotherapy for borderline personality disorder: Randomized trial of schema-focused therapy vs. transference-focused psychotherapy. *Archives of General Psychiatry, 63,* 649–659.
Green, H., Barkham, M., Kellett, S., & Saxon, D. (2014). Therapist effects and IAPT psychological wellbeing practitioners (PWPs): A multilevel modelling and mixed methods analysis. *Behaviour Research and Therapy, 63,* 43–54.
Grenyer, B. F. S. (2007). Hope for sustaining a positive 3-year therapeutic relationship with borderline personality disorder. *Archives of General Psychiatry, 64*(5), 609.

Huppert, J. D., Bufka, L. F., Barlow, D. H., Gorman, J. M., Shear, M. K., & Woods, S. W. (2001). Therapists, therapist variables, and cognitive-behavioral therapy outcome in a multicenter trial for panic disorder. *Journal of Consulting and Clinical Psychology, 69,* 747–755.

Jørgensen, C. R., Freund, C., Bøye, R., Jordet, H., Andersen, D., & Kjølbye, M. (2013). Outcome of mentalization-based and supportive psychotherapy in patients with borderline personality disorder: A randomized trial. *Acta Psychitrica Scandinavica, 127,* 305–317.

Jørgensen, C. R., Bøye, R., Andersen, D., Blaabjerg, A.-H. D., Freund, C., & Kjølbye, M. (2014). Eighteen months post-treatment naturalistic follow-up of mentalization-based therapy and supportive group treatment for borderline personality disorder: Clinical outcomes and functioning. *Nordic Psychology, 66*(4), 254–273.

Kiesler, D. J. (1966). Some myths of psychotherapy research and the search for a paradigm. *Psychological Bulletin, 65,* 110–136.

Kim, D.-M., Wampold, B. E., & Bolt, D. M. (2006). Therapist effects in psychotherapy: A random-effects modeling of the national institute of mental health treatment of depression collaborative research program data. *Psychotherapy Research, 16,* 161–172.

Kivlighan, D. M., Goldberg, S. B., Abbas, M., Pace, B. T., Yulish, N. E., Thomas, J. G., et al. (2015). The enduring effects of psychodynamic treatment vis-a-vis alternative treatments: A longitudinal meta-analysis. *Clinical Psychology Review, 40,* 1–14.

Kraus, D. R., Castonguay, L., Boswell, J. F., Nordberg, S. S., & Hayes, J. A. (2011). Therapist effectiveness: Implications for accountability and patient care. *Psychotherapy Research, 21,* 267–276.

Lambert, M. J. (2013a). Introduction and historical overview. In M. J. Lambert (Ed.), *Bergin and Garfield's handbook of psychotherapy and behavior change* (6th ed., pp. 3–21). New York, NY: Wiley.

Lambert, M. J. (2013b). The efficacy and effectiveness of psychotherapy. In M. J. Lambert (Ed.), *Bergin and Garfield's handbook of psychotherapy and behavior change* (6th ed., pp. 169–219). New York, NY: Wiley.

Luborsky, L., McLellan, T., Woody, G. E., O'Brian, C. P., & Auerbach, A. (1985). Therapist success and its determinants. *Archives of General Psychiatry, 42,* 602–611.

Luborsky, L., McLellan, A. T., Diguer, L., Woody, G., & Seligman, D. A. (1997). The psychotherapist matters: Comparison of outcomes across twenty-two therapists and seven patient samples. *Clinical Psychology: Science and Practice, 4,* 53–65.

Lutz, W., Leon, S. C., Martinovich, J. S., & Stiles, W. B. (2007). Therapist effects in outpatient psychotherapy: A three-level growth curve approach. *Journal of Counseling Psychology, 54,* 32–39.

Nathan, P. E., & Gorman, J. M. (Eds.). (2015). *A guide to treatments that work* (4th ed.). New York, NY: Oxford University Press.

Nissen-Lie, H. A., Monsen, J. T., Ulleberg, P., & Rønnestad, M. H. (2013). Psychotherapists self-reports of their interpersonal functioning and difficulties in practice as predictors of patient outcome. *Psychotherapy Research, 23,* 86–104.

Nissen-Lie, H. A., Goldberg, S. B., Hoyt, W. T., Falkenström, F., Holmqvist, R., Nielsen, S. L., et al. (2016). Are therapists uniformly effective across patient outcome domains? A study on therapist effectiveness in two different treatment contexts. *Journal of Counseling Psychology, 64*(4), 367–378.

Normann, N., Van Emmerik, A. A. P., & Morina, N. (2014). The efficacy of metacognitive therapy for anxiety and depression: A meta-analytic review. *Depression and Anxiety, 31,* 402–411.

Okiishi, J., Lambert, M. J., Nielsen, S. L., & Ogles, B. M. (2003). Waiting for supershrink: An empirical analysis of therapist effects. *Clinical Psychology and Psychotherapy, 10,* 361–373.

Okiishi, J. C., Lambert, M. J., Eggett, D., Nielsen, L., Dayton, D. D., & Vermeersch, D. A. (2006). An analysis of therapist treatment effects: Toward providing feedback to individual therapists on their clients' psychotherapy outcome. *Journal of Clinical Psychology, 62,* 1157–1172.

Owen, J., Drinane, J. M., Idigo, K. C., & Valentine, J. C. (2015). Psychotherapist effects in meta-analyses: How accurate are treatment effects? *Psychotherapy, 52,* 321–328.

Ricks, D. F. (1974). Supershrink: Methods of a therapist judged successful on the basis of adult outcomes of adolescent patients. In D. F. Ricks, M. Roff, & A. Thomas (Eds.), *Life history research in psychopathology* (Vol. 3, pp. 275–297). Minneapolis: University of Minnesota Press.
Roth, A., & Fonagy, P. (2006). *What works for whom? A critical review of psychotherapy research*. New York, NY: Guilford.
Saxon, D., & Barkham, M. (2012). Patterns of therapist variability: Therapist effects and the contribution of patient severity and risk. *Journal of Consulting and Clinical Psychology, 80,* 535–546.
Soldz, S. (2006). Models and meanings: Therapist effects and the stories we tell. *Psychotherapy Research, 16,* 173–177.
Tolin, D. F. (2010). Is cognitive-behavioral therapy more effective than other therapies? A meta-analytic review. *Clinical Psychology Review, 30,* 710–720.
Tyrrell, C. L., Dozier, M., Teague, G. B., & Fallot, R. D. (1999). Effective treatment relationships for persons with serious psychiatric disorders: The importance of attachment states of mind. *Journal of Consulting and Clinical Psychology, 67,* 725–733.
Von Wyl, A., Tschuschke, V., Crameri, A., Koemeda-Lutz, M., & Schulthess, P. (Eds.). (2016). *Was wirkt in der Psychotherapie? Ergebnisse der Praxisstudie ambulante Psychotherapie zu 10 unterschiedlichen Verfahren* [What works in psychotherapy? Findings of a practice study of day-patient psychotherapy with 10 different methods]. Gießen: Psychosozial-Verlag.
Wampold, B. E., & Bolt, D. M. (2006). Therapist effects: Clever ways to make them (and everything else) disappear. *Psychotherapy Research, 16,* 184–187.
Wampold, B. E., & Imel, Z.-E. (2015). *The great psychotherapy debate: The evidence for what makes psychotherapy work* (2nd ed.). London, England: Routledge.
Wampold, B. E., Budge, S. L., Laska, K. M., Del Re, A. C., Baardseth, T. P., Flückiger, C., et al. (2011). Evidence-based treatments for depression and anxiety versus treatment-as-usual: A meta-analysis of direct comparisons. *Clinical Psychology Review, 31,* 1304–1312.
Wampold, B. E., Flückiger, C., Del Re, A. C., Yulish, N. E., Frost, N. D., Pace, B. T., et al. (2017). In pursuit of truth: A critical examination of meta-analyses of cognitive behavior therapy. *Psychotherapy Research, 27,* 14–32.
Weisz, J. R., Kuppens, S., Ng, M. Y., Eckshtain, D., Ugueto, A. M., Vaughn-Coaxum, R., et al. (2017). What five decades of research tells us about the effects of youth psychological therapy: A multilevel meta-analysis and implications for science and practice. *American Psychologist, 72,* 79–117.
Yeomans, F. E. (2007). Questions concerning the randomized trial of schema-focused vs. transference-focused psychotherapy. *Archives of General Psychiatry, 64,* 609–610.

Chapter 7
The Good Therapist

> What, then, are the basic requirements as to the personality and the professional abilities of a psychiatrist? […] The psychiatrist must be able to listen. […] To be able to listen and to gather information from another person in this other person's own right, without reacting along the lines of one's own problems or experiences, of which one may be reminded, perhaps in a disturbing way, is an art of interpersonal exchange which few people are able to practice without special training (Fromm-Reichmann 1960:7).

As outlined in the previous chapter, there may be quite substantial differences between individual therapists' treatment outcomes—differences that cannot be attributed to their choice of treatment method but which instead seems to reflect their more personal qualities, including their ability to provide a secure base for the patient and to display competence, relational skills and other features that influence the development of trust and a sustainable therapeutic relationship and alliance. Meta-analyses of the contribution of common factors to treatment effect suggest that forming a good therapeutic alliance, including consensus about the goal of the treatment, is key to treatment outcome (average effect sizes around 0.5–0.6) (Wampold and Imel 2015:209). The impact of the therapeutic alliance on outcome may stem from the fact that forming a good working alliance can be presumed to strengthen the patient's epistemic trust in the therapist and in what happens in the therapeutic space. This in turn makes it easier for the patient to accept what the therapist brings to the interaction, and to generate new experiences in the therapeutic space (with the power to revise fixed perceptions of self and others), instead of merely experiencing everything that happens in the therapeutic relationship as either variations on previous (mostly negative) experiences or as experiences with no particular significance for the self (Fonagy et al. 2015:593). Similarly, numerous studies have found that the therapist's empathy, genuineness in the contact with the patient and positive regard and affirmation of the patient have a significant impact on treatment outcome (with respective effect sizes around 0.6, 0.5 and 0.55) (Wampold and Imel 2015:209).

There is also some empirical support for the claim that the therapist's ability to adapt the treatment to the individual patient's (sub)culture and create positive expectations has an influence on effectiveness (Wampold and Imel 2015:209). Finally, meta-analyses have found that the number of patients who drop out of the treatment

C. R. Jørgensen, *The Psychotherapeutic Stance*,
https://doi.org/10.1007/978-3-030-20437-2_7

is markedly lower for experienced therapists, independent of their theoretical and therapeutic orientation (Swift and Greenberg 2012). This may be because experienced therapists are more responsive and better at reading and managing problems in the therapeutic relationship than younger and less experienced therapists (Swift and Greenberg 2012:556). On the other hand, it is also possible that therapists with good relational skills are more likely to remain in the profession, while those who are less suited for practising psychotherapy are more likely to leave. Finally, it may be that less successful senior therapists are less likely to take part in empirical studies, just as it may generally be difficult to ensure that the therapists participating in empirical studies are representative of the profession at large. The published meta-analyses do not shed light on any potential correlations between specific therapist characteristics and the risk of patient drop-out.

7.1 The Ability to Form an Alliance, Relational Skills and Treatment Outcome

As mentioned earlier, the correlation between the quality of the therapeutic alliance (typically as rated by the patient at an early stage of the therapy) and treatment outcome (typically self-reported post-treatment symptom relief) is one of the most robust findings in empirical psychotherapy research (around 0.25) (Wampold and Imel 2015:179f; Horvath et al. 2011:47), just as, across treatment methods, the therapeutic alliance is estimated to account for around 7% of outcome variance (Flückiger et al. 2012:10f; Horvath et al. 2011:49). It remains unclear, however, what the causal link is between alliance and treatment outcome; one possibility is of course that forming a good therapeutic alliance is in itself an important mechanism of change. It is also possible that the development of a good alliance is in part a product of the patient's perceived improvement; there is no doubt that the link between alliance and treatment outcome is complex (Zilcha-Mano and Barber 2014:65).

Recent studies and meta-analyses (Del Re et al. 2012:646) suggest that there are big differences in individual therapists' ability to form a good alliance with their patients, and that the therapist's contribution to the alliance has a bigger impact on treatment outcome than the patient's contribution (Baldwin et al. 2007). From a clinical perspective, the latter makes sense, as more poorly functioning patients often lack some of the psychological resources and the trust that are key conditions for entering into a therapeutic alliance. Thus, especially in the early stages of the treatment it is a key aspect of the therapy to deal with the issues that make it difficult for the patient to enter into an alliance. The more severe the patient's pathology is, the greater the demands on the therapist's ability to develop and repair ruptures in the therapeutic alliance—and the more variation will there be in different therapists' ability to help these patients. Some studies find that problems in the therapeutic alliance grow more pronounced, the more severe and chronic the patient's condition is—problems that are manifest, among other ways, in frequent misunderstandings between patient and therapist or in the patient explicitly questioning the purpose of the treatment, threatening to walk out, attacking or provoking the therapist and showing signs of profound resistance to the treatment (Von Wyl et al. 2016:114f). These issues may dominate the therapeutic space for long spans of time in work with patients with more severe personality disorders.

It is often quite demanding to remain empathic and understanding, warm and tolerant in interactions with patients who have attachment disorders and, more generally, severe conditions. On the other hand, less severely disturbed patients who have a basic trust in others and a fairly well-developed relational capacity will often be able to enter into a good alliance with most therapists (Baldwin et al. 2007), in which case the demands on the therapist's relational skills will be different and much lighter. In extension of this point, research has found that patients working with therapists who form particularly good therapeutic alliances with their patients are, on average, more likely to have a good treatment outcome (Del Re et al. 2012:647). Similarly, therapists who on average develop good alliances with their patients have significantly better treatment outcomes than therapists who form less strong alliances (Baldwin et al. 2007:849). In relation to this point, however, it should be noted that some therapists are presumably better at forming alliances with certain types of patients, while other therapists excel with other types of patients. Most therapists are more responsive in their meeting with some patients than with others. Generally, however, one would expect that patients with severe relational difficulties and attachment disorders are more likely to benefit from working with therapists with strong relational skills, including special skills for forming a sustainable therapeutic alliance, remaining empathic and maintaining a psychotherapeutic stance in conflict situations with high emotional arousal.

Many empirical studies suggest that different personal characteristics in the therapist and the use of a range of specific techniques increase the likelihood of forming a good therapeutic alliance across specific therapeutic methods (Ackerman and Hilsenroth 2003). Although it is, naturally, not without problems to list such general correlations between therapist characteristics, technical interventions and the forming of an alliance, as alliances always depend on patient characteristics too—far from all patients need the same from the therapist to help them enter into an alliance—they can still offer some pointers as to what is likely to influence the alliance in a positive direction.

Among other aspects, therapist characteristics such as flexibility, experience, honesty, credibility, kindness, warmth, openness, interest, respectfulness and taking an interest in the patients have been found to make a positive contribution to the therapeutic alliance. The therapist's experience, however, mostly seems to matter for those aspects of the alliance that deal with reaching consensus on the goals and method of the treatment, not for forming the emotional bond between patient and therapist that appears to play a crucial role for the therapeutic process (Ackerman and Hilsenroth 2003). On the other hand, patients (with less severe disorders) working with therapists who are comfortable with emotional closeness in relationships (and who have a perceived supportive social network) perceive the emotional bond of the alliance to be stronger than do patients in treatment with therapists who are less comfortable with emotional closeness (Dunkle and Friedlander 1996:58). Similarly, active, understanding, supportive, explorative and reflective interventions typically, where the patient is met with recognition, help to form and maintain a good working alliance, just as interventions that support the verbalization of affects and the patient's subjective experiences as well as interventions that promote the sense that the patient and therapist are working together on a common problem—establishing a 'we-feeling' in the therapeutic space (Jørgensen 2000:664)—and communicate a sense of hope that the patients can achieve their goals appear to contribute positively to the alliance (Ackerman and Hilsenroth 2003:13). This also includes a balanced response to criticism and ruptures in the alliance, including that the therapist acknowledges his contribution to the rupture (Ackerman and Hilsenroth 2003:29). None of these fairly general findings concerning correlations between therapist characteristics, interventions and the ability to form a good therapeutic alliance appear particularly surprising.

Similarly, certain therapist characteristics have been identified that diminish the likelihood of forming and maintaining a good alliance; these include being rigid, uncertain, avoidant, aloof and critical in interactions with the patient, tense, unfocused and exploitive (Ackerman and Hilsenroth 2001:182). As for the therapist's interventions, failure to structure the therapeutic work or, conversely, rigidly overstructuring it, inappropriate self-disclosure, unyielding transference interpretations, inappropriate use of silence, superficial, incompetent or intrusive interventions and interventions that are moralistic, belittling or seek to impose the therapist's values on the patient have been found to correlate with a poorer working alliance (ibid.).

It is of course debatable how informative these very general links between what must be characterized as broad characteristics of competent and less competent—bordering on incompetent—therapists and the therapeutic alliance are for practice. Although it can easily be argued that many of listed qualities of competent versus less competent therapists are so general, predictable and, to some extent, vague that they border on the inane and trivial, they still lend support to the assumption that the therapist's personal characteristics and specific behaviour in the therapeutic space actually have a considerable impact on the psychotherapeutic process and the likelihood of a good outcome. Besides, there is some empirical basis for assuming that the therapist's ability to deal with negative therapeutic processes—ruptures in the alliance—affect the course and outcome of the therapy (Safran et al. 2011:231). It should be noted that the patient, for many different reasons (see, e.g., Chap. 8 on transference) often has ambivalent or negative feelings towards the therapist and the therapy. It is up to the therapist to create a space where the patient can express these negative feelings—before they develop into serious ruptures in the alliance or cause the patient to terminate the treatment—without fear of revenge, sanctions or other negative and countertherapeutic reactions from the therapist. As much as possible, the therapist should offer an open, non-defensive response (rather than becoming defensive and adopting a victimized position) and explicitly accept responsibility for his contribution to the patient's perceived frustration and dissatisfaction.

In his response to the patient's articulation of dissatisfaction, the therapist must be empathic and validating, assessing whether the stated dissatisfaction may be used in an in-depth exploration of the possible dynamic background of the patient's frustration and dissatisfaction, including pointing out possible connections to recurring patterns in the patient's past and current relationships (Safran et al. 2011:235f). Crucially, the therapist must avoid giving the patient the impression that her current experience of the therapist and the therapeutic relationship are denied reality, because they are simply seen as a recurring pattern in her life and thus as something that is solely related to her and her disorder; that would typically be received as an invalidation and dismissal of her subjective experience. The therapist has to meet the patient's stated dissatisfaction and frustration with a stance that signals openness and tolerance and which validates her subjective experience. Only then can the therapist, perhaps, invite a common exploration of the background of the experience, whether that primarily concerns the therapist's own missteps, recurring relational dynamics in the patient's life or (most likely) a combination of both.

This psychotherapeutic stance and approach to the patient's implicitly or explicitly expressed frustration and dissatisfaction with the therapist and the therapy requires the therapist to be able to strike the right balance between, on the one hand, seeing the patient's dissatisfaction as a reflection of misattunement in the therapy and the need to adjust the therapeutic strategy and, on the other hand, viewing it as therapeutic material that contains valuable information about some of the patient's recurring problems in interpersonal relationships. The frustrations expressed by the patient also convey how she typically attempts to handle such situations, and how she typically reacts when these problems arise, for example by becoming aggressive, taking on the role of helpless victim, withdrawing from contact ('fleeing'), activating self-loathing and negative self-perceptions ('it's my own fault/because there's something wrong with me that others always ignore/misunderstand me' and so on).

The Therapist's Relational Skills

As mentioned, there is growing empirical documentation that the strongest predictors of outcome relate to therapist factors, not least relational skills, in a broad sense (Nissen-Lie et al. 2013:87; Baldwin and Imel 2013). Corresponding to the therapist factors mentioned above that correlate with a good therapeutic alliance, a range of interpersonal therapist characteristics have been proposed as possible predictors of good treatment outcomes, including empathy, being a good communicator, communicative attunement, warm and trusting interpersonal style, responding thoughtfully and appropriately to patient hostility, being sensitive to and aware of developments in the therapeutic process and ability to address ruptures in the therapeutic alliance (Schöttke et al. 2017:643). Similarly, rigidity, an anxious attachment style and impulsivity and a tendency to be hostile, excessively controlling, become emotionally overwhelmed and withdraw from the patient have, to varying degrees, been found to correlate with poorer treatment outcomes (Beutler et al. 2004:274ff; Castonguay et al. 2010; Rønnestad and Skovholt 2013:108; Najavits and Weiss 1994:685). Therapists' demographic characteristics (sex, age, training) do not generally appear to influence treatment outcome (Beutler et al. 2004:291), while it remains uncertain whether—and if so, exactly how—the therapist's experience level influences outcome.

There is far from consensus on how best to operationalize the therapist's experience level (Hill and Knox 2013:802)—a simple definition based on number of years spent practising psychotherapy is hardly adequate, just as there is reason to assume that experience matters more in therapy with certain patient groups (patients with more severe pathology) than with others. A few studies, including a large-scale naturalistic study in Switzerland (Von Wyl et al. 2016:115f), thus find that more disturbed patients in particular benefit far more when they are treated by more experienced therapists (based on number of years spent practising psychotherapy), while another study (Berglar et al. 2016) finds that experience generally correlates with a better treatment outcome across all patients, including those with less severe conditions.

It has further been argued that empirical studies are usually dominated by trainee and novice therapists treating patients with relatively mild disorders, while there is an underrepresentation of very experienced therapists; this leads to a weak basis for assessing the importance of experience. This point should be seen in light of the fact that it takes years to develop in-depth psychotherapeutic expertise (cf. Skovholt et al. 1997), and there is reason to assume that expert therapists' special competences will mainly be manifest in the treatment of more severely disturbed patients. However, there are indications that the therapist's experience level may have some, albeit generally no more than moderate, positive influence on treatment outcome (Beutler et al. 2004:239; Willutzki et al. 2013:431), although some studies find a marginal deterioration in individual therapists' outcomes over time (Goldberg et al. 2016) and suggest that therapists either fail to improve their treatment outcomes over the course of a years-long training course (Hill et al. 2015) or only achieve marginal improvements and only for less disturbed patients (Owen et al. 2016). In this discussion, it is important to consider the professional setting the therapists work in, for example, whether it provides a trusting environment that encourages therapists to speak openly about and continuously reflect on their work, including their less successful treatments (Goldberg et al. 2016).

The field is, however, somewhat dominated by studies that have serious methodological limitations and are based on vaguely defined patient groups in short-term therapy, just as there are substantial variations between therapists, some of whom improve during training, while others fail to improve or actually become less successful over time. There is thus considerable variation in the effectiveness of therapeutic training across the participating therapists, which presumably has more to do with individual personal qualities, which are fairly unaffected by traditional therapeutic training. Further, some studies suggest that therapists improve their ability to retain patients in treatment (decreasing drop out rates) with growing experience (Goldberg et al. 2016), although some studies contradict this (Hill et al. 2015:189). These studies too, however, have methodological limitations and are based on short-term treatment of patients with (very inadequately diagnosed) less severe pathology. Finally, it has been proposed that psychotherapists with superior outcomes take a more psychological, rather than a biological approach in their clinical work, in the sense that they operate with more psychologically oriented concepts of aetiology and are less likely to focus on medical and other non-psychotherapeutic treatments; they also have a higher level of education (Ph.D.) (Blatt et al.1996).

Generally, however, the area is characterized by a lack of substantial empirical data and by studies with a weak methodology (see, e.g., Powell et al. 2010).

Several experimental studies have looked at the predictive value of fully trained and trainee therapists' interpersonal skills in regard to subsequent treatment outcomes. The most interesting aspect of this effort may be the attempts at operationalizing interpersonal skills and defining key elements of the therapist's relational competence. Thus, researchers (Anderson et al. 2009) have developed an instrument aimed at documenting therapists' interpersonal skills based on independent raters' structured evaluations of therapists' responses to video recordings of standardized interpersonal interactions from a therapy session ('Facilitative Interpersonal Skills', FIS). The instrument describes seven dimensions of therapists' interpersonal skills (Anderson et al. 2009:759, 2016a:58; Uhlin 2011):

(1) Verbal fluency; ease and capability of the therapist's verbal communication of what is going on in the therapy—ability to express oneself without signs of anxiety.
(2) Emotional expression, engagement and involvement, including the ability to attune this to the therapeutic context and the patient's current state.
(3) Ability to convey a clear, structured and persuasive understanding of the patient's situation, ability to communicate understanding and acceptance—expressing certainty and authority.
(4) Conveying warmth, acceptance and understanding—the therapist's ability to challenge the patient's (self-)perception in a non-judging way.
(5) Communicating hope, optimism and positive expectations of the treatment—the therapist's ability to promote the development of the patient's agency.
(6) Ability to communicate a precis, empathic and nuanced understanding of the patient's thoughts, emotions and other mental states.
(7) Ability to form an emotional bond with the patient and a collaborative atmosphere in the therapeutic space; the therapist's ability to respond to and repair ruptures in the alliance.

Therapists' Relational Skills and Treatment Outcomes

The first study to use the FIS instrument finds that therapists' interpersonal skills on the seven dimensions have some predictive value in relation to outcome, in the sense that patients who work with therapists with better interpersonal skills, as measured in a rating of their responses to standardized therapeutic situations on the seven dimensions, are likely to report greater outcomes (Anderson et al. 2009:762f, 2016a:62f). Despite methodological limitations—including that the study is naturalistic, only uses a single measure for treatment outcome and is based on a somewhat vaguely described group of mildly disturbed patients—the findings may be seen as confirmation that the described interpersonal skills can be assumed to capture and specify some of the therapist effects that have been identified in traditional efficacy studies (Anderson et al. 2009:764), just as they naturally also support the important role of the therapist's more personal qualities—relational skills—in psychotherapy.

Finally, the study confirms the need to focus on interpersonal skills in the selection and training of new psychotherapists.

We should assume that it will be fairly difficult to develop therapists' basic interpersonal skills and their ability to form and maintain a good therapeutic alliance, particularly with patients who have an attachment disorder. Hence, persons who intend to work with psychotherapy should possess these skills at a certain level even before they are offered therapeutic training (Del Re et al. 2012:647), just as we should acknowledge that far from everybody has what it takes to develop the interpersonal skills that are a necessary condition for successful psychotherapy. Not everyone has the necessary skill set to become an effective therapist, not even everyone who thinks they do. Hence, it may be helpful to test interpersonal skills using FIS or similar instruments when selecting prospective psychotherapists rather than relying on psychometric tests or questionnaires that simply map personality features and cognitive skills (Schöttke et al. 2017).

In two subsequent studies, Anderson et al. (2016a, b) investigated whether interpersonal skills (measured using FIS) in clinical trainees and in students without any clinical training can predict the effect of brief 'therapy courses' which these students subsequently conduct with low-severity patients. This study, too, found that the students' interpersonal skills are somewhat predictive of the effect of the 'therapy courses'. That finding only applies to brief therapy lasting less than eight sessions, while the 'therapist's' interpersonal skills do not predict the effect of (the relatively few) 'treatments' lasting more than 16 sessions (Anderson et al. 2016a). Here, other conditions seem to outweigh the importance of the 'therapist's' interpersonal skills, as documented by the FIS instrument.

Patients in 'treatment' with the 'therapists' who have the best interpersonal skills rate the alliance as being clearly better from the outset of the treatment, and these alliances improve more over time, compared to 'therapy processes' with 'therapists' with poorer interpersonal skills (Anderson et al. 2016b:13). It might be considered whether one of the factors distinguishing therapists with good relational skills from therapists with poorer relational skills is the ability to be aware of and deal with the inevitable ruptures in the alliance that occur in all therapy, albeit to varying degrees and particularly in working with patients with personality disorders and other attachment disorders. Although these studies, too, have obvious limitations—including that most of the participating 'therapists' are not (yet) fully trained psychotherapists, that they only 'treat' one patient, and that most of patients have very mild difficulties, which makes it unclear whether the findings can be generalized to the treatment of more severe psychological disorders—they do confirm the importance of the therapist's interpersonal skills for the formation of the alliance and for the effectiveness of the treatment. The therapist's interpersonal skills are clearly a key aspect of the common therapeutic factors across treatment methods.

A German study with a somewhat similar design, where trainee therapists discuss fragments of a therapy session in groups, and independent raters subsequently assess their contributions to these group discussions, also finds that therapists who demonstrate the best interpersonal skills have the best treatment outcomes, independent of the specific treatment method (cognitive or psychodynamic) (Schöttke et al.

2017:7f). Here, the focus of the assessment of the therapists' interpersonal skills is clear and positive communication, empathy and communicative attunement to 'the other', respectful and warm interpersonal behaviour, respectful management of criticism and willingness to cooperate (Schöttke et al. 2017:5), that is, dimensions related to the FIS instrument—and dimensions that can help us specify some of the skills to look for and seek to develop in (prospective) psychotherapists.

A series of studies of connections between therapist characteristics, elements of the therapeutic process and treatment outcome identified factors in the therapist's interactions with the patient that correlate with patient outcome (Henry et al. 1986, 1990; Najavits and Strupp 1994). The studies are based on short-term (up to 25 sessions) interpersonal therapy for patients with medium-severity, mainly interpersonal, pathology. A number of therapy courses with both good and poor outcomes are selected, and the interpersonal process in selected therapy sessions is analysed in detail. The researchers find, among other results, that in effective (high change) therapy courses, therapist behaviours include much more affirming, understanding, helping and protecting and less belittling and blaming, compared to ineffective (low change) therapies (Henry et al. 1986). Moreover, effective processes generally have more positive interaction (positive complementarity) between patient and therapist, while less successful processes have a much higher share of patient-therapist interactions characterized by poor attunement and hostility, so-called negative complementarity and complex communication, where patient and therapist send each other multiple contradictory messages at once (ibid.). Finally, the study finds a strong correlation between hostile, controlling behaviours from the therapist and a tendency for the patient to become self-blaming and self-critical (Henry et al. 1990:771f), which, all things being equal, will have a negative influence on the patient's self-image (introject) and treatment outcome, as the patient presumably internalizes the interpersonal process during the therapy as part of her inner object relations and thus her perceptions of self, others and interpersonal relationships.

Most of these findings are replicated in a later study (Von der Lippe et al. 2008), which also finds that in less effective therapies, the therapist engages in self-intensifying negative interactions, where the patient rejects the therapist's attempts at helping, and the therapist in turn responds with various forms of hostile, countertherapeutic behaviour (belittling, rejecting or ignoring what the patient is trying to communicate—failing to maintain the psychotherapeutic stance towards the patient). In successful treatment courses, the interaction between patient and therapist is like a dance, where they continuously attune to one another; in ineffective processes, this connection is absent or is gradually lost (Von der Lippe et al. 2008:429).

Therapist Characteristics, Interpersonal Behaviour and Outcome

Further, therapists with more negative introjects (negative self-perception and a tendency towards self-hostility and lack of self-nurturing behaviour) are more likely to be hostile in their interactions with the patient (Henry et al. 1990:772), which may be interpreted to mean that these therapists carry unprocessed issues from previous relationships, which they act out and otherwise express in the countertransference. This interpretation finds some support in a later study from the same research group, which concludes that seemingly unprocessed negative experiences from the therapist's early relationships influence his perception of—and (indirectly shapes) his ability to establish a constructive interpersonal process with—his patients (Hilliard et al. 2000:129f), which in turn impacts the treatment effect (Hilliard et al. 2000:130). This correlation between the therapist's negative introjects and correspondingly negative contributions to the interpersonal process in the therapy—and thus, indirectly, to the effectiveness of the treatment—appears to persist even after intensive training in interpersonal psychotherapy, which should raises a serious issue (Henry et al. 1993, Castonguay et al. 2010:40). A newer, related study (Safran et al. 2014) finds that systematic training of CBT-therapists' ability to register and handle ruptures in the alliance can increase the individual therapist's positive contribution to—and ability to reflect on—the interpersonal process in the therapeutic space. However, this study also does not find that therapeutic training 'eliminates' or even significantly changes the participating CBT therapists' negative contribution to the interaction with the patient (Safran et al. 2014:276).

In extension of these observations, it is worth noting that some studies find indications to suggest that compared to therapists with an insecure attachment, therapists with a secure attachment style are better able to attune to the relational needs in patients with a range of different attachment styles (disorders) and relational needs, including needs that the patients cannot communicate effectively, or which differ from the needs the patient appears to communicate (Dozier et al. 1994:797f; Schauenburg et al. 2010:198; Martin et al. 2007:54; Willutzki et al. 2013:432). Thus, the therapist's ability to act in the therapeutic space in ways that disprove the patient's maladaptive perceptions of herself and others, framed by a secure base (cf. corrective emotional experiences)—also in work with more severely disturbed patients, where there may be considerable interpersonal pressure for countertransferences that are destructive to the therapy—seems to depend on the organization of the therapist's own attachment system. This dynamic is also related to the therapist's ability to suspend his own relational needs and regulate his countertransferences, including any tendencies or urges to act on the anxiety that may be activated by the therapist's own attachment system.

A related study Najavits and Strupp (1994:119f) finds that one of the factors that most clearly distinguish the least successful from the most successful therapists—as measured on average treatment outcomes and drop-out rates—in a group of fairly inexperienced (on average just over five years' psychotherapeutic practice) therapists is that the least effective therapists' behaviour during shorter or longer sequences of their treatment courses are explicitly hostile to the patient (attacking, belittling and blaming the patient). The most successful therapists are more critical of their own practice (Najavits and Strupp 1994:119), even if it may not, to a casual observer, appear that they have any reason to be so—despite the fact that the capacity for healthy self-criticism and balanced questioning of one's own therapeutic abilities seems to be a characteristic of effective therapists (cf. Nissen-Lie et al. 2016). There are few intensive process-effect studies of this type, but overall, they clearly confirm that the therapist's relational skills and his ability to manage countertransference play an important role for patient outcomes.

As Henry et al. (1990:773) conclude in their classic study of the psychotherapeutic process, the absence of negative interpersonal processes in the interaction between therapist and patient is hardly in itself sufficient to generate lasting change in the patient, but the presence of even a fairly low amount of negative therapist behaviour in the therapeutic space may be sufficient to render it impossible. The therapist's psychotherapeutic stance and his ability to take a step back and regulate his reactions in the interaction with the patient—and thus the therapeutic space—collapse, which undermines the prospects of a good treatment outcome, especially if it is not just a one-time occurrence, and the therapist fails to quickly and competently manage these breakdowns of his therapeutic capacity.

Patients who struggle with difficulties that are rooted in earlier maladaptive interactions with significant others (including parents and caregivers) are likely to project their negative past experiences with significant others onto the therapist in the present moment and thus—unconsciously—act in ways that invite the therapist to play his part in re-enacting the patterns in the therapeutic relationship. It can be a challenge for the therapist to register when this is about to happen and thus to avoid contributing too much to a re-enactment that, on the one hand, has the potential to undermine the therapeutic process and, on the other hand, contains important therapeutic potentials if it is handled competently and from a psychotherapeutic stance (see Part II). Psychotherapists therefore need systematic training in spotting how recurring maladaptive interaction patterns from the patient's life may be re-enacted in the therapeutic relationship, and how they can be incorporated into the therapeutic process. The training should aim to enhance therapists' sensitivity to the complexities of the therapeutic process and their awareness of the significant impact for the therapeutic process of even brief incidents of negative and hostile interactions and ruptures in the alliance, especially if they are not subsequently explicitly acknowledged (by the therapist), thematized and processed with the patient.

7.2 Master Therapists

A team of researchers in Norway and the United States, led by Thomas Skovholdt, Helge Rønnestad and Helene Nissen-Lie, have investigated what characterizes exceptional therapists, master therapists and expert psychotherapist, that is, what sets them apart from novices and more average therapists. To the extent that the therapist's personal characteristics have major impact on the formation of the alliance and on treatment outcome, it is of course interesting to determine what sets exceptional therapists apart. In one of the first, now classic, studies of this topic Ricks (1974) compares what he calls the supershrink and the pseudoshrink, based on long-term treatment outcomes with at-risk adolescents. In his study, the supershrink stands out by investing more time in his more disturbed patients, drawing on resources outside the therapy, developing a stronger therapeutic relationship (alliance) with his patients and supporting the development of autonomy in his patients, while the pseudoshrink is afraid of his more disturbed patients' pathology, tends to withdraw from them and is susceptive to being 'infected' by their depression and hopelessness. Thus, what appears to set the two categories of therapists apart is their relational skills and their ability to establish balanced emotional boundaries in relation to the patient and manage their own countertransference (self-regulation).

Generally, the single most important factor for the master therapist is his ability to establish emotional contact and form a sustainable therapeutic alliance—also with patients with severe attachments disorders, who at times (or more consistently) attack, devalue, 'test' and 'sabotage' the therapist and the therapy (Skovholt et al. 1997:362). This ability cannot be developed solely by completing a theoretical academic training programme; it takes emotional stability, psychological maturity and relational and reflective skills that are typically developed over many years of clinical experience, therapeutic training and supervision.

Although there remains some disagreement about the key characteristics of the therapeutic relationship, including how active, structuring and directive the therapist should be (which may vary a great deal across patients), some studies suggest that the ability to establish and maintain an effective therapeutic relationship has more to do with what might be called, for lack of a better term, general psychotherapeutic expertise; thus it has more do to with the therapist's more personal qualities than with training in any specific treatment method. In an older and fairly primitive study, Fiedler thus finds that expert therapists from different therapeutic orientations agree more among themselves as to what characterizes the ideal therapeutic relationship than they do with novice therapists who pursue the same treatment model as they do (Fiedler 1950a). Similarly, expert therapists' actual therapeutic relationships are closer to what is defined as the ideal therapeutic relationship (Fiedler 1950b:439f), compared to novice therapists'. Further, expert therapists working in different treatment traditions form therapeutic relationships that are more closely aligned than any of them are with the therapeutic relationships formed by novice therapists working within their own therapeutic tradition (Fiedler 1950b:440f). A few later studies that closely analyse the actual therapy process find that master therapists from different treatment traditions (cognitive-behavioural and psychodynamic) are very similar in their approach to the therapeutic work; they are far less likely to adhere rigorously to 'their' method and any manuals than less experienced therapists (Goldfried et al. 1998).

Jennings and Skovholdt (1999) used semi-structured interviews with ten therapists who had been characterized as exceptional by their colleagues to attempt to define what sets these therapists apart. The study finds the following characteristics, among others, of master therapists:

- They are voracious learners with an insatiable appetite for professional development and new learning.
- Accumulated experiences have become a major resource for master therapists. They draw on their accumulated experience while always remaining open to learning from new experiences.

- They value cognitive complexity and the ambiguity of the human condition; they not only tolerate ambiguity and complexity but actively seek it out. They associate psychotherapy with complexity and the meeting with the unknown, which they view as a positive quality.
- They appear to have emotional receptivity, defined as being self-aware, reflective, nondefensive, and open to feedback; they are reflective, do not resort to defensiveness when they encounter criticism and constantly strive to learn more about their work and themselves.
- They seem to be mentally healthy and mature individuals who attend to their own emotional well-being in interactions with their patients. They also appear humble and are not self-centred and grandiose in presentation. They have a healthy balance between confidence and humility in relation to the complexity of the therapeutic work (Nissen-Lie et al. 2016).
- They are aware of how their emotional health affects the quality of their work and thus of the need to look out for themselves, perhaps dealing with their own unresolved conflicts and so on.
- They possess strong relational skills and are good at listening, observing and caring for the welfare of others. They have a high degree of sensitivity to and empathy with others, and based on a genuine interest in their patients they manage to make them feel special and important.
- They believe that the foundation for therapeutic change is a strong working alliance, and they believe firmly in their patients' ability to change and develop, which strengthens the patients' hope and faith in change.
- They are experts at using their exceptional relationship skills in therapy; they manage to challenge their patients and face tough and emotionally painful issues in an atmosphere that combines challenge with support. They have no fear of their patients' or their own strong emotions but are able to 'be with' the patient, even when it is emotionally difficult.

Later, these characteristics have been supplemented with a number of paradoxical characteristics of master therapists (Jennings et al. 2013:221). Thus, master therapists are typically able both to 'give of their self' in the interaction with their patients and to nurture their self; they are open to feedback about their own contributions without being emotionally destabilized by criticism; they can integrate their personal and professional selves while maintaining clear boundaries between the two; they have a clear awareness of the strengths in their therapeutic skills while maintaining a humble self-perception and of the limits of their own capabilities; they are able to enter deeply into another's world, while often preferring solitude; and they are able to create a therapeutic setting that provides a safe space for the patient, while also at times challenging and confronting the patient with undesirable or split-off parts of her psyche; they are curious, have a nuanced ethical compass, are highly reflective, enjoy life and have a sense of humour that helps counteract heaviness and pain (Jennings et al. 2013:238ff). Several of these characteristics will also, to varying degrees, characterize experienced therapists in general. It is worth noting that the growing ability to integrate one's personal and professional selves—and appear authentic in the meeting with the patient—is only an advantage for psychologically well-functioning therapists, while it is not necessarily helpful for the patients when less well-functioning therapists become more authentically 'themselves' in the therapeutic space and in their contact with the patient (Rønnestad and Skovholt 2013:107).

There have also been attempts at defining what 'therapeutic wisdom' more specifically implies. Generally, wisdom is associated, among other things, with a deeper understanding of reality, self awareness, psychological understanding of others, an ability to reframe information, maturity (high level of ego development), qualified intuition, appreciation of ambiguity, ability to learn from experience, to resist the automatization of thought and think beyond the immediately given and obvious (Levitt and Piazza-Bonin 2016; Hanna and Ottens 1995:196f; Sternberg 1998). Wisdom is also related to an ability to make competent choices, to act only after considering both factual and procedural knowledge, knowledge about different aspects of human life, insight into different possible values, goals and priorities and knowledge about one's own limitations (ibid.). Finally, wisdom may be associated with an ability to integrate knowledge from multiple sources and perspectives, including cognitive, emotional and experiential knowledge and a complex and nuanced coherent understanding of specific problems, situations and reality in general. Wisdom is frequently domain-specific in the sense that a person may have a high level of wisdom in certain areas but not in others, just as academic expertise within a given area is no guarantee of practical wisdom within the same area, and vice versa (Sternberg 1998:356f).

Published material from qualitative interviews with expert psychotherapists (Råbu and McLeod 2016) and psychotherapists who were nominated by their peers as possessing particular clinical wisdom (Levitt and Piazza-Bonin 2016) can help us specify how clinical wisdom is manifested. Among the qualities mentioned by the interviewed therapists as being associated with clinical wisdom was the awareness that no theory contains the whole truth about psychological disorder and psychotherapy, and that one should therefore avoid an excessive identification with a specific theory or method, combined with an understanding of how different theories and methods can be helpful in various contexts and with different patients (Råbu and McLeod 2016:8ff). In reference to this point, the German psychoanalyst Gerhard Schneider (2003:233ff) writes that the experienced therapist can adopt what Schneider calls an atopical position where the therapist draws on fragments of various theories and treatment approaches without embracing the typical theory's totalizing ambition (demand for universal validity and applicability). This atopical position contains a strong element of not knowing (a priori) but seeing it as an important task to be openly explorative and thus discovering (what is going on) together with the patient. Clinical wisdom is also manifest in a refined sensitivity to interpersonal interactions, an ability to be spontaneous and present as a person without crossing into the private sphere and to liberate oneself from notions or expectations of needing to understand everything and being 'smart', including handling uncertainty, vulnerability, intimacy, intense affects and the limits to one's own capabilities (Råbu and McLeod 2016:8ff). Therapists with a high degree of clinical wisdom remain curious about their patients (rather than seeking to confine them quickly into pre-defined categories), do not cling to standardized methods in an attempt to avoid uncertainty but emphasize relational attunement to the individual patient over the use of standardized interventions (Levitt and Piazza-Bonin 2016:37ff). Finally, they are characterized by enthusiasm for the therapy and manage to stay hopeful and optimistic, utilize humour and remain aware of the individual patient's resources (ibid.).

Overall, exceptional therapists combine a well-developed (cognitive and emotional) understanding of complex psychological and relational dynamics and unique relational skills with an ability to contain severe pathology, intense affects and a wide range of mental states. They have an inner sense of calm and stability (they feel 'comfortable in the chair') and are able to contain and manage critical feedback, conflicts and aspects that do not initially make sense, combined with a well-developed sensitivity and nuanced understanding of themselves, others and interpersonal interactions. In terms of personality, they are characterized by considerable maturity and integrity (internal integration). The master therapist thus brings together advanced cognitive, emotional, self-regulatory and relational skills, which all therapists may strive for, but far from everyone will be fully able to attain.

Professional Humility

Several studies of correlations between therapists' self-perception, therapeutic alliance and treatment outcome suggest that the therapist's professional humility generally has a positive influence on the course and outcome of the psychotherapeutic work. Nissen-Lie et al. (2010, 2017) have compared a large group of fairly experienced therapists' self-reported professional self-perception and introject (how they perceive and treat themselves) with their patients' perception of the therapeutic alliance and with a number of measures of the patients' benefit from fairly long therapeutic treatments (on average a little over 50 sessions). These studies find a correlation between the therapist's well-balanced doubt about his own professional capability—which may also be viewed as a healthy awareness of the limitations of his own skills and of the complexity of the therapeutic process, which may reflect a balanced professional humility—and positive patient-ratings of the alliance at an early stage of the therapy (Nissen-Lie et al. 2010:638ff). Further, it finds that therapists who have both 'healthy self-critical evaluation' of their professional skills (rather than omnipotent notions of infallibility) and a positive (friendly, non-judging, nurturant) introject that lets them forgive their own errors and shortcomings achieve substantially better treatment outcomes, as reflected in measures of their patients' interpersonal functioning, than therapists with lower scores on measures of professional self-doubt (Nissen-Lie et al. 2017:56ff).

Therapists with exaggerated self-confidence, an insufficient capacity for realistic and balanced self-criticism and inadequate self-reflection are unlikely to display an optimal therapeutic stance, which affects their outcomes negatively. In addition, there is reason to consider how these therapists will handle criticism from their patients and other ruptures in the therapeutic alliance, which, as mentioned earlier, should be met with humility and a genuine readiness to acknowledge one's own contribution to the problems that arise in the therapeutic relationship—not with a tendency to place all the blame on the patient (misattribution) or, perhaps, to see the patient's criticism and the ruptures as reflective of the patient's transference or general pathology. In some cases, excessive confidence in one's own excellence as a therapist may also serve as a defence against underlying feelings of incompetence and inadequacy, just as the disinclination to doubt one's own ability to handle situations that arise in the therapeutic space may reflect a somewhat maladaptive reduction of the complexity of the therapeutic process (Nissen-Lie et al. 2017:57) and a lack of sensitivity in the meeting with the patient. When the therapist responds to criticism from the patient with explicitly critical self-reflection, the patient may perceive this as a reflection of the therapist's respect for the patient's self. On the other hand, in some situations, the patient may perceive excessive self-reflection and, not least, self-criticism on the part of the therapist as a sign of insecurity and incompetence (which it may in fact be), which will undermine the therapist's professional authority and increase the patient's anxiety and insecurity in the therapeutic space (cf. Jaspers 1942:667).

There is reason to assume that therapists with a friendly introject will convey this to their patients, who during the treatment will be able to internalize the therapist's more empathic, kindly accepting and forgiving approach to own mistakes and shortcomings. In a sense, the therapist thus models a different way of being with oneself and dealing with one's own inadequacies, mistakes and, perhaps, less desirable qualities. Researchers have also found that therapists with constructive strategies for managing problems in the therapeutic space—therapists who try to see problems from different perspectives, seek supervision, reflect on the issues and actively seek to resolve them in a dialogue with the patient—have better treatment outcomes than therapists with less constructive strategies for managing problems that arise during the therapy (Nissen-Lie et al. 2017:55f).

It does not appear, however, that the extent of therapeutic training in itself has a positive impact on the participating therapists' ability to manage the problems that arise in the alliance; in fact, there seems to be a negative correlation between the extent of their (mainly psychodynamic) therapeutic training and the patients' rating of the therapeutic alliance at different times (after sessions 20–120) in long-term treatment (Hersoug et al. 2009:105). That may, of course, have many different explanations, including that certain types of therapeutic training probably does not correct or, in some cases, may even exacerbate unhelpful behaviour in the therapist (the 'neutral', emotionally detached therapist). It is also conceivable that therapists who have personal and professional problems seek more training (Hersoug et al. 2009:108). The authors conclude their study with a thought-provoking general recommendation to psychotherapists: 'Love yourself as a person, doubt yourself as a therapist' (Nissen-Lie et al. 2017:48). Thus, the therapist should abandon any (in practice delusional) notions of the ideal, perfect therapist and instead strive to be the good-enough therapist (cf. Treurniet 1997:623), who will inevitably make mistakes but avoids being overwhelmed by shame and destructive self-criticism, and who maintains a balanced ability to take a step back, reflect on and maintain a psychotherapeutic stance towards his own missteps in the therapeutic space.

7.3 The Experienced Professional Therapist

The professional therapist has a highly differentiated and scientifically based conceptual framework for the nuanced categorization and understanding of and reflections on human psychology and psychological disorders. He has integrated an ability to give of himself and to use his own reactions and subjective experiences in the therapeutic process, and he has a wide range of therapeutic tools which he knows exactly when and how to use (Rønnestad and Skovholt 2013:46f). He is able to match his use of different treatment methods to the individual patient, unlike novice therapists or effective, but narrow-minded 'technicians', who often have nothing but a hammer at their disposal and hence tend to see most issues as nails. In addition, he has a well-developed ability to get fairly quickly to the core of the patient's problem and to develop a nuanced, complex and contextualized understanding of it—an understanding that is not merely descriptive but functional and dynamic-psychological (what are the patient's symptoms about, what dynamic function do they serve, what meaning do they have from the patient's point of view?) (Oddli 2014:73). This is of particular importance in work with patients who have more complex and comorbid disorders. On the other hand, the professional therapist must also be able to resist the urge to categorize the patient too quickly, maintaining an open and curious mind and the ability to see what is unique about the individual patient and her difficulties.

One of the challenges in the psychotherapeutic work is the need to alternate between, on the one hand, empathic involvement and interaction with the patient in the present moment and, on the other hand, taking a step back from the patient, oneself and the interaction in order to reflect on 'what is happening right now,' how it can aid one's understanding of the patient, and what would be the most appropriate intervention. While the experienced professional therapist is well equipped to meet these requirements, a less experienced, non-professional or, for various reasons, personally overburdened therapist (in addition to the risk of emotional detachment from the patient and her difficulties driven by an urge for self-protection) risks overidentifying with the patient and the difficulties she is facing—possibly based on profound sympathy for and empathy with the patient—which may jeopardize the ability to take a step back and adopt a more analytical perspective (Rønnestad and Skovholt 2013:49). When that happens, it increases the risk of acting out the countertransference and being overwhelmed by the urge to act without due consideration instead of maintaining the psychotherapeutic stance and reflective position in relation to the patient.

The professional therapist has the personal qualities and empathic capacity that are needed to empathize with, understand and help the patient. In addition, he or she has the ability to adopt and maintain a therapeutic stance, which is a crucial condition for ensuring, first, that the treatment is not simply reduced to 'a nice experience' for the patient or, alternatively, to a long sequence of unacknowledged repetitions of maladaptive patterns from the patient's life, with serious ramifications for outcome, and, second, that the therapist does not get trapped in unconscious acting out of countertransferences, which would compromise the necessary variation between experiencing and analysing what is happening in the therapeutic relationship.

It may be a necessary step in the novice therapist's professional development to acquire a set of fairly simple methods for the treatment of specific disorders and to try to follow certain standardized guidelines for working with patients with specific problems. With growing experience, however, the professional therapist will gradually loosen the reins of the strict adherence to standardized methods, discarding the sense of security that comes with following specific instructions and ground rules, and develop a more creative use of guidelines and specific treatment methods. The methods are then internalized, personalized and individualized and implemented in ways that are more closely attuned to the individual patient and to the therapist's own personal style or voice. Generally, it is only after developing a thorough grasp of a given therapeutic method that one is in a position to begin to 'forget' it, only to 'rediscover' it in a more personalized form (cf. Ogden 2009:3).

With therapeutic experience, the therapist develops a qualified intuition that gives him a nuanced ability to notice and understand recurring patterns in the patient's relationships and behaviour in the therapeutic space and to apply general theories, abstract principles, conceptual models and specific intervention methods in ways that are attuned to the individual patient. Based on clinical experience and acquired theoretical knowledge, the therapist develops a sense for 'where to look, what to look at, and how to look at it' (Bollas 1993:89) and for how best to handle what he sees, without necessarily needing to consider long (Binder 2004:268). That makes it possible to move from a predominantly technical-mechanical approach to a more personally integrated and context-sensitive use of specific conceptual models and therapeutic methods, where the therapist increasingly uses himself as an instrument in the therapeutic process, and where it often simply seems 'natural' to act in certain ways in the therapeutic space. This is a practice approach that contains elements of what Schön (1983:50) described as 'knowing-in-action', where knowledge that is not necessarily fully articulated is manifested in intelligent acts that are attuned to the given situation and context—and which are based on a nuanced understanding of the patient in the moment. This is reflection-in-action that is related to the artistic creative process, where common principles and regularities are used in the given situation in ways that are attuned to the unique nature of the individual person in the current situation and context. Such an approach requires thorough knowledge of common regularities and principles (scientific psychology and specific treatment methods) as well as good judgment and a capacity for nuanced analysis and understanding of the given patient and situation, here and now. In a sense, the experienced and competent therapist develops his own unique theory of or working model for understanding the individual patient's unique difficulties and way of functioning. This marks an approach to psychological understanding and therapy that is quite different from the use of authorized diagnostic categories complete with standardized treatment methods aimed at patients with specific psychiatric diagnoses (Klöpper 2014:68f).

7.4 Handling Countertransference

There is only very limited empirical data on the possible correlations between countertransference, the therapist's handling of countertransference and treatment outcome, and the few studies that do exist are limited by (in some cases severe) methodological problems. Perhaps of most interest in this context are the studies attempting to describe and operationalize certain elements of the countertransference and how countertransference is manifested in the therapeutic space (Hayes et al. 2011). A meta-analysis of the existing studies in this area finds a small (negative), yet significant, correlation between manifestations of the therapist's countertransference—here defined fairly narrowly as manifestations of the therapist's own unresolved conflicts in his behaviour in the therapeutic space (see Chap. 10 for a more in-depth treatment of the concept of countertransference)—and treatment outcome, just as these manifestations of countertransference also appear to have a negative impact on the therapeutic alliance (Hayes et al. 2011:249ff).

Conversely, research lends some support to the notion that the therapist's processing of countertransferences both diminishes their manifestations in the therapeutic space and has a positive effect on treatment outcome (Hayes et al. 2011:252ff), although this finding is based on a very small number of studies. It is far from clear how we should specify exactly what it involves for the therapist to process and get better at containing his countertransferences—as opposed to acting them out—except that it requires him to remain continuously aware of his own reactions in the interaction with the patient and to pause and reflect on how these reactions might be understood, possibly with the help of a supervisor. Moreover, it must be assumed that therapists who are not overburdened by an excessive caseload with too many very disturbed patients will be better able to find the necessary space to reflect on and process their countertransferences and thus diminish the risk of harming the therapeutic process by acting them out. In extension of this point, it should be noted that the therapist's countertransference cannot, inherently, be examined and understood without considering the patient, since, all things being equal, the character and severity of her pathology will have a major influence on the development and manifestations of the therapist's countertransferences.

Manifestations of Countertransference

Betan et al.'s (2005) study of countertransference contains interesting attempts at crystallizing key elements of countertransference, including various forms of countertransference manifestations. In the study, 181 psychotherapists were asked to describe the last patient they saw the previous week and to fill out a questionnaire to chart their countertransferences in therapy with this patient. A factor analysis of the therapists' replies revealed eight typical factors in the manifestation of countertransferences (Betan et al. 2005:892f):

(1) Feeling overwhelmed, disorganized—accompanied by an urge to avoid the patient and the strong negative feelings that are actualized in the interaction, including dread, repulsion and resentment as well as fantasies about terminating the treatment.
(2) Feeling helpless, inadequate—feelings of hopelessness and incompetence. The therapist imagines that the patient would be better off with another therapist.
(3) Experiencing a positive relationship, alliance and close connection with the patient—enjoying working with the patient. The therapist imagines that he could be friends with the patient, if he or she were not his patient.
(4) Overinvolvement—an experience that the patient is special (compared with other patients), accompanied by problems in maintaining boundaries with the patient, including inappropriate self-disclosure and feeling excessively responsible and concerned for the patient.
(5) Sexualization—the therapist has sexual feelings for and fantasies about the patient or experiences sexual tension in the therapeutic space, is in love with the patient.
(6) Disengaging—feels easily distracted, detached, bored (frequently checking the time and so on) or annoyed in sessions with the patient. The therapist withdraws from the emotional contact with the patient.
(7) Feeling protective—adopts a parental role with the patient, desires to protect and care for the patient. The therapist has unrealistic ideas about being able to give the patient what she never had in life.
(8) Feeling criticized, mistreated, unappreciated, devalued or dismissed by the patient, possibly accompanied by an urge to 'go on the counterattack' against the patient.

It is worth noting that most of these factors (especially 1, 5, 6 and 8) have been found to correlate with a dimensional measure for cluster-B personality disorder (borderline, histrionic, narcissistic and dissocial/antisocial) in the patient. Only one of the listed countertransference manifestations has no association with dimensional measures for cluster-B personality disorders: feeling overinvolved and feeling the urge to take a parental role in relation to the patient, while the feeling of having a positive relationship with the patient is significantly negatively correlated to measures of cluster-B personality disorders (Betan et al. 2005:894). Other studies have similarly found that (especially fairly inexperienced) therapists are far more likely to perceive that patients with a borderline personality disorder react negatively to them (feeling criticized, rejected and so on by the patient). With this patient group, they are also more likely to withdraw from the contact or otherwise react in ways that are negative (and countertherapeutic; acting out what must be considered as problematic countertransferences) than when they work with depressive patients (Bourke and Grenyer 2010). After the fact, the therapists are more likely to feel incompetent and to feel that they lack positive influence on the patient; they also find it an ongoing effort to attempt to control their emotional reactions in interactions with borderline patients (Bourke and Grenyer 2010:686).

This may reflect that psychotherapeutic work with patients with certain personality disorders—especially borderline—often leads to strong and, for some therapists, intensely negative countertransference. Hence, one should seek to select competent therapists with good (possibly specialized) training to help patients with borderline and other cluster-B personality disorders, where the ability to read and handle what plays out in the therapeutic relationship is of particular importance. However, the most interesting aspect of the proposed factors in the present context is the contribution they can make to specifying some of the possible manifestations of countertransference in the therapeutic space, which may jeopardize the psychotherapeutic stance, both generally and, perhaps in particular, in the work with more severely disturbed patients.

The Therapist's Ability to Contain Countertransference

There can be substantial differences in individual therapists' ability to contain and manage various countertransference manifestations and thus in whether and how countertransferences are reflected in the therapist's actual performance in the therapeutic space. Even if the therapist feels criticized and devalued by his patient—and feels the urge to defend himself or counterattack—it is far from given that he is going to 'take it in' and take it very personally. The art is to take a step back from one's immediate feelings, urges and other experiences in the interaction with the patient and to reflect on how these reactions may be understood in light of the patient's difficulties, actualized object relations and recurring patterns in the patient's interpersonal interactions. The therapist also needs to remain aware of his own contribution to the relationship with the patient and the current interaction—remembering that his own unresolved conflicts and needs may colour his perception of and reactions to what happens in the therapeutic space. The countertransferences that are actualized in the interaction with the patient may offer vital clues about the patient's difficulties and mental states, which she finds it hard to verbalize and accept; in that sense, the therapist's countertransferences should be seen as a form of communication with the patient. A constructive management of, especially, more primitive countertransferences requires an inner sense of calm in the therapist; he has to be able to draw on considerable affect tolerance, the ability to contain and regulate a wide range of mental states and strong affects in himself and others.

It seems that it is not sufficient merely to contain one's countertransferences, without otherwise reflecting on or trying to decode their meaning, and that therapists who consistently remain aware of their (inner) subjective experiences in the therapeutic space are more likely to achieve good treatment outcomes (Hayes et al. 2015:131). On the other hand, there is reason to assume that acting out or self-disclosure of unresolved and insufficiently processed—especially more primitive—countertransferences will typically have a negative influence on the therapeutic process, the working alliance and, ultimately, the treatment outcome (cf. Yeh and Hayes 2011).

Generally, however, there is little empirical data, both because it can be difficult, as mentioned earlier, to operationalize the therapist's countertransference, and because there is no consensus on how to define therapeutic self-disclosure (of countertransferences, among other elements). That makes it difficult to have a qualified discussion of the potential pros and cons of the therapist's use of self-disclosure (cf. Farber 2006). Moreover, it must be assumed that not only the character of the self-disclosure but also the character of the therapeutic relationship (the alliance) at the time of the therapist's self-disclosure will influence its effect on the patient, including the patient's subsequent perception of the therapist and of the therapeutic relationship (cf. Myers and Hayes 2006).

Among the possible benefits of the disclosing more subjective experiences and selected elements from one's personal life in the therapeutic space, some have proposed that it may in some cases strengthen the therapeutic alliance, help to normalize the patient's painful and shameful experiences ('you are not the only one who feels that way'; this may help to break the social isolation and, in some cases, stigma associated with certain experiences or acts) and provide the patient with alternative perspectives on reality (Farber 2006:139). Overall, however, therapists should be cautious to include elements from their personal life outside the therapy in the therapeutic process, in part because it may blur the professional boundaries of the therapeutic relationship and shift the focus away from the patient. Nevertheless, there is reason to assume that especially more experienced and generally well-functioning therapists may successfully disclose selected aspects of their more subjective experiences in the therapeutic space without burdening or invading the patient with elements from their personal lives outside the therapy. It should be noted, however, that although the psychotherapeutic process plays out in the intersubjective field within and between patient and therapist, thus involving the therapist's subjectivity and subjective experiences, the patient's psychology and development must always remain the object and focus of the psychotherapy (cf. Bonaminio 2008:1135).

A series of Norwegian studies have investigated how aspects of the therapist's life can influence what happens in the therapeutic space. Based on self-reported forms completed by experienced therapists the researchers find that therapists' perceived social support in their private relationships correlates positively with the patients' perception of the therapeutic alliance (Nissen-Lie et al. 2013:490), while therapists' reported level of burden in their personal lives, on the other hand, correlates negatively with the development of the therapeutic alliance over time, as perceived by the patient (Nissen-Lie 2013:489). This may be because therapists who are emotionally or otherwise burdened have less mental energy to contain and attune to their patients and thus may get trapped in countertransferences shaped by unresolved experiences, burdens and conflicts from their personal lives outside the therapy (Nissen-Lie et al. 2013:491).

7.5 Summary—Should We Abandon the Medical Model of Psychotherapy?

Overall, the medical understanding of psychotherapy seems, at best, to rest on a weak foundation and to align poorly with a large number of important findings from empirical psychotherapy research, while a more dynamic and relationally oriented model of psychotherapy that is focused on the individual therapist's more personal qualities, relational skills and therapeutic stance seems to be more in tune with key insights from empirical research. From the perspective of a traditional model of psychotherapy and based on important insights from empirical research, the medical model of psychotherapy and some of the related research within this conceptual framework seem somewhat reductionist and appear to understate the complexities of psychotherapy. Roughly put, they have the wrong focus—the outcome of specific therapeutic methods—while common therapeutic factors and therapist factors at best receive insufficient attention, if they are not outright ignored.

Nevertheless, there is no basis for a simplistic rejection of the medical approach to psychotherapy, with its related research programmes, both because many of the questions raised by empirical therapy research remain open, and because the medically framed research does make important contributions, even if it rests on a highly simplified and, in some regards, erroneous concept of psychotherapy. However, there are clearly grounds for challenging and abandoning the current near-hegemonic position of the medical model of psychotherapy in the field.

As has been laid out in the previous chapters, there does not seem to be any real difference in the effectiveness of the widely approved psychotherapeutic methods. Naturally, specific therapeutic methods influence the effectiveness of psychotherapy, but with a few possible exceptions, it makes little difference whether one chooses one or another of the approved methods that have been developed for the treatment of the major categories of psychological disorders, provided the therapist chooses (and receives intensive training in) one method rather than resorting to a confusing arbitrariness in his choice of specific interventions. On the other hand, therapist factors seem to have a major impact on treatment outcome—an impact that appears to be at least as big as, and in some cases probably bigger than, the impact of the specific choice of therapeutic method. Common therapeutic factors are more important for outcome than specific technical factors related to standardized and manualized treatment methods, although in practice, it is close to impossible to separate these elements in psychotherapy.

The therapist's more personal qualities and stance and his way of meeting the patient, handling the therapeutic relationship and implementing the various therapeutic methods in relation to the individual patient in the therapeutic space, here and now, are crucial for the process and outcome of therapy. The more structural elements and the therapist's specific application of the various therapeutic interventions and methods carry more weight than the specific choice of method. Taken together, these points suggest that the dynamic relational model of psychotherapy should have a far more prominent place in our general understanding of psychotherapy, in the training of psychotherapists and in psychotherapy research, while the medically oriented approach to psychotherapy should be toned down. One key aspect that we need to explore and develop further is the psychotherapeutic stance: how the psychotherapist meets the patient and the material the patient presents in the therapeutic space in a way that maximizes the effect of the de common therapeutic factors and what we know about key elements of the psychotherapeutic relationship from classical and contemporary psychoanalytic theory. That is the main focus of Part II.

References

Ackerman, S. J., & Hilsenroth, M. J. (2001). A review of therapist characteristics and techniques negatively impacting the therapeutic alliance. *Psychotherapy, 38,* 171–185.

Ackerman, S. J., & Hilsenroth, M. J. (2003). A review of therapist characteristics and techniques positively impacting the therapeutic alliance. *Clinical Psychology Review, 23,* 1–33.

Anderson, T., Ogles, B. M., Patterson, C. L., Lambert, M. J., & Vermeersch, D. A. (2009). Therapist effects: Facilitative interpersonal skills as a predictor of therapist success. *Journal of Clinical Psychology, 65,* 755–768.

Anderson, T., McClintock, A. S., Himawan, L., Song, X., & Patterson, C. L. (2016a). A prospective study of therapist facilitative interpersonal skills as a predictor of treatment outcome. *Journal of Consulting and Clinical Psychology, 84,* 57–66.

Anderson, T., Crowley, M. E., Himawan, L., Holmberg, J. K., & Uhlin, B. D. (2016b). Therapist facilitative interpersonal skills and training status: A randomized trial on alliance and outcome. *Psychotherapy Research, 26*(5), 511–529.

Baldwin, S. A., & Imel, Z. E. (2013). Therapist effects: Findings and methods. In M. J. Lambert (Ed.), *Bergin and Garfield's handbook of psychotherapy and behavior change* (6th ed., pp. 258–298). New York, NY: Wiley.

Baldwin, S. A., Wampold, B. E., & Imel, Z. E. (2007). Untangling the alliance-outcome correlation: Exploring the relative importance of therapist and patient variability in the alliance. *Journal of Consulting and Clinical Psychology, 75,* 842–852.

Berglar, J., Crameri, A., Von Wyl, A., Koemeda-Lutz, M., Köhler, M., Staczan, P., et al. (2016). Therapist effects on treatment outcome in psychotherapy: A multilevel modelling analysis. *International Journal of Psychotherapy, 20,* 61–80.

Betan, E., Heim, A. K., Conklin, C. Z., & Westen, D. (2005). Countertransference phenomena and personality pathology in clinical practice: An empirical investigation. *American Journal of Psychiatry, 162,* 890–898.

Beutler, L. E., Malik, M., Alimohamed, S., Harwood, T. M., Talebi, H., Noble, S., et al. (2004). Therapist variables. In M. J. Lambert (Ed.), *Bergin and Garfield's handbook of psychotherapy and behavior change* (5th ed., pp. 227–306). New York, NY: Wiley.

Binder, J. L. (2004). *Key competencies in brief dynamic psychotherapy: Clinical practice beyond the manual.* New York, NY: Guilford.

Blatt, S. J., Sanislow, C. A., Zuroff, D. C., & Pilkonis, P. A. (1996). Characteristics of effective therapists: Further analyses of data from the national institute of mental health treatment of depression collaborative research program. *Journal of Consulting and Clinical Psychology, 64*(6), 1276–1284.

Bollas, C. (1993). *Being a character: Psychoanalysis and self experience.* London, England: Routledge (Original work published 1992).

Bonaminio, V. (2008). The person of the analyst, interpreting, not interpreting, and countertransference. *Psychoanalytic Quarterly, 77,* 1105–1146.

Bourke, M. E., & Grenyer, B. F. S. (2010). Psychotherapists' response to borderline personality disorder: A core conflictual relationship theme analysis. *Psychotherapy Research, 20*(6), 680–691.

Castonguay, L. G., Boswell, J. F., Constantino, M. J., Goldfried, M. R., & Hill, C. E. (2010). Training implications of harmful effects of psychological treatments. *American Psychologist, 65,* 34–49.

Del Re, A. C., Flückiger, C., Horvarth, A., Symonds, D., & Wampold, B. E. (2012). Therapist effects in the therapeutic alliance-outcome relationship: A restricted-maximum likelihood meta-analysis. *Clinical Psychology Review, 32,* 642–649.

Dozier, M., Cue, K. L., & Barnett, L. (1994). Clinicians as caregivers: Role of attachment organization in treatment. *Journal of Consulting and Clinical Psychology, 62,* 793–800.

Dunkle, J. H., & Friedlander, M. L. (1996). Contribution of therapist experience and personal characteristics to the working alliance. *Journal of Counseling Psychology, 43,* 456–460.

Farber, B. A. (2006). *Self-disclosure in psychotherapy.* New York, NY: Guilford.

Fiedler, F. E. (1950a). The concept of an ideal therapeutic relationship. *Journal of Consulting and Clinical Psychology, 14,* 239–245.

Fiedler, F. E. (1950b). A comparison of therapeutic relationships in psychoanalytic, non-directive and Adlerian therapy. *Journal of Consulting and Clinical Psychology, 14*(6), 436–445.

Flückiger, C., Del Re, A. C., Wampold, B. E., Symonds, D., & Horvath, A. O. (2012). How central is the alliance in psychotherapy? A multilevel longitudinal meta-analysis. *Journal of Counseling Psychology, 59,* 10–17.

Fonagy, P., Luyten, P., & Allison, E. (2015). Epistemic petrification and the restoration of epistemic trust: A new conceptualization of borderline personality disorder and its psychosocial treatment. *Journal of Personality Disorders, 29,* 575–609.

Fromm-Reichmann, F. (1960). *Principles of intensive psychotherapy*. Chicago, IL: University of Chicago Press.

Goldberg, S. B., Rousmaniere, T., Miller, S. D., Whipple, J., Nielsen, S. L., & Hoyt, W. T. (2016a). Do psychotherapists improve with time and experience? A longitudinal analysis of outcome in a clinical setting. *Journal of Counseling Psychology, 63,* 1–11.

Goldberg, S. B., Babins-Wagner, R., Rousmaniere, T., Berzins, S., Hoyt, W. T., Whipple, J. L., et al. (2016b). Creating a climate for therapist improvement: A case study of an agency focused on outcomes and deliberate practice. *Psychotherapy, 53,* 367–375.

Goldfried, M. R., Raue, P. J., & Castonguay, L. G. (1998). The therapeutic focus in significant sessions of master therapists: A comparison of cognitive-behavioral and psychodynamic-interpersonal interventions. *Journal of Consulting and Clinical Psychology, 66*(5), 803–810.

Hanna, F. J., & Ottens, A. J. (1995). The role of wisdom in psychotherapy. *Journal of Psychotherapy Integration, 5,* 195–219.

Hayes, J. A., Gelson, C. J., & Hummel, A. M. (2011). Managing countertransference. Evidence-based psychotherapy relationships. In J. C. Norcross (Ed.), *Psychotherapy relationships that work: Evidence-based responsiveness* (2nd ed., pp. 239–260). New York, NY: Oxford University Press.

Hayes, J. A., Nelson, D. L., & Fauth, J. (2015). Countertransference in successful and unsuccessful cases of psychotherapy. *Psychotherapy, 52,* 127–133.

Henry, W. P., Schacht, T. E., & Strupp, H. H. (1986). Structural analysis of social behavior: Application to a study of interpersonal process in differential psychotherapeutic outcome. *Journal of Consulting and Clinical Psychology, 54,* 27–31.

Henry, W. P., Schacht, T. E., & Strupp, H. H. (1990). Patient and therapist introject, interpersonal process, and differential therapy outcome. *Journal of Consulting and Clinical Psychology, 58,* 768–774.

Henry, W. P., Strupp, H. H., Butler, S. F., Schacht, T. E., & Binder, J. L. (1993). Effects of training in time-limited dynamic psychotherapy: Changes in therapist behavior. *Journal of Consulting and Clinical Psychology, 61,* 434–440.

Hersoug, A. G., Høglend, P., Havik, O., Von der Lippe, A., & Monsen, J. (2009). Therapist characteristics influencing the quality of alliance in long-term psychotherapy. *Clinical Psychology and Psychotherapy, 16,* 100–110.

Hill, C. E., & Knox, S. (2013). Training and supervision in psychotherapy. In M. Lambert (Ed.), *Bergin and Garfield's handbook of psychotherapy and behavior change* (6th ed., pp. 775–812). New York, NY: Wiley.

Hill, C. E., Baumann, E., Shafran, N., Gupta, S., Morrison, A., Rojas, A. E. P., et al. (2015). Is training effective? A study of counseling psychology doctoral trainees in a psychodynamic/interpersonal training clinic. *Journal of Counseling Psychology, 62,* 184–201.

Hilliard, R. B., Henry, W. P., & Strupp, H. H. (2000). An interpersonal model of psychotherapy: Linking patient and therapist developmental history, therapeutic process, and types of outcome. *Journal of Consulting and Clinical Psychology, 68,* 125–133.

Horvath, A. O., Del Re, A. C., Flückiger, C., & Symonds, D. (2011). Alliance in individual psychotherapy. Evidence-based psychotherapy relationships. In J. C. Norcross (Ed.), *Psychotherapy relationships that work: Evidence-based responsiveness* (2nd ed., pp. 25–69). New York, NY: Oxford University Press.

Jaspers, K. (1942). *Allgemeine psychopathologie* [General psychopathology] (4th ed.). Berlin, Germany: Springer.

Jennings, L., & Skovholt, T. M. (1999). The cognitive, emotional, and relational characteristics of master therapists. *Journal of Counseling Psychology, 46,* 3–11.

Jennings, L., Skovholt, T. M., Goh, M., & Lian, F. (2013). Master therapists: Explorations of expertise. In M. H. Rønnestad & T. M. Skovholt (Ed.), *The developing practitioner* (pp. 213–246). London, England: Routledge.

Jørgensen, C. R. (2000). Den tilstrækkeligt gode terapeuts håndtering af brud på den terapeutiske alliance. *Et kvalitativt enkeltcasestudie. Psyke & Logos, 21,* 631–675.

Klöpper, M. (2014). *Die Dynamik des Psychischen. Praxishandbuch für das Verständnis der Beziehungsdynamik.* Stuttgart, Germany: Klett-Cotta Verlag.

Levitt, H. M., & Piazza-Bonin, E. (2016). Wisdom and psychotherapy: Studying expert therapists' clinical wisdom to explicate common processes. *Psychotherapy Research, 26,* 31–47.

Martin, A., Buchheim, A., Berger, U., & Strauss, B. (2007). The impact of attachment organization on potential countertransference reactions. *Psychotherapy Research, 17,* 46–58.

Myers, D., & Hayes, J. A. (2006). Effects of therapist general self-disclosure and countertransference disclosure on ratings of the therapist and session. *Psychotherapy: Theory, Research, Practice, Training, 43,* 173–185.

Najavits, L. M., & Strupp, H. H. (1994). Differences in the effectiveness of psychodynamic therapists: A process-outcome study. *Psychotherapy, 31,* 114–123.

Najavits, L. M., & Weiss, R. D. (1994). Variations in therapist effectiveness in the treatment of patients with substance use disorders: An empirical view. *Addiction, 89,* 679–688.

Nissen-Lie, H. A., Monsen, J. T., & Rønnestad, M. H. (2010). Therapist predictors of early patient-rated working alliance: A multilevel approach. *Psychotherapy Research, 20,* 627–646.

Nissen-Lie, H. A., Monsen, J. T., Ulleberg, P., & Rønnestad, M. H. (2013a). Psychotherapists self-reports of their interpersonal functioning and difficulties in practice as predictors of patient outcome. *Psychotherapy Research, 23,* 86–104.

Nissen-Lie, H. A., Havik, O. D., Høglend, P. A., Monsen, J. T., & Rønnestad, M. H. (2013b). The contribution of the quality of therapists personal lives to the development of the working alliance. *Journal of Counseling Psychology, 60,* 483–495.

Nissen-Lie, H. A., Goldberg, S. B., Hoyt, W. T., Falkenström, F., Holmqvist, R., Nielsen, S. L., et al. (2016). Are therapists uniformly effective across patient outcome domains? A study on therapist effectiveness in two different treatment contexts. *Journal of Counseling Psychology, 64*(4), 367–378.

Nissen-Lie, H. A., Rønnestad, M. H., Høglend, P. A., Havik, O. E., Solbakken, O. A., Stiles, T. C., et al. (2017). Love yourself as a person, doubt yourself as a therapist? *Clinical Psychology & Psychotherapy, 24*(1), 48–60.

Oddli, H. W. (2014). Klinisk ekspertise: Hvordan bruker erfarne terapeuter kunnskap? (Clinical expertise. How do experienced therapists use knowledge?] In A. Von der Lippe, H. A. Nissen-Lie, & H.W. Oddli (Eds.), *Psykoterapeuten. En antologi om terapeutens rolle i psykoterapi* (pp. 70–93). Oslo, Norway: Gyldendal Akademisk.

Ogden, T. H. (2009). *Rediscovering psychoanalysis: Thinking and dreaming, learning and forgetting.* London, England: Routledge.

Owen, J., Wampold, B. E., Kopta, M., Rousmaniere, T., & Miller, S. D. (2016). As good as it gets? Therapy outcome of trainees over time. *Journal of Counseling Psychology, 63,* 12–19.

Powell, J. L., Hunter, H. L., Beasley, L. O., & Vernberg, E. M. (2010). Using fine-grained indexes of therapists experience and training to predict treatment outcomes in a university-based training clinic for children and families. *Training and Education in Professional Psychology, 4,* 138–144.

Råbu, M., & McLeod, J. (2016). Wisdom in professional knowledge: Why it can be valuable to listen to the voices of senior psychotherapists. *Psychotherapy Research* (ahead of print). https://doi.org/10.1080/10503307.2016.1265685.

Ricks, D. F. (1974). Supershrink: Methods of a therapist judged successful on the basis of adult outcomes of adolescent patients. In D. F. Ricks, M. Roff, & A. Thomas (Eds.), *Life history research in psychopathology* (Vol. 3, pp. 275–297). Minneapolis: University of Minnesota Press.

Rønnestad, M. H., & Skovholt, T. M. (2013). *The developing practitioner: Growth and stagnation of therapists and counselors*. London, England: Routledge.

Safran, J. D., Muran, J. C., & Eubanks-Carter, C. (2011). Repairing alliance ruptures. *Psychotherapy, 48,* 80–87.

Safran, J. D., Muran, J. C., Demaria, A., Boutwell, C., Eubanks-Carter, C., & Winston, A. (2014). Investigating the impact of alliance-focused training on interpersonal process and therapists' capacity for experimental reflection. *Psychotherapy Research, 24,* 269–285.

Schauenburg, H., Buchheim, A., Beckh, K., Nolte, T., Brenk-Franz, K., Leichsenring, F., et al. (2010). The influence of psychodynamically oriented therapists' attachment representations on outcome and alliance in inpatient psychotherapy. *Psychotherapy Research, 20,* 193–202.

Schneider, G. (2003). Die Zukunft? Plädoyer für eine atopische Grundhaltung in der Psychoanalyse – mit einem Exkurs zu Melvilles Bartleby [The future? Plea for an atopic basic attitude in psychoanalysis-with a digression on Melville's Bartleby]. *Psyche, 57,* 226–248.

Schön, D. A. (1983). *The reflective practitioner: How professionals think in action*. Aldershot, England: Arena.

Schöttke, H., Flückinger, C., Goldberg, S. B., Eversmann, J., & Lange, J. (2017). Predicting psychotherapy outcome based on therapist interpersonal skills: A five-year longitudinal study of a therapist assessment protocol. *Psychotherapy Research, 27*(6), 642–656. https://doi.org/10.1080/10503307.2015.1125546.

Skovholt, T. M., Rønnestad, M. H., & Jennings, L. (1997). Searching for expertise in counseling, psychotherapy, and professional psychology. *Educational Psychology Review, 9,* 361–369.

Sternberg, R. J. (1998). A balance theory of wisdom. *Review of General Psychology, 2,* 347–365.

Swift, J. K., & Greenberg, R. P. (2012). Premature discontinuation in adult psychotherapy: A meta-analysis. *Journal of Consulting and Clinical Psychology, 80,* 547–559.

Treurniet, N. (1997). On an ethic of psychoanalytic technique. *Psychoanalytic Quarterly, 66,* 596–627.

Uhlin, B. D. (2011). *Therapist in-session rated Facilitative Interpersonal Skills (FIS-IS) in the psychotherapy process*. Dissertation presented to the Faculty of the College of Arts and Sciences, Ohio University, Athens.

Von der Lippe, A., Monsen, J. T., Rønnestad, M. H., & Eilertsen, D. E. (2008). Treatment failure in psychotherapy: The pull of hostility. *Psychotherapy Research, 18*(4), 420–432.

Von Wyl, A., Tschuschke, V., Crameri, A., Koemeda-Lutz, M., & Schulthess, P. (Eds.). (2016). *Was wirkt in der Psychotherapie? Ergebnisse der Praxisstudie ambulante Psychotherapie zu 10 unterschiedlichen Verfahren* [What works in psychotherapy? Findings of a practice study of day-patient psychotherapy with 10 different methods]. Gießen: Psychosozial-Verlag.

Wampold, B. E., & Imel, Z.-E. (2015). *The great psychotherapy debate: The evidence for what makes psychotherapy work* (2nd ed.). London, England: Routledge.

Willutzki, U., Reinke-Kappenstein, B., & Hermer, M. (2013). Ohne Heiler geht es nicht. Bedeutung von Psychotherapeuten für Therapieprozess und -ergebnis [Nothing works without the healer. Impact of psychotherapists on the process and outcome of psychotherapy]. *Psychotherapeut, 58,* 427–437.

Yeh, Y. J., & Hayes, J. A. (2011). How does disclosing countertransference affect perceptions of the therapist and the session? *Psychotherapy, 48*(4), 322–329.

Zilcha-Mano, S., & Barber, J. (2014). Learning from well-trained and experienced dynamic psychotherapists: Research on the efficacy of dynamic psychotherapy and its mechanisms of change. *Contemporary Psychoanalysis, 50,* 58–88.

Part II
The Psychotherapeutic Stance

Chapter 8
The Basis of the Psychotherapeutic Stance

In the Danish encyclopaedia *Den Store Danske Encyklopædi*, Boye Katzenelson defines the Danish 'holdning'—attitude or stance—as 'a fairly persistent orientation, acquired throughout life, towards people, things, ideas, ideologies, values and social events, accompanied by a disposition or a prior inclination to hold certain opinions about these and react to them in certain ways' (Katzenelson 2010). The meaning of the Danish word 'holdning' is closely related to both 'attitude' and 'stance' in English and so cannot be translated unambiguously to either of these two words; a similar issue pertains to the German word 'Haltung'. Dictionaries associate *attitude* and *stance* with, among other things, body posture or position, which may express certain feelings and contain an element of action, just as they are also both associated with a person's feelings towards someone or something, a person's inclination to think and act in certain ways and, not least, with a mental disposition, that is, a way of meeting and engaging with experiences, other people and the world in general. The latter aspect in particular lies close to the intended meaning of the psychotherapeutic stance.

In social psychology, 'attitude' and, to some extent, 'stance' are often used to refer to a complex, fairly stable cognitive and emotional identification with certain values and orientations in one's approach to the world, which is closely related to one's sense of identity (Löchel 2013:1169). Similarly, the psychotherapeutic stance is closely related to, especially, more experienced therapists' professional and, to varying degrees, personal and social identity (Jørgensen 2008), just as the psychotherapeutic stance contains both a set of values and understandings of humanity and the world and an inclination to act and react in certain ways in the therapeutic space. In a sense, especially the more technical aspects of the psychotherapist's professional identity are vaguely or loosely delimited and defined, as it is far from given a priori what the therapist 'should do', in concrete terms, in the therapeutic space—which places him or her in a vulnerable position. This may also be considered an important strength in the therapeutic process, as it leaves the therapist open to what the individual patient brings into and needs in the session and allows him to attune his strategy accordingly (Zwiebel 2007:194).

C. R. Jørgensen, *The Psychotherapeutic Stance*,
https://doi.org/10.1007/978-3-030-20437-2_8

As Katzenelson (2010) goes on to add, 'the cognitive factor of our attitude/stance affects the way we perceive reality' and will often cause us 'to perform certain acts rather than others' (*Den Store Danske Encyklopædi*). 'Attitudes/stances are mental factors that influence and, to varying degrees, strengthen our perceptions and convictions, and thus they constitute part of the basis for explaining a person's behaviour and predicting future behaviour' (ibid.). Although this largely social psychological definition of 'attitude' or 'stance' does not overlap fully with the implications of 'stance' in relation to the psychotherapist's being and work in the therapeutic space, it does point to key structural aspects of the concept of the psychotherapeutic stance, related to a set of (humanistic) values, a certain emotional and mental inclination and a certain way of meeting the patient and what unfolds in the therapeutic space.

More psychoanalytically oriented authors in particular have sought to define the psychotherapeutic stance. The English-language literature refers to both psychotherapeutic or psychoanalytic 'attitude' (Schafer 1983) and 'stance' (Druck 1994; Bloom-Feshbach and Bloom-Feshbach 1996); of these, 'attitude' may be perceived as being slightly more cognitive and deliberately chosen, while 'stance' may also be said to include more moral aspects. It can be difficult to determine which of the two terms is more apt. In German, the main term is the psychotherapeutic 'Haltung' (Kutter 1988), a term that is also associated with the ability to stand firm and to hold on to oneself and one's norms and values under pressure or the quality of having 'backbone' and character.

The psychotherapeutic stance refers to fundamental attitude towards psychotherapeutic work and to the therapist's basic psychological understanding of aetiology, human psychology, treatment theory and theory of psychotherapeutic efficacy factors and, not least, how these elements are enacted in the therapist's actual meeting with the patient. In that sense, the effort to define the concept of the psychotherapeutic stance can be said to be about discerning the core of psychotherapeutic work. The psychotherapeutic stance has received remarkably little attention and remains largely unspecified in the contemporary therapy literature, which more or less presupposes the existence of a tacit consensus on what it means to adopt a psychotherapeutic stance or position or that the specific implications of the concept are somehow self-explanatory within a given treatment theory and method, which is far from the case. Informed by the writings of the German psychoanalyst Kutter (1988:19, 2003:371f), we may discern at least three levels of the therapeutic stance:

(1) The basic psychotherapeutic stance, which remains largely invariable across patients, independent of the individual patient's diagnosis, functioning level and specific treatment needs. Kutter also refers to this as the therapist's inner stance.
(2) Those aspects of the therapist's attitude towards and way of meeting his or her patients that may vary either over the course of the therapy or with the individual patient's specific disorder, current functioning level and needs.
(3) The therapist's specific use of interventions, elements from specific therapeutic methods and aspects of one or more therapeutic theories, including the use of psychoanalytic theory as a hermeneutic method.

In the present context, the term will mainly be used about the first two levels in Kutter's analysis, as his third level has more to do with the practical applications of specific elements of given treatment model and theory. This third level is the focus of various treatment manuals and is not relevant in the present context. Further, it may be argued that Kutter's second level should really be seen as an aspect of his first, as it is part of the basic psychotherapeutic stance (as it is defined in the following) that the therapist continuously assesses what the patient needs and attunes his chosen strategies and interventions accordingly. The specific attunement of subtle nuances in the psychotherapeutic stance to the characteristics and specific difficulties of the individual patient also lie outside the scope of the present book (however, see Chap. 10).

8.1 Dynamic Relational Understanding of Pathology and Psychotherapy

The psychotherapeutic stance is based on more or less fundamental beliefs about humanity, human psychology (personality and development theory), the core of psychopathology, normality and the essence of the psychotherapeutic work (therapeutic theory). The present context does not allow for an exhaustive discussion of these aspects, but the following offers a brief outline of some of the main elements of what could be called a dynamic-relational understanding of pathology and psychotherapy (Mentzos 2009; Jørgensen 2009). The dynamic-relational approach primarily defines a certain way of thinking about and understanding the patient, what unfolds between patient and therapist in the therapeutic space and of oneself, one's role and one's reactions in the interaction with the patient (cf. Gabbard 2014:4).

It is a basic characteristic of human psychology that our past experiences influence our current experiences, perceptions and behaviour as well as our thoughts about the future. Early interactions with significant others are internalized and serve as the basis for the development of mental representations of the self ('who am I?'), others ('what are other people like?'), interpersonal relations ('what happens between people') and the world in general—mental representations and internal working models or object relations that play an important role in shaping our subsequent perceptions of ourselves, others and interpersonal interactions. These internal object relations are 'activated' and have a major influence on our behaviour in interpersonal interactions. Aspects of these perceptions of self, others and the world are conscious—or are fairly easy to render conscious—while others are more non-conscious sensations, implicit norms, implicit relational knowledge and non-conscious inclinations to act in certain ways (stored in procedural memory, see Chap. 11) that we are not readily able to verbalize, let alone modify, via conscious, intentional decisions. Our self-perception is founded in interactions with important others and in our perception of their perception of us. In a sense, we find ourselves by seeing ourselves mirrored in the eyes of important others. Similarly, our self-perception may later be revised if the image of ourselves that we see in the eyes of important others is altered, for example when we enter into new relationships with people who see us in new and different ways from the way we were perceived by our parents and other people close to us in early life. In extension of this point, the image of herself that the patient sees in the therapist's perception is important. The image of the patient and her inner life that the therapist constructs and continuously revises in light of his experiences with the patient may thus have a big impact on the development of the patient's self-image (cf. Bateman and Fonagy 2016:182f).

On the other hand, the establishment of mental representations (the development of the declarative and the procedural memory) provides an aspect of predictability but also of inertia and a tendency towards self-fulfilling prophecies, in the sense that once we have developed a certain self-image—an image of who we are, our identity—we tend to appear and act in ways that match the image; this in turn increases the likelihood that others affirm and reinforce that image. Similarly, our perceptions of others—our ideas about what other people are like—can cause us to engage in interpersonal interactions in ways that invite others to act in accordance with these perceptions and thus affirm or even reinforce our established ideas about reality. Broadly speaking, the longer the patients has held these perceptions, and the more times they have been confirmed and thus reinforced, the harder they can be to change. Over time, they become increasingly ingrained in our psychology, and we tend to interpret all new experiences in light of these pre-established notions of self, others and the world in general, which thus become a sort of self-fulfilling prophecies. Hence, disorders in our early relationships, including the way important caregivers mirror the self, can contribute to the establishment of self-fuelling negative processes in a person's self-perception and engagement with the world.

On this basis we can offer the following relational concept of the core of psychopathology: psychopathology originates in and is continually maintained and manifested in disorders in the interaction with others, including negative, simplistic, rigid and often distorted perception of self, others, the world and what happens in interpersonal interactions. This typically involves a reduced capacity for holding nuanced and context-sensitive thoughts about psychological processes (mental states) and possible connections between one's own and others' internal subjective perceptions and behaviour (mentalizing capacity), that is, an impaired capacity to have psychological and nuanced perceptions of self and others. This capacity is further compromised when the person is under pressure and in connection with emotional arousal (activation of the attachment system and so on). We should also note that disturbed relationships always involve at least two persons, and that the basis of dysfunctional interactions with others, including the patient's interaction with the therapist, never pertains exclusively to the patient but also, always, involves the others who interact with the patient (including the therapist).

With regard to the psychotherapeutic process and the psychotherapeutic mechanisms of change, the relational concept of pathology implies that the core of the patient's difficulties—persistent (simplistic and negative) perceptions of self, others and relationships and recurring maladaptive patterns interpersonal interactions—is also persistently actualized and manifested in the patient's interactions with the therapist, here and now, and in the patient's psychological functioning in the therapeutic space. This dynamic not only contains the potential for the therapist to observe the core of the patient's difficulties but also offers important possibilities for modifying the patient's basic perception of self, others and interpersonal relationships (the core of the patient's pathology). Among the ways this may occur is when the therapist acts in a way that defies the patient's expectations and previous experiences (avoiding the repetition of otherwise recurring interaction patterns) and when the therapist sees something other and more in the patient than caregivers and significant others have seen and mirrors this in an adaptive (congruent and marked) manner. Together, these experiences can lead to changes in the patient's self-perception and thus in her basis for relating to others—modifying her internal object relations, working models and procedural memory. The underlying assumptions driving the dynamic-relational concept of pathology and its related therapy model can briefly be summarized in the following main points:

- Past experiences influence current psychological functioning—and current experiences and ideas about the future.
- Recurring patterns in relationships are often a key factor in the development, maintenance and manifestation of psychopathology. The patient's symptoms and, to an immediate observer, 'disturbed' behaviour may, to varying degrees, be seen as manifestations of the patient's 'failed' attempts at managing perceived difficulties—or at adapting to a perceived reality—in the present via strategies developed earlier in life (when they would typically also have been maladaptive, to varying degrees). These patterns will also manifest themselves in the patient's interactions with the therapist (in the transference, see Chaps. 9 and 11) and in the therapist's mental states and reactions in the therapeutic space (via countertransferences, possibly projective identification, see Chap. 11). The therapeutic relationship—what unfolds in the treatment relationship—thus has a key role in the psychotherapeutic process.
- One cannot expect the patient to be able to verbalize what constitutes the core of his or her difficulties (possibly because it has never been mentally represented and articulated, or because it is stored exclusively in the procedural memory), but it will often be evident in the way the patient acts in the therapeutic space and in the interaction with the therapist. This includes the patient's unconscious activation of various defensive strategies and attempts at avoiding painful or shameful emotions and experiences. It is therefore important for the therapist to register what the patient may avoid bringing up, says 'between the lines' or communicates via other channels besides explicit verbal communication (see Chap. 11).
- Psychopathology is often associated with a reduced ability to think in psychological terms and to understand one's own and others' reactions in light of psychological processes and internal mental states. Hence, developing the patient's ability to think with psychological nuance, to make connections between internal (mental states, psychological processes) and external reality (behaviour, interpersonal processes) and to view reality from different perspectives (mentalize) is an important element of the psychotherapeutic process.

- Psychopathology may also be associated with a lack of internal integration, meaning that certain experiences, needs, aspects of the self, emotions and other mental states are split off or repressed.

The dynamic-relational model of pathology and therapy is based on what might be called a contemporary two-person psychology, which differs in certain regards from a more classical one-person psychology. The main elements of contemporary two-person psychology are outlined in Table 8.1.

The dynamic-relational model of pathology implies that the therapist has to direct his attention at the therapeutic process, that is, what is happening in the therapeutic relationship here and now, the structure of the patient's narrative (what is told, when and how) and developments in the patient's and the therapist's own mental states. The focus is on what the patient says and does in the therapeutic space and in the interaction with the therapist as a way to uncover key aspects of the patient's difficulties, including recurring relational patterns, symptomatology, maladaptive behaviours, emotional reactions and defensive strategies. This focus is used to understand the patient's psychology and difficulties and as a basis for working with (observing, verbalizing and thinking about) psychological, interpersonal and mental processes in the patient and in the therapeutic space. It is a joint effort that gradually enables the patient to do the same on her own after internalizing the therapeutic process, which develops the patient's alpha function (ability to verbalize, think about and process perceptions), mentalizing capacity, ability to think in psychological terms and to process emotional experiences. All things being equal, this also gives the patient a series of corrective emotional experiences, that is, experiences of being seen, taken seriously and understood as a human being, a subject, who matters (see Chap. 10).

From the Traditional One-Person Psychology to the Contemporary Two-Person Psychology

> We have often heard it maintained that sciences should be built up on clear and sharply defined basic concepts. In actual fact no science, not even the most exact, begins with such definitions. The true beginning of scientific activity consists rather in describing phenomena […] Even at the stage of description it is not possible to avoid applying certain abstract ideas to the material in hand […] [t]hey must at first necessarily possess some degree of indefiniteness […] strictly speaking, they are in the nature of conventions […] The advance of knowledge, however, does not tolerate any rigidity even in definitions. […] A conventional basic concept of this kind, which at the moment is still somewhat obscure but which is indispensable to us in psychology, is that of an "instinct" (Freud 1915/1957:117f).
>
> It is true that Individual Psychology is concerned with the individual man and explores the paths by which he seeks to find satisfaction for his instinctual impulses; but only rarely and under certain exceptional conditions is Individual Psychology in a position to disregard the relations of this individual to others. In the individual's mental life someone else is invariably involved, as a model, as an object, as a helper, as an opponent; and so from the very first individual psychology, in this extended but entirely justifiable sense of the words is at the same time social psychology as well (Freud 1921/1955:69).

Just a few years after the birth of psychoanalysis, and thus psychotherapy, in the circle around Freud, the first internal disagreements began to emerge, about whether our understanding of human psychology, psychopathology and psychotherapy

Table 8.1 Key differences between one-person and two/multiple-person psychology that are relevant to the dynamic-relational psychotherapeutic stance (Levenson 1995:32f; Köhler-Weisker 1986:148)

One-person psychology classical psychoanalytic stance	Contemporary two/multiple-person psychology dynamic-relational stance
The therapist is primarily viewed as a neutral (personally and emotionally detached or withdrawn) observer in a clearly asymmetrical relationship; 'objective' mirroring of the patient is a core task. The therapist's main role is to serve as a transference object	The therapist is a participating observer, is present as a subject and influences the patient's behaviour ('the observed') in a largely symmetrical relationship; the therapist's interpersonal reactions and feedback to the patient are more important than 'objective' mirroring. The therapist should also serve as a self-object that, to varying degrees, satisfies some of the patient's (primarily relational) needs
Focus on internal psychological dynamics in the patient and on past experiences	Focus on recurring interpersonal patterns and processes in the present moment
The psychotherapeutic stance is mainly applied to the patient's narratives, transferences and other acts in the therapeutic space	The psychotherapeutic stance is applied to the patient's narratives and acts (transference), the therapist's reactions and acts (countertransferences) and on the interaction between patient and therapist in the therapeutic space
Uncovering repressed unconscious experiences (from the declarative memory) and achieving insight are key efficacy factors	Corrective emotional experiences, modifying the procedural memory in the meeting with the therapist and internalizing the therapist's psychological functions (mentalizing capacity) are key efficacy factors; the therapist contains—'holds'—the patient
The therapist verbalizes, 'alphabetizes' and offers mental representations of what has so far remained unrepresented, with a main focus on internal psychological reality	The therapist verbalizes, 'alphabetizes' and offers mental representations of what has so far remained unrepresented, with a main focus on relational dynamics (stored in the procedural memory)
The therapist attempts (in the style of a detective or an archaeologist) to uncover hidden or repressed meanings behind the patient's symptoms	The therapist works with the patient in an attempt to understand the meaning of the patient's symptoms (their psychological functions) and to shape a narrative that can contribute to greater understanding and link the patient's subjective experiences, symptoms and behaviour together
The therapeutic process aims to uncover meaning, 'the truth' about the origins of the patient's difficulties	The therapeutic process aims primarily to generate meaning, a coherent self-narrative and conditions basis for a higher level of integration, especially in poorly functioning patients (integration of excluded aspects of the self)
Transference distorts the patient's perception of the therapist	Transference is seen, in part, as the patient's attempt to understand and manage the interaction with the therapist and the therapist's behaviour, which contribute to the generation of certain transferences
The therapist should strive to control his countertransference as much as possible and avoid to communicate it to the patient (because countertransference leads to the 'wrong' focus)	At times, the therapist will inevitably act out parts of the countertransference; the therapist should therefore communicate parts of his countertransferences to the patient and use them and the way they are acted out as therapeutic material

should be focused predominantly on the specific individual's internal psychological dynamics, or whether we should, to a much higher degree, view human beings as fundamentally social and contact-seeking and hence devote more attention to interpersonal interactions and their impact on the individual person's psychology. This represents a conflict between a one-person psychology, rooted in the mainly instinct/drive-oriented theoretical elements of classical psychoanalysis, versus a two-person psychology, which may take its origins in some of Freud's papers on the technical aspects of therapy (including the concept of transference), but which also moves gradually further away from classical psychoanalysis, especially Freud's theory of instincts or drives and his concept of psychological development.

Historically, there has thus not only been a clash between the medical and the dynamic-relational model of psychotherapy (see Chap. 3), but also at times intense disagreements between different representatives of a broadly defined dynamic concept of therapy. In that regard, it should be noted that there is no indisputable link between classical psychoanalytic theory on motivations and development (drive theory) and the psychoanalytic therapeutic method, in the sense that Freud and his followers' technical recommendations are automatically rendered invalid or useless because certain core elements of Freud's metapsychology prove untenable (cf. Bowlby 1969:16f) (see Chap. 9). Besides, Freud himself considered his drive theory a preliminary and hypothetical model for understanding human psychology, which might later be refuted by empirical findings and would therefore have to be abandoned (see the quotation above). Finally, it should be noted that Freud's theory—including, especially, his writings on technical aspects—contain clear relational elements and thus, at least, the beginnings of a two-person model of psychology; hence, we should not overstate the differences and polarization between classical and contemporary psychoanalysis (cf., e.g., Mills 2012).

In developing psychoanalysis Freud indisputably founded a new humanistic science. Freud, however, to some extent viewed psychoanalysis as a medical science (part of the health and natural sciences), and indeed, certain aspects of classical one-person psychoanalysis do have features with obvious affinities to the medical model of therapy (see Chap. 2), including the notion of the objective and neutral therapist, who from a position of an uninvolved authority figure can observe and understand the patient's internal psychological conflicts, as they are manifested in the patient's transference and symptoms, and whose role is to communicate this understanding to the patient in the form of psychoanalytic interpretations. In relation to this issue, Habermas (1987:246ff) speaks of the scientistic self-misunderstanding of classical psychoanalysis, referring to the inability or unwillingness of Freud and some of his immediate successors (mostly doctors) to acknowledge the obvious link between psychoanalysis and the humanities and to their determination, for various reasons, to associate psychoanalysis with the medical science. This self-misunderstanding had negative consequences for the development of the psychoanalytic method and also meant that notoriously untenable aspects of classical psychoanalytic theory and method were maintained for far too long (for example the rule of abstinence, see Chap. 10). This may also be seen as evident of the internal tension or rift in Freud's theory and classical psychoanalysis, which contains both a clinical method, where psychological disorders are interpreted in light of the patient's individual history, interpersonal interaction and the meaning of the manifested symptoms or their origin in potentially understandable causes (intentional processes that can be uncovered via hermeneutic methods), and the beginnings of a general theory of human psychology, where the focus is on physical-material (drives-based) causes of psychological disorders.

In recent decades, however, object relations theory, relational and intersubjective theory and, especially, attachment theory have gained such prominence that there is some justification for arguing that in major sections of the psychotherapeutic culture (perhaps especially in North America) a certain consensus has emerged concerning the fundamental aspects of the dynamic-relational two-person model of psychology (Mitchell 1988; Mills 2012), although, for example, more cognitively oriented therapists naturally use slightly different concepts and models for handling relational dynamics than psychotherapists with a psychoanalytic orientation. In parallel with this relational turn, the classical one-person features of psychoanalysis, which are rooted in drive theory, nomadic concepts of humanity and other, more speculative, ideas (including the notion of the oedipal conflict as a universal dynamic with crucial impact on human psychological development), have gradually lost most of their practical role in clinical psychology and psychotherapeutic practice, even if they may be said to live on in new guises, for example in Lacanian psychoanalysis, just as parts of the German-speaking psychoanalytic scene has also maintained closer ties to parts of Freud's original work (Mertens 2004, 2015).

On the other hand, more radical representatives of relational and intersubjective theory have, rightly, been criticized for going so far in their relational understanding of human psychological development and function that the individual (the individual's subjectivity, intentionality, free will and so on) is de facto dissolved or reduced to his or her relationships (see, e.g., Mills 2012), which risks jeopardizing the bodily components of human psychology and its links to human biology, brain processes and so on. Moreover, more radical representatives of the intersubjective approach may be criticized for a nearly sacral view of the interpersonal meeting, where the use of a therapeutic method and a psychotherapeutic stance tends to be seen as an obstacle to the patient's meeting with the therapist, while the importance of the patient's awareness of the therapist's and, thus, other people's separate subjectivity and otherness is overlooked (cf. Bohleber 2012). Importantly, this is not a matter of either searching for meaning or establishing an authentic interpersonal meeting characterized by psychological closeness and emotional contact, but a both/and proposition, where the two elements will often be interdependent. The therapist's psychological and emotional contact with the patient thus serves as the basis for a new and deeper understanding of the patient, while the therapist's ability to maintain a psychotherapeutic stance, take a step back from what is playing out in the contact with the patient in the present moment and intervene in light of the understanding that has developed over time can help the patient relate to the therapist as a new object (in contrast to a contact dominated by transference where the patient mainly experiences the therapist as a variation on persons from her past) and achieve corrective emotional experiences in the therapeutic space.

This is not the place for an in-depth discussion of how psychoanalysis and, thus, the psychotherapeutic culture have historically moved from a predominantly one-person psychology to a two-person psychology—a transition that also involves a gradually growing openness to the idea that psychotherapeutic work should generally be informed by empirical research and rest on scientifically founded theory as well as a growing scepticism of highly speculative and abstract theories and concepts (for example Freud's notion of an inherently human quasi-somatic death drive), which in practice defy any attempt at reaching a common understanding and application. Among others, Greenberg and Mitchell (1983) and Wallerstein (1995) have presented detailed analyses of this movement. The development of contemporary two-person relational psychoanalysis begins, in part, with psychoanalyst Sandor Ferenczi's technical therapy experiments from the 1920s (Ferenczi 1985; Ferenczi and Rank 1924) and gains momentum during the 1940 and 1950s with, among others, the American psychoanalyst Horney (1939), the British psychoanalyst Fairbairn (1952) and the American psychiatrist Sullivan (1953), Greenberg and Mitchell (1983) have argued quite convincingly that the British psychoanalyst Melanie Klein can, in many ways, be seen as a key transitional figure from the one-person psychology, rooted in drive theory, to the relational two-person-psychology in psychoanalysis. Klein thus holds on to the drive theory but also (in some of her writings) abandons the original solipsistic concept of drives and views human drives as fundamentally object-oriented (human beings pursuing contact/attachment as a goal in itself) and thus as an element of basic human sociality (Jørgensen 1999).

Attachment theory and its later involvement in psychotherapy, in part in the form of mentalization-based psychotherapy (Bateman and Fonagy 2016), have played a key role in opening the psychotherapeutic culture to incorporating and conducting empirical research—an opening that has naturally not been without problems, and which continually gives cause for balanced reflections on the validity of empirical research findings and on which features of the psychotherapeutic work can be made the object of quantitative research in ways that are meaningful and do not lead to unreasonable simplifications of the complexities of the psychotherapeutic process (cf. Part I of the present book).

Freud's classical one-person psychology, which is rooted in drive psychology, rests on a view of humanity (clearly defined, drive-motivated individuals) that is fundamentally different from the underlying view of contemporary dynamic-relational therapeutic theory, based on two-person psychology—two different perceptions of humanity with respective links to liberalism and communitarianism in political philosophy (interested readers are referred to Greenberg and Mitchell 1983:400f; Kymlicka 1990), each of which is characterized by an exaggerated focus on one of the two fundamental human needs: self-definition (self-identity, self-determination) and relatedness in social communities (attachment, internalization of shared ideas and beliefs), as they have been described by, among others, Blatt (2008). Liberalism is primarily focused on the individual's self-realization and how to minimize internal and external obstacles to this, while communitarianism insists that self-realization is only possible in community with others; it occurs in social relationships, and in that sense it depends on the individual's relatedness and ability to function in social communities.

While liberalism is based on the idea that every individual has his or her own truth about what is a good life, and that others (including therapists) should therefore not interfere (they should remain neutral and avoid trying to convey any specific goals and values to the patient), communitarianism believes that unlimited freedom only leads to painful confusion, and that in order to preserve our freedom, we need to relate in social communities with a common frame of reference, a set of common supra-individual norms and values (a horizon of meanings where something has greater value than something else), which must thus be conveyed (for example by the therapist) to and internalized by the individual (the patient) (cf. Taylor 1991). Broadly speaking, the shift from a one-person to a two-person psychology implies a similar shift from an understanding of human psychology as developing from pre-determined structures in the individual to the much more interactional understanding, where human psychology is seen to develop in interpersonal interactions (Mitchell 1988:17f). With this shift, the intersubjective meeting, approval, common meaning-making and the therapist's authenticity and more personal qualities take on far greater importance in the therapeutic process, while the therapist's neutrality and the attainment of insight are toned down or reinterpreted.

Just as the conflict between liberalism and communitarianism seems timeless and universal, presumably because it relates to a conflict between two fundamental but also partially contradictory human needs (freedom versus security; autonomy versus social approval/community and so on), we should expect that psychology will always be characterized by an internal struggle between theories that focus mainly on processes in the individual versus theories insisting that human beings develop and exist in social relationships, and that those should therefore be our main focus. We should not, however, resort to dichotomous either/or thinking and thus lose sight of how human psychological development and functioning unfold in a continuous interaction between internal (individual) and external (relational, contextual) factors. As individuals, we are something other and more than our interpersonal relationships. At the same time, we are also social beings with an individuality and an inner life that, to varying degrees, are the result of past (relational and other) experiences. A person's separation, individuation and development of an own (unique) individuality always occur in interaction with others; an interaction between individual (in part constitutional) and social (relational and cultural) factors. This is thus not a question of either/or but of the relative importance of internal (purely individual) and external (relational, cultural) for human psychology.

The classical psychoanalytic one-person approach to psychopathology and psychotherapy is focused on the delimited, well-defined individual and concerns itself solely or predominantly with internal psychological processes, including the individual's striving to satisfy biological needs, while approaches based on a two-person psychology view people as fundamentally social beings driven by needs for emotional contact, attachment and approval from important others. What therapists hear the patient say, what they choose to focus on in the therapeutic space, how it is interpreted and, not least, how it is addressed in the psychotherapeutic process will always be coloured or informed by their fundamental view of human psychology, psychopathology and the core of psychotherapy, including their basic perception of humanity—regardless whether they are consciously aware of this basic understanding and have made it explicit.

For example, the therapist's way of relating to his patients and his perception of the psychotherapeutic process may be profoundly influenced by whether he views psychopathology as a result of pent-up urges and internal conflicts about satisfying drives, or whether he views psychopathology as a result of disturbed past and current interpersonal relationships. A therapist who bases his work on a classical one-person psychology views therapeutic change as largely the result of the patient's attainment of cognitive insight into her internal psychological (drive) conflicts and the strengthening of her ego, catalysed by analytical interpretations from a neutral or emotionally withdrawn therapist; on the contrary, the dynamic-relational therapist will focus much more on forming an effective therapeutic relationship where the patient can acquire new corrective emotional experiences that challenge and have the capacity to modify the patient's established perceptions of self, others and the world in general. That is also why the transition away from the largely untenable (cf. Bowlby 1969; Stern 1985; Fonagy et al. 2002) one-person psychology to the contemporary two-person-psychology has been so crucial for the development of psychotherapeutic practice and our understanding of the psychotherapeutic stance.

Arguably, the psychoanalytic and psychotherapeutic community still contains remnants of the historical disagreements between, among others, ego psychology (one-person psychology) and object relations and attachment theory (two-person psychology) in the distinction between pathology stemming from less severe (or later founded, oedipal) conflict and pathology stemming from more severe (or earlier founded, pre-oedipal) deficiency that is often—and with some justification—applied in relation to the understanding and psychotherapeutic treatment of personality disorders and other pathologies (see Chap. 11).

8.2 How Should We Understand the Patient's Symptoms?

A young woman presents at the psychiatric emergency ward accompanied by a friend after a serious suicide attempt. She shows intense self-loathing and self-blame. She apologizes for the trouble and is sorry that she shocked and upset her mother. At the same time, one senses an underlying anger and irritation, especially directed at the mother, but also at the receiving doctor at the emergency ward, who in her opinion does not understand her, let alone give her what she needs. She is referred to psychotherapy, where she appears as a young woman who for much of her life has felt that she was in the way, difficult and 'a burden on mother', who herself struggles with psychological difficulties and therefore lacked the necessary resources to take care of her daughter. 'You ruined my life,' the mother said repeatedly to the patient. The patient describes how, during her childhood and youth, she often had to take care of her mother after she had drunk herself into a stupor. And how the mother became annoyed, angry or, alternatively, tired and exhausted when the patient hurt herself or came home from school upset because she had been bullied, felt excluded or kept to herself in class. She has previously received treatment for depression, with little effect, and has initiated several courses of psychotherapy, but soon dropped out because she did not feel that the therapist understood her or gave her what she needed.

During the first phase of the therapy the patient finds it difficult to 'take up room' and to tell the therapist how she feels and what she needs. She is worried about being a burden and taking the therapist's time when other patients surely 'need your help more than I do.' She also finds it hard to understand why the therapist would take the time to talk to her, but 'I guess you're just doing it because you get paid to.' At the same time, there is an undercurrent of irritation that the therapist fails to understand immediately (intuitively) what her problem is and what she needs—although she has not been able to articulate it. In order to prevent the patient from dropping out again, the therapist seizes on the pattern that appears to be actualized, and which would repeat itself in their relationship, lest they attend to it. Her experience from earlier relationships is that she is in the way and a burden if she expresses her needs. She has learned that she ought to remain invisible, and that it serves no purpose to tell others how she feels, since they are not going to understand or take any interest anyway. They are mostly focused on their own needs, which makes her angry. But she dares not express her anger directly, for fear that she will be abandoned. Instead she responds with sarcasm or withdraws from contact. These fundamental perceptions of self, others and what is at stake in relationships are activated and present as an undercurrent in the way the patient relates to the therapist. To the extent that the therapist realizes this, he can avoid taking part in a full re-enactment and thus break the pattern that has characterized the patient's relationships and in turn initiate changes in the patient's perception of self, others and what she expects to gain from relationships with others.

The Meaning of Pathology and Interpersonal Manifestations

What is the therapist's role, and how should the therapist meet and relate to the difficulties presented by this patient? During the initial conversations the therapist is expected to make a formal diagnosis—does she have a depression, or should her depressive symptoms rather be seen as secondary manifestations or the consequences of a personality disorder? Next, he is supposed to assess the patient's general functioning level, personality organization and any needs for other types of assistance: does she need somatic examinations or treatment, counselling from a social worker, physiotherapist, dietitian or other professional? However, the psychotherapist's first main tasks together with the patient are:

(1) To examine the meaning of the patient's core symptoms—when they emerge and in what contexts and how the patient views her own difficulties.

(2) To examine what patterns appear to be at play in the patient's relations with others—how she perceives self and others, how she feels and acts in interpersonal interactions, including whether there are any signs that these patterns are recurring in the therapeutic relationship.

Their common attention is directed at how 'we' can understand the patient's symptoms and behaviour—it is a shared task, hence 'we'—how the patient's difficulties are embedded in relational patterns, and the various ways in which these patterns are re-enacted in the treatment relationship.

Another focal point is whether any of the patient's original attempts at problem-solving (for example to avoid emotional contact to prevent new experiences of abandonment) have in themselves become a key part of the patient's current problems. How does the patient generally feel about asking for and accepting help, and how does she feel that she has been met when she has asked for help? If she has learned that she cannot trust the people who are supposed to help her, one should expect that she would initially be sceptical and guarded in her contact with the therapist. If she has grown accustomed to getting by on her own, appearing strong and trivializing her difficulties in order to avoid being a burden to others, or if she has, by contrast, learned that she needs to dramatize her problems and make perceived difficulties appear as major disasters in order to be seen at all and have any hope of getting help, we should expect her to, unconsciously, either understate or overstate her current problems in a re-enactment of these strategies for managing perceived problems in an interpersonal relationship.

How are the patient's difficulties manifested in the transference and in the therapist's experiences in the interaction with the patient (the countertransference)? How does the therapist respond to the fact that the patient appears a little vague and has trouble describing what her problem is, and that she suddenly reacts with biting sarcasm to his well-intended (but, from her point of view, stupid) questions? Does he get annoyed ('what a demanding and difficult woman'), offended or hurt ('she has no right to be so nasty, I'm doing my best to help her'), startled and insecure ('ooh, wow, I'd better be careful what I say here, or she's going to get mad') or maybe concerned and unsure of his own competence ('I hope she doesn't go right home and kills herself, just because I don't know enough to help her')? Does he feel the urge to quit or to punish the patient, or is he more likely to be curious and keen to understand and establish contact with the patient? All the reactions that occur in the meeting between the patient and the therapist tells us something about them both. However, to the extent that the therapist has a reasonable grasp of his normal reactions to his patients, these reactions can also serve as indications of the reactions the patient typically evokes in others and thus of the maladaptive patterns that characterize the patient's interpersonal relationships and which are activated or re-enacted, especially when she is under pressure.

What the therapist sees and how he understands what he sees play a big role for what he thinks should be done, and how. Unlike contemporary checklist psychiatry and our authorized, largely descriptive diagnostic systems—where the focus is on formal diagnostic criteria, symptom duration and the patient's functioning level on specific parameters, with no real formalized interest in the meaning of symptoms and possible individual causes in the individual patient—the patient's symptoms are not primarily interesting as potential indications of specific disorders, as described in our diagnostic systems (Teising 2014:202). The primary topic is not how the patient and the patient's difficulties match what is found in other patients (with the same diagnosis) or the formal criteria for different diagnoses; instead, the focus is more on what is unique about this particular individual and the difficulties he or she is experiencing. That also includes an interest in how the patient perceives and relates to her own difficulties, as she is not viewed as merely a cluster of symptoms to be categorized but as a person, a subject, who is always already relating to herself and her difficulties (cf. Fuchs 2013:88, 2010).

Psychiatric diagnoses are clusters of symptoms that are found frequently to coincide, but in themselves they do not say a great deal about what is at the root of the individual's specific symptoms and difficulties. Thus, we should not forget to distinguish between our constructs—our diagnostic categories—and the underlying phenomena that these constructs (with varying degrees of success) represent and attempt to capture. That would mean reifying our patients. The diagnostic categories in our authorized diagnostic systems may give the impression of a degree of specificity that is unfounded, viewed from a more dynamic-relational perspective, in the sense that it is far from always possible to trace specific symptoms unambiguously back to a specific disorder, issue or 'disease' (Küchenhoff 2001), just as disorder-specific treatment methods are often based on a somewhat simplified (decontextualized) perception of individual psychological difficulties.

The interesting question, and psychotherapeutically crucial, question is what the underlying cause is of the perceived or observed symptoms in this particular patient. The same symptoms in persons who meet the formal criteria of the same diagnosis may have very dynamic relational backgrounds. Symptoms of depression and anxiety may stem from a wide range of causes. Symptoms and behaviours that appear superficially similar may spring from fundamentally different psychological processes and dynamics. An excessive focus on how best to eliminate specific symptoms quickly via concrete action may cause us to overlook how symptoms and disturbed behaviour may constitute compromise formations, reflecting the individual patient's attempts to manage anxiety, inner turmoil and painful experiences that do not go away simply because the patient learns to act slightly differently in certain situations (Ogden and Gabbard 2010) or receives medical treatment for specific symptoms. The vast majority of the people who request help to understand and overcome psychological difficulties need emotional—not just instrumental, factual—contact with a therapist who is genuinely interested in understanding what it is like being him or her, and who is prepared to work with the person to consider how his or her difficulties can best be understood. Thus, the patient needs something other and far more than tallying how many diagnostic criteria in formalized diagnostic manuals are met, even though it is typically also meaningful and possibly necessary to make one or more formal diagnoses as part of a qualified professional assessment of the patient's difficulties, and of what is the best way to help the patient.

Different Approaches to Psychopathology

As a professional discipline, psychopathology can be broadly defined as knowledge about the core mechanisms or the processes and causes leading to psychological disorder. Our knowledge about the specific causes of specific psychological disorders remains fairly limited. In most cases, psychopathology develops as the result of an interaction between a wide range of factors, none of which is in itself sufficient or even necessary for developing a specific disorder. Similar genetic dispositions, stressors and incidents affect different people differently and have different specific consequences for a person's psychological balance and development. Similarly, the aetiology of most psychological disorders is very heterogeneous in the sense that the development of one and the same disorder (as defined by our formal diagnostic criteria) may follow many different paths. Broadly speaking, we can distinguish at least three fundamentally different approaches to psychopathology with related concepts of pathology and of human psychology (Hoff 2011:197ff):

1. A biological view of psychological disorders as brain disorders that are not fundamentally different from traditional somatic diseases. Based on this—reductionist—perception of human psychology we might dream that at some point in the future it would be possible to develop objective tests and methods to make psychiatric diagnoses, and that neuroscience will make it possible to supplant more dynamic, hermeneutic and psychological approaches to diagnostics and pathology models with a purely neurobiological approach, abandoning 'mentalist' concepts, such as the patient's personality, intentionality and self-understanding, and no longer viewing the individual patient as a subject that interprets him/herself and the world, but as a collection of brain processes. This represents a naturalistic, eliminative, materialist model of pathology.
2. A nominal understanding, as seen in our current authorized diagnostic systems (DSM-5, ICD-11), which focuses primarily on quantifiable and operationalizable diagnostic criteria without any explicit assumptions about the aetiology and underlying processes of the psychological disorders. Here, the emphasis is on developing specific and precise descriptive criteria for well-defined (categorical) psychiatric diagnoses, minimizing the use of in-depth interpretations of the observed symptoms in order to maximize the reliability of the diagnostic evaluations.
3. A biographical-heuristic approach, where psychological disorders are understood as individual reactions to or results of the interaction between diverse events and psychological processes. The patient is viewed as an inherently free and autonomous subject with agency and personal judgment, and psychological disorders are seen as potentially restricting the person's autonomy (freedom), judgment and capacity for rational behaviour. Here, the main emphasis is on charting and understanding the patient's individual history and self-narrative and, not least, the patient's subjective experiences, self-understanding, interpersonal relationships and the dynamic-relational processes behind the patient's symptoms and dysfunctional behaviour.

The psychotherapeutic stance and approach to the patient is closely associated with the biographical-hermeneutic understanding of psychopathology and is easily compatible with an undogmatic nominal model of pathology, while it is farther removed from a narrow neuroscientific understanding that, to varying degrees, reduces psychopathology to biochemical imbalances in the patient's brain and, accordingly, prioritizes medical treatment. This naturalistic approach to human psychology offers deterministic-causal explanations of human behaviour (reducing it material brain processes) and does not attribute any meaning to the patient's symptoms and behaviour, besides viewing them as concrete manifestations of underlying biochemical dysfunctions. It is incompatible with humanistic views and the human sciences, which, although they view human beings as (bodily) natural beings and, as such, causally determined, also view them as rational beings, capable of acting as free subjects (cf. Nida-Rümelin 2013:52ff). Human behaviour is, to varying degrees, determined by conscious deliberations on various options, urges and reasons. That also applies to people with psychological disorders, whose behaviour cannot be reduced to primitive acts determined by (causal) brain processes or simple stimulus response links.

Regardless which approach to psychopathology one embraces, it is important not to contribute to any unnecessary pathologization of normal and temporary psychological reactions to stress. Essentially, many psychologically painful experiences and states should thus be considered as normal parts of human existence that should not lead to a psychiatric diagnosis, let alone be made the object of psychotherapy. Someone who has a serious, potentially life-threatening physical illness, or who recently lost an emotionally important person in their life, will naturally be sad and function more poorly than normal for some time. Those are not in themselves symptoms of a psychological disorder to be diagnosed and treated. A person who recently divorced, lost their job or has a close relative who suffers from serious mental or physical illness may also feel psychological pain and have a reduced functioning level for some time, without this being an indication of a psychological disorder. Similarly, most people will encounter existential challenges at various times in their life that may cause their attention to shift and lead to what may, at first glance, seem like a reduced functioning level at work and in other contexts.

A therapist should always be alert to when a person's perceived challenges, pain and difficulties are evidence of a psychological disorder, and when that is not the case (Jørgensen 2014:27–38), that is, when it is relevant to apply a psychotherapeutic perspective and adopt a psychotherapeutic stance, and when one should mainly focus on listening empathically to the other person's story—hear their pain and existential challenges. Subsequently, the therapist should communicate his professional opinion that the current situation does not constitute a disorder that requires treatment, even if it is painful and may seem difficult to deal with, hard to handle on one's own, and so on. The therapist may encourage the person to seek help and support in other settings and explain that there is no basis for actual psychotherapeutic treatment. This is not merely important in order to avoid pathologizing and overtreatment, but also in order to reserve our notoriously limited psychotherapeutic resources for the persons who are in serious need of and stand to benefit from psychotherapy.

Understanding Psychopathology

With inspiration from the prominent German psychiatrist Karl Jaspers's understanding psychopathology (Jaspers 1942; Küchenhoff 2013) and Edmund Husserl's phenomenology, the patient's symptoms and (to an outside observer) dysfunctional behaviour should not merely be seen as epiphenomena, that is, as concrete manifestations of biochemical imbalances in the brain or other 'objective' findings in the patient but as inherently meaningful expressions of the patient's condition (the patient's subjective experience) and of the patient's attempts at managing her difficulties. Essentially, symptom behaviour should be seen as manifestations of the patient's subjectivity and (typically, to varying degrees, failed) attempts at protecting the self or satisfying basic needs and not just as the otherwise meaningless manifestations of a disorder, non-specific deficiency or a psychological defect. Generally, symptom behaviour should be seen as originally (potentially) adaptive (or at least understandable and in that sense meaningful) attempts at handling perceived difficulties or threats to the self (painful experiences, conflicts, failure to have basic needs met) that subsequently took on a life of their own and got out of control. Such an understanding of psychopathology goes beyond the purely descriptive diagnostic systems (DSM-5, ICD-11) and insists on the need for a theoretically informed interpretation of the patient's symptoms and their functionality and meaning to the patient.

This is seen, for example, in the woman who has been subjected to sexual abuse and has learned that she can avoid further abuse by appearing 'as a sexless grey mouse' or by withdrawing (fleeing) every time she comes close to establishing emotional contact with a man. Alternatively, she has learned that the only way she can achieve any form of contact is by making herself sexually available to varying men. As a result, she may 'have the problem' that she is incapable of establishing the loving, enduring relationship she yearns for, because she is compelled, for various reasons, to break off her relationship with men after a short amount of time (because she flees, feels like a slut, does not feel that the other sees her and wants her as she is and so on). Or the woman who has been subjected to sexual abuse and now works as a prostitute, in part because it involves repeating elements from the original situations of abuse over and over again, but now in a way where she—mostly—feels in control of the sex act. Here, working as a prostitute may be viewed as an unconscious attempt at processing and handling the earlier perceived abuse, just as it may offer an experience of profiting, in a sense, from what is perceived as inevitable: 'I've been a slut my whole life, I may as well get paid for it.' If the goal is to get her out of prostitution, it makes no sense simply to ban prostitution or to meet her work as a prostitute with various forms of sanctions or morals condemnation. It is necessary to understand the psychological background for her to seek out and remain in the prostitution environment.

If we disregard psychotic states (the interested reader is referred to Küchenhoff et al. 2017; Küchenhoff and Warsitz 2017) and psychological disorders with predominantly organic causes (dementia, autism, certain forms of manic-depressive disorders, consequences of traumatic brain injury or long-term abuse, certain forms of severe impulse regulation disorder) the basic assumption is that there are meaningful reasons for the patients to act the way they do; reasons that have to do with internal psychological processes, subjective experiences and intentional choices. Human behaviour cannot be attributed, let alone reduced to, more or less mechanical causes, including brain processes. In some cases, of course, it takes time, patience and genuine interest to investigate the patient's reasons for acting the way she does and for understanding how the patient's symptoms are meaningfully linked to her subjective perception of herself, interpersonal interactions and reality in general. Naturally, such an understanding invites a different kind of meeting with the patient and a different attitude—a psychotherapeutic stance—towards the patient. Human behaviour is structured by meaning—related to subjectively perceived meaning—and any attempt at attributing (reducing) human behaviour to 'objective' brain processes or other 'objective causes' alone represents a category error.

The psychotherapeutic view of the symptoms presented by the patient and her deviant behaviour thus directs our attention to the meaning and functions of the symptoms in the patient's inner universe and psychology, including the (to some extent unconscious) psychological processes underlying the patient's symptoms. Unlike our categorical diagnostic systems, which operate with an inherently clear-cut distinction between normality and pathology, psychotherapy regards the transition between normal and pathological as more fluid. Many of us will recognize or, at the very least, empathize with many of the experiences and reactions we see in persons who have been diagnosed with psychological disorders, because to varying degrees, we know them from our own life, only to a lesser and less debilitating degree. That includes the defensive strategies the patient typically develops in an attempt to escape the internal or external conflicts and painful experiences, emotions and other mental states.

A distinction is drawn between different levels of defence mechanisms, from the more mature and functional, such as humour, intellectualization, repression and effective coping strategies, to the less mature, which do not cause any actual distortion of the experience, such as splitting, idealization and devaluing, to the severely immature and reality-distorting mechanisms that are seen, for example, in severely paranoid and manic states (Mentzos 2009:45f). These defensive strategies will often also be activated in the therapeutic space in the form of various forms of resistance to getting into contact with painful experiences and mental anguish. For example, when the patient misses sessions, changes the focus of the conversation, withdraws from contact with the therapist, shuts down emotionally or tries to take control of the therapeutic space, this should generally be seen as the patient's (mostly unconscious) attempt at self-protection and avoiding contact with, for example, feelings of anger, guilt, shame, hate, sexuality, envy, grief, anxiety, emptiness, loneliness or other painful—and, for the patient, possibly forbidden or completely unbearable—mental states. The patient seeks to self-regulate, so to speak, by trying to avoid being overwhelmed or showing the therapist aspects of herself that she is convinced will cause him to despise her and break off their relationship, or which she fears may harm her in other ways. In some cases, this may also be seen as a manifestation of the patient's attempt to protect the therapist and their relationship against overwhelming experiences and mental states that she imagines will be more than the therapist and their relationship can sustain.

References

Bateman, A., & Fonagy, P. (2016). *Mentalization-based treatment for personality disorders: A practical guide*. Oxford, England: Oxford University Press.

Blatt, S. J. (2008). *Polarities of experience: Relatedness and self-definition in personality development, psychopathology, and the therapeutic process*. Washington, DC: American Psychological Association.

Bloom-Feshbach, J., & Bloom-Feshbach, S. (1996). The related-autonomous position: Psychological freedom, mourning, and the psychoanalytic stance. *Psychoanalytic Psychology, 13,* 531–545.

Bohleber, W. (2012). *Was Psychoanalyse heute leistet* [What psychoanalysis does today]. Stuttgart, Germany: Klett-Cotta Verlag.

Bowlby, J. (1969). *Attachment*. London, England: Hogarth Press.

Druck, A. B. (1994). Multiple models and the psychoanalytic stance. *Psychoanalytic Inquiry, 14,* 243–260.

Fairbairn, W. R. D. (1952). *Psychoanalytic studies of the personality*. London, England: Routledge.

Ferenczi, S. (1985). *The clinical diary of Sandor Ferenczi*. Cambridge, MA: Harvard University Press.

Ferenczi, S., & Rank, O. (1924). *Entwicklungsziele der Psychoanalyse* [The developmental aims of psychoanalysis]. Vienna, Austria: Turia + Kant.

Fonagy, P., Gergely, G., Jurist, E. L., & Target, M. (2002). *Affect regulation, mentalization, and the development of the self.* New York, NY: Other Press.

Freud, S. (1955). Group psychology and the analysis of the ego. In J. Strachey (Ed. and Trans.), *The standard edition of the complete psychological works of Sigmund Freud* (Vol. 18, pp. 65–144). London, England: Hogarth (Original work published 1921).

Freud, S. (1957). Instincts and their vicissitudes. In J. Strachey (Ed. and Trans.), *The standard edition of the complete psychological works of Sigmund Freud* (Vol. 14, pp. 109–140). London, England: Hogarth (Original work published 1915).

Fuchs, T. (2013). Personalisierte Psychiatrie? Eine Kritik und Gegendarstellung [Personalized psychiatry? A critique and counterstatement]. In M. Heinze, J. E. Schlimme, & C. Kupke (Eds.), *Personalisierte Psychiatrie*. Zur Kritik eines Konzepts: BerlIn Parodos Verlag.

Gabbard, G. O. (2014). *Psychodynamic psychiatry in clinical practice* (5th ed.). Washington, DC: American Psychiatric Press.

Greenberg, J., & Mitchell, S. A. (1983). *Object relations in psychoanalytic theory*. Cambridge, MA: Harvard University Press.

Habermas, J. (1987). *Knowledge & human interests*. Cambridge, England and Malden, MA: Polity Press.

Hoff, P. (2011). Über die zukünftige Rolle der Psychopathologie: Grundlagen- oder Hilfswissenschaft? [The future role of psychopathology: Basic or ancillary science?] In T. Fuchs, K. Vogely, & M. Heinze (Eds.), *Subjektivität und Gehirn* (pp. 195–211). Berlin, Germany: Parados Verlag.

Horney, K. (1939). *New ways in psychoanalysis*. New York, NY: Norton.

Jaspers, K. (1942). *Allgemeine psychopathologie* [General psychopathology] (4th ed.). Berlin, Germany: Springer.

Jørgensen, C. R. (1999). Den interpersonelle psykoanalyse. *Nordisk Psykologi, 51,* 279–305.

Jørgensen, C. R. (2008). *Identitet. Psykologiske og kulturanalytiske perspektiver* [Identity. Psychological and culture analysis perspectives]. Copenhagen, Denmark: Hans Reitzels Forlag.

Jørgensen, C. R. (2009). *Personlighedsforstyrrelser. Moderne relationel forståelse og behandling af borderlinelidelse* [Personality disorders. Modern relational understanding and treatment of borderline disorder] (2nd ed.). Copenhagen, Denmark: Hans Reitzels Forlag.

Jørgensen, C. R. (2014). *ADHD. Bidrag til en kritisk psykologisk forståelse* [ADHD. Contributions to a critical psychological understanding]. Copenhagen, Denmark: Hans Reitzels Forlag.

Katzenelson, B. (2010). Holdning [Stance/attitude]. In *Den Store Danske Encyklopædi*. Retrieved from www.denstoredanske.dk.

Köhler-Weisker, A. (1986). Zum Begriff der Haltung des Psychoanalytikers am Beispiel einer Fokaltherapie [On the concept of the psychotherapist's stance as an example of focal therapy]. *Jahrbuch der Psychoanalyse, 18,* 143–173.

Küchenhoff, J. (2001). Störungsspezifität und psychoanalytische Psychotherapie – ein Widerspruch? [Disorder specificity and psychoanalytic psychotherapy—a contradiction?] *Psychotherapie. Psychosomatik, Medizinische Psychologie, 51,* 418–424.

Küchenhoff, J. (2013). *Der Sinn im Nein und die Gabe des Gesprächs. Psychoanalytisches Verstehen zwischen Philosophie und Klinik* [The meaning of no and the gift of conversation. Psychoanalytic understanding between philosophy and clinic]. Weilerswist. Germany: Velbrück Wissenschaft.

Küchenhoff, J., & Warsitz, R.-P. (2017). *Labyrinthe des Ohres. Vom therapeutischen Sinn des Zuhörens bei psychotischen und anderen Erfahrungen* [The labyrinth of the ear. Of the therapeutic meaning of listening in relation to psychotic and other experiences]. Gießen. Germany: Psychosozial-Verlag.

Küchenhoff, J., Prause, K., & Schulz, G. (2017). Engagement und Respekt. Psychotherapeutische Haltung und Bezieungsarbeit in der Psychotherapie mit psychotisch erlebenden Menschen [Commitment and respect: Psychotherapeutic attitude and work on analyst-patient relationships in psychotherapy for individuals with psychotic experience]. *Psyche, 71,* 60–81.

Kutter, P. (1988). Grundhaltung, professionelle Einstellungen und psychoanalytische Methode. In P. Kutter, R. Paramo-Ortega, & P. Zagermann (Eds.), *Die psychoanalytische Haltung* (pp. 17–29). Munich, Germany: Verlag Internationale Psychoanalyse.

Kutter, P. (2003). Psychoanalytische Haltung – Klein, Bion und Selbstpsychologie – Basiskonflikt, Laios und Iokaste [Psychoanalytic Stance—Klein, Bion and self-psychology—basic conflict, Laius and Jocasta]. *Zeitschrift für Individualpsychologie, 23*, 371–382.

Kymlicka, W. (1990). *Contemporary political philosophy.* Oxford, England: Clarendon Press; New York, NY: Oxford University Press.

Levenson, H. (1995). *Time-limited dynamic psychotherapy: A guide to clinical practice*. New York, NY: Basic Books.

Löchel, E. (2013). Ringen um psychoanalytische Haltung [Achieving the analytic attitude]. *Psyche, 67,* 1167–1190.

Mentzos, S. (2009). *Lehrbuch der Psychodynamik. Die Funktion der Dysfunktionalität psychischer Störungen* [Handbook of psychodynamics. The function of dysfunctionality of psychological disorders]. Göttingen, Germany: Vandenhoeck & Ruprecht.

Mertens, W. (2004). *Einführung in die psychoanalytische Therapie. Bd.2* [Introduction to psychoanalytic therapy. Vol. 2]. Stuttgart, Germany: Kohlhammer.

Mertens, W. (2015). *Psychoanalytische Behandlungstechnik. Konzepte und Themen psychoanalytisch begründeter Behandlungsverfahren* [Psychoanalytic treatment technique. Concepts and themes of psychoanalytically motivated treatment methods]. Stuttgart, Germany: Kohlhammer.

Mills, J. (2012). *Conundrums: A critique of contemporary psychoanalysis*. London, England: Routledge.

Mitchell, S. A. (1988). *Relational concepts in psychoanalysis: An integration*. Cambridge, MA: Harvard University Press.

Nida-Rümelin, J. (2013). *Philosophie einer humanen Bildung* [The philosophy of a humane education]. Hamburg, Germany: Edition Körber-Stiftung.

Ogden, T. H., & Gabbard, G. O. (2010). The lure of the symptom in psychoanalytic treatment. *Journal of the American Psychoanalytic Association, 58,* 533–544.

Schafer, R. (1983). *The analytic attitude*. New York, NY: Basic Books.

Stern, D. N. (1985). *The interpersonal world of the infant*. New York, NY: Basic Books.

Sullivan, H. S. (1953). *The interpersonal theory of psychiatry*. New York, NY: Tavistock Publications.

Taylor, C. (1991). *The ethics of authenticity*. Cambridge, MA: Harvard University Press.

Teising, M. (2014). Überlegungen zur Krankheitslehre der Psychoanalyse – heute [Some thoughts on pathology in psychoanalysis—today]. *Jahrbuch der Psychoanalyse, 69,* 187–208.

Wallerstein, R. S. (1995). *The talking cures: The psychoanalyses and the psychotherapies*. New Haven, CT: Yale University Press.

Zwiebel, R. (2007). *Von der Angst Psychoanalytiker zu sein* [On the fear of being a psychoanalyst]. Stuttgart, Germany: Klett-Cotta Verlag.

Chapter 9
The Historical Bedrock of Psychotherapy. Freud's Contribution—and Contemporary Corrections

Particularly in his papers on technique in particular, Freud offers a number of recommendations for how we can understand and manage what plays out in the therapeutic relationship, which also helps us define what characterizes the psychotherapeutic or, more specifically, the psychoanalytic stance in the therapeutic process. Although Freud to some extent motivates his technical recommendations with reference to classical psychoanalytic theory, which must be considered untenable and obsolete from a contemporary perspective—including, especially, his drive theory—his understanding of psychotherapy still contains many important contributions to a nuanced conceptualization of psychotherapeutic work. Moreover, Freud is perhaps the most important figure in modern psychotherapy. For that reason too, it remains interesting and relevant to consult his technical guidelines in any effort to specify the fundamental elements of the psychotherapeutic stance. His writings should be read with respect and understanding for the fact that they were written at a time when our knowledge of human psychology was highly imperfect, compared to today, as the first empirical psychological studies had only begun to appear from the fairly recently founded psychological laboratories, and psychotherapy was an unknown phenomenon. Finally, Freud's technical papers also contain the first seeds to an alternative to the model of psychopathology and psychotherapy that was based on the drive-oriented one-person psychology; an alternative that places a greater emphasis on internal psychological integration and interpersonal experiences (in the transference and in the therapeutic relationship), while the role of the drive theory is toned down (see, e.g., Friedman 1991).

Still, when reading Freud's papers on technique, one should bear in mind that the cultural context surrounding the therapeutic space and the psychotherapeutic relationship has changed considerably in the one hundred years or so that have passed since Freud developed the psychoanalytic method. Similarly, the most common psychological disorders we see in the clinic today are different from the ones that were prevalent in early 20th century—identity and self-regulation/impulse disorders, loneliness/unfulfilled attachment needs and disorders related to an inadequate ability to build mental representations (Jørgensen 2002, 2012, 2014). Thus, the foundation of the psychotherapeutic work is not quite the same as it was when Freud presented

C. R. Jørgensen, *The Psychotherapeutic Stance*,
https://doi.org/10.1007/978-3-030-20437-2_9

his technical recommendations, and certain elements of the psychotherapeutic stance should be modified to match the changing settings and conditions for psychotherapy.

A key goal of classical psychoanalytic treatment is (descriptively) to fill the patient's memory gaps and (dynamically) overcome repression resistance (Freud 1958c[1914]:148), based on the notion that psychopathology can be attributed, in part, to repressed past experiences that have weakened the ego and narrowed its scope and to unfulfilled drives and drive conflicts that determine the patient's psychological function on an unconscious level. Today, this must be considered, at best, an incomplete understanding of pathology, just as uncovering (recollecting) specific past event is no longer seen, in itself, as a key condition for psychological recovery. Nevertheless, some of the key elements of Freud's descriptions of dynamics in the psychotherapeutic space and his recommendations for how they can be applied in the therapeutic process, remain current and inspire respect, particularly in light of the fact that they were published about a century ago, when the knowledge of psychopathology was so limited, and psychotherapy de facto did not exist. On the other hand, his more theoretical understanding of the background for what happens in the therapeutic space and the theoretical explanations for his technical recommendations are somewhat incomplete and, in some regards, clearly untenable. His recommendations thus form an important part of the foundation for a contemporary description of the psychotherapeutic stance, although the original theoretical explanations behind them may have proven largely unfounded.

Perhaps Freud's most important contribution to psychotherapeutic practice is his discussions of the phenomenon of transference, which is both a key part of the basis for contemporary relational and psychodynamic psychotherapy (Jørgensen 2009) and forms the basis for some of his most important technical guidelines, requiring that the treatment must be conducted under a rule of abstinence, that the patient should engage in free association in the therapeutic space, and that the therapist should remain neutral and meet the patient with evenly suspended attention. Uncovering the patient's unconscious and handling the patient's resistance to this uncovering are no longer regarded as the main drivers of psychotherapeutic work, although some, more psychoanalytically oriented, therapists still consider the unconscious to hold special importance for the therapeutic process—albeit in some cases in a broader and more interpersonal sense than in Freud. However, any form of psychotherapeutic work requires the therapist to maintain a consistent focus on the dynamic psychological processes underlying the individual patient's symptoms and immediately observable maladaptive behaviour. Another focus of continuous attention in the effort to understand the patient is how core elements of the patient's difficulties are repeated and played out in the therapeutic space and in the therapeutic relationship in the here and now, including considering what dynamic psychological functions the observed symptoms and behaviours may serve. As mentioned earlier, with few exceptions (severely psychotic states, dementia and so on), symptoms and pathological behaviour are not mere (predominantly) arbitrary or meaningless manifestations of biochemical imbalances in the bran. They serve a function and hold meaning for the patient, which it may be part of the therapeutic task to verbalize or (re)construct. Here, parts of Freud's theory and technical recommendations are still relevant.

Especially many older psychotherapists have witnessed in the early stages of their career how psychoanalytic theory and psychoanalytic practice guidelines were used in a rigid, fairly unreflective and authoritarian manner to prescribe a certain approach to the patient and to exclude dissidents, which to some extent undermined the legitimacy of psychoanalysis. That is unfortunate for several reasons, one reason being that it can block the affected persons' ability to see and benefit from the considerable potentials of the psychoanalytic culture and tradition, not least with regard to the psychotherapeutic stance. Moreover, contemporary culture and modern humanity are seized by a powerful notion—and hope—of unstoppable (rapid) scientific progress and search for 'newness', accompanied by a somewhat unreflective tendency to devalue or view the status quo (whatever has been thought, seen and described by others before us), which in increasingly short order is defined as 'old', obsolete and without any real value.

These dynamics can also be observed in clinical psychology and among psychotherapists as a constant search for new and seemingly ground-breaking psychotherapeutic theories, methods and claims about what constitutes the core of the psychotherapeutic process, while older theories and methods tend to fall into oblivion, so that we risk losing the often quite significant knowledge and understanding that these theories contain. This often happens in a fairly unreflective excitement with the latest new therapeutic method, which is rarely decidedly better than older theories and methods and in some regards are often has less power of explanation or nuance in its understanding of human psychology (although it may be easier to grasp and translate into specific procedures). The present book insists that we should not uncritically join this mindless quest for fatuous innovation; instead we should preserve our appreciation of the invaluable insights into psychotherapeutic work that have been presented by prominent researchers and therapists before us and keep our eyes open to the contributions that both older and newer, not least, psychoanalytic literature can make to a contemporary understanding and concretization of the psychotherapeutic stance. For that reason too, we begin with Freud.

9.1 Abstinence

The classical psychoanalytic rule of abstinence says, among other things, that patient and therapist cannot use each other to satisfy their respective relational needs. Broadly speaking, needs that are actualized in the therapeutic space should not be satisfied but made the object of analysis and thus serve to understand the patient and her difficulties. As Freud (1955[1919]:163) puts it, the relationship with the therapist and the therapy should not become a source of substitutive satisfaction for the patient, even if the patient may unconsciously seek this in the transference. 'The treatment must be carried out in abstinence. […] the patient's need and longing should be allowed to persist in her, in order that they may serve as forces impelling her to do work and to make changes, and that we must beware of appeasing those forces by means of surrogate' (Freud 1958d[1915]:165). Theoretically, Freud thus motivates the rule of abstinence with reference to the idea that the patient will unconsciously seek substitutive or surrogate satisfaction for frustrated drives (unmet needs) in the therapy, and that the possibilities of this should be minimized so that they may instead be manifested in the transference, where they can be made the object of therapeutic work (analysis).

According to Freud, the therapist should thus also frustrate the patient's actualized needs in order to maintain the patient's treatment motivation-based on the idea that immediate gratification might lead to a temporary (but only temporary) improvement in the patient's condition, which may cause the patient to terminate the treatment or create a maladaptive dependency on the therapist, as the patient expects the therapist to continue to satisfy certain elementary (emotional and relational) needs, preventing the patient from developing other, more mature and adaptive strategies for satisfying her needs outside the therapy. The therapist should represent reality, including, for example, that adults cannot expect to have their more infantile needs met by others (needs for unlimited, asymmetrical, unreciprocated nurture, attention and so on), even if the patient never had these needs met and hence, in part quite understandably, may feel a certain entitlement to the delayed satisfaction of these needs (cf. Killingmo 1997:154f). Similarly, the therapist should seek to prevent the patient from seeking substitutive satisfaction outside the treatment, for example when the male patient 'seeks prematurely to attach himself to a woman' (Freud 1955[1919]:163) and is likely to repeat previous maladaptive patterns in this fixation or relationship.

In line with his rationalist view of humanity (Strenger 1989) and the concept of enlightenment, Freud believes that it is 'the truth'—the attainment of insight—that cures psychological disorder, not the satisfaction of previously frustrated needs—needs that he often refers to as 'infantile'. His recommendations are framed by a somewhat vague distinction between 'real' or 'mature' needs satisfaction and 'false' surrogate satisfaction. Moreover, he argues that the satisfaction of painful (frustrated) needs springing from internal conflicts do not bring actual relief. These are, however, notions that are rooted in a misguided or, at best, far too narrow understanding of psychopathology centred on internal psychological conflicts (cf. Killingmo 1997:147), which also involves the notion that confronting the patient with feared, shameful and painful parts of herself and of the human existence and increasing her self-insight will make a crucial contribution to the development of an autonomous subject with agency that is the goal of the treatment.

Freud's notion, rooted in drive theory, that the patient's frustrated drive-related needs may be the key mechanism of change in the therapy, must be viewed as quite untenable today. That raises questions about the appropriateness of a more conservative interpretation of Freud's rule of abstinence and suggest that to some extent and in certain contexts, the therapist should be prepared to gratify some of the patient's relational and emotional needs (needs for contact and psychological closeness), as they are expressed in the transference and in the therapeutic space. This is particularly relevant in work with severely disturbed poorly functioning patients (deficit pathology), where one of the key issues may be that they have, for various reasons, lost confidence that their needs for emotional contact and psychological closeness that does not violate their boundaries can ever be seen, acknowledged and satisfied (cf. Pflichthofer 2010:54). Freud (1955[1919]:165) appears to make the same suggestion when he writes that 'various forms of disease cannot all be dealt with by the same technique', and that 'Some concessions [needs gratification] must of course be made to him [the patient], greater or less, according to the nature of the case and the patient's individuality' (Freud 1955[1919]:164). He does warn, however, that too many such concession are not helpful: 'Any analyst who out of the fullness of his heart, perhaps, and is readiness to help, extends to the patient all that one human being can hope to receive from another [...] [aims] to make everything as pleasant as possible for den patient, so that he may feel well there' (ibid.)—a strategy that, in Freud's (ibid.) opinion 'they make no attempt to give him [the patient] more strength for facing life and more capacity for carrying out his actual tasks in it'.

According to Freud, the patient's ego, functioning and autonomy are not strengthened by what Freud perceives as substitutive gratification in the therapeutic relationship; that can only be achieved through the attainment of insight. He is right in insisting that the therapist must avoid 'spoiling' the patient (Freud 1955[1919]:164) and thus increasing the risk of immature dependence on part of the patient through excessive needs gratification. On the other hand, such a recommendation risks causing the therapist to go too far in frustrating the patient's relational needs through unreflective adherence to Freud's admonition that 'It is expedient to deny him [the patient] precisely those satisfactions which he desires most intensely and expresses most importunately' (Freud 1955[1919]:164). Patients with particularly severe attachment disorders will often perceive the anonymous and abstinent (frustrating) therapist as expressing a form of authorized indifference that only perpetuates what they have encountered, in their past, from significant others (Pflichthofer 2010:56). The therapist has to register how the patient consciously and unconsciously communicates certain needs in the therapeutic relationship and continuously consider what this might reveal about the patient's history and, not least, about recurring patterns in the patient's relationships. On this basis, the therapist should then consider what is the most appropriate strategy.

Generally, it would thus be unhelpful to adhere to rigid guidelines positing that the patient's relational needs should never be gratified, including the particular emphasis on not meeting the patient's most intensely felt needs. The patient's most intensely communicated relational needs in the transference will typically contain valuable information about the patient's difficulties. The therapist has to decide on a case-by-case basis and in a holistic assessment how the communicated needs can most appropriately be handled. An adequate response may involve both specific and limited gratification of these needs and an invitation to shared reflection on the needs the patient comes into contact with in the therapeutic space. The task is to strike the right balance between emotional closeness and distance and between frustrating and gratifying the patient's needs in order to promote the therapeutic process and the patient's development in the best possible manner (cf. Treurniet 1997:599).

In its more conservative and dogmatic interpretations, the rule of abstinence thus contains a number of obvious problems. It may, however, also be viewed as part of the therapeutic setting that protects the therapist from being blinded by the patient's transferences and thus confusing the patient's transference phantasies with aspects of the real relationship, where the therapist might otherwise, for example, be tempted to accommodate and take part in acting out the patient's eroticized transference. That would constitute a serious transgression of the therapeutic relationship and bring about the collapse of the therapeutic space—and thus the possibility of performing therapy. The rule of abstinence aims to prevent the therapeutic relationship from devolving into an everyday, non-therapeutic interpersonal relationship, where we seek to satisfy needs and act out impulses rather than making them objects of the therapeutic work and understanding.

Today, we must regard the rule of abstinence as a kind of (imagined) ideal that can and should only be realized to a certain, varying, degree. A less conservative interpretation of the rule is a necessity in the work with, especially, patients with more severe pathology, where the therapist has to accommodate some of the patient's expressed needs, particularly relational and emotional needs (attachment, being seen and feeling contained and understood) and, to varying degrees, at times should take on and act out the role or position in the patient's actualized object relations he is unconsciously assigned by the patient. This accommodation should serve both to secure the formation of a sustainable therapeutic alliance, provide access to the therapeutic material this effort uncovers and enable the patient to attain corrective emotional experiences in the therapeutic relationship, where the frustration of fundamental emotional needs in the patient's earlier relationships is not repeated, and where she has an opportunity to feel seen, accepted and accommodated in ways that go beyond her previous experiences. That experience may in itself contribute to the patient's recovery process, including changing the patient's often negative and defeatist perception of her own self(-worth), others and the possibility of having a positive outcome of interpersonal contact.

In therapy with more severely disturbed patients in particular it may be necessary to go farther in accommodating some of the patient's (emotional and relational) needs in order to form and maintain an effective therapeutic relationship (therapeutic alliance) (Balint 1968:196). On the one hand, a moderate version of the abstinence rule can be an important element in the way the therapist handles countertransferences, regulates closeness and distance in the therapeutic relationship and prevents countertherapeutic acting out in the therapeutic space, where the therapeutic relationship turns into a private intimate relationship. On the other hand, it should not be applied rigidly, without regard for the individual patient's needs and in ways that in practice prevent the therapist from being present as a fellow human being and thus causes him to be inhuman in his interactions with the patient (cf. Cremerius 1984:790). Hence, the psychotherapist should invite the patient into a relationship where he is also personally and emotionally present; he should encourage the contact and emotional closeness in the therapeutic space that is a necessary condition for processing the patient's disturbed attachment, recurring maladaptive relational patterns (implicit relational knowledge) and emotional difficulties. This is moving towards the opposite of a more conservative interpretation of Freud's original recommendations about therapist abstinence.

Evenly Suspended Responsiveness

Generally, one should bear in mind that the therapeutic relationship always will and should be asymmetrical in the sense that the goal of the therapy is to understand and cure the patient, and thus, the therapist's task is to help the patient—not to satisfy his own conscious or unconscious needs. At the same time, both patient and therapist may have an urge to establish a more symmetrical, reciprocal and 'ordinary' relationship. If that happens in a manner where the psychotherapeutic aim (which has to remain in the foreground at all times) is lost, the relationship is no longer therapeutic, but has become an ordinary interpersonal relationship, and the therapeutic space will collapse (Hoffer 1993). It is crucial that the therapist acknowledges his potential urge to step out of his role as a therapist and abandon the fundamental psychotherapeutic stance; on the other hand, the urge must under no circumstances be acted out for long.

It is part of the therapist's responsibility to tolerate and adopt an analytic-therapeutic approach to the tensions that may arise (also in the therapist), when the urge to convert the therapeutic relationship into an ordinary reciprocal relationship is actualized in the therapeutic space. At the same time, the therapist has to be prepared to engage in the kind of relationship and interaction that the patient more or less unconsciously invites in the therapeutic space; he has to respond to the role he is assigned in patient's actualized object relations and meet the patient with an evenly suspended readiness to take on the role she assigns him in the interpersonal interaction (cf. Sandler 1976). If the therapist is not ready to allow himself to be influenced by the patient's actualized object relations and the invitation to take on certain roles, he will not be able to understand and catalyse any in-depth therapeutic work with the patient's recurring relational patterns and thus the core of the patient's difficulties. This may involve briefly gratifying some of the patient's more regressive interpersonal needs, for example to lean on the therapist as an idealized authority. The therapist has to act out a role-responsiveness that is another key aspect of the psychotherapeutic stance (Körner 2002:1402), while always balancing this role-responsiveness and readiness to be influenced by the patient (the therapist's perceiving ego) with a persistently analytical awareness of what is playing out in the therapeutic space.

We may also speak of the therapist's free-flowing responsiveness, where parts of the therapist's behaviour in the therapeutic space springs from a compromise between, on the one hand, the role that the patient places him or her in and, on the other hand, the therapist's own (conscious and unconscious) intentions (Klüver 1983:137). At the same time, he has to take an analytic-reflecting attitude to the same interaction. This role as a participating observer (see later) demands that the therapist's has a high level of self-awareness (insight into his own needs, reaction dispositions and so on), good judgment and capacity for nuanced self-reflection (cf. Killingmo 1997:151). It is neither realistic nor desirable for the therapist to suppress all his own wishes and needs that are activated in the interaction with the patient, as that would impair his sensitivity to what is playing out in the patient and in the therapeutic relationship. Instead, the therapist should be open to and register what desires, needs and action impulses are actualized in him or her, tolerate that they cannot be realized—or only to a very limited extent—and refrain from acting them out but instead regard them as reactions to what is happening in the interaction with the patient in the present moment (Zwiebel 2013:153).

9.2 Evenly Suspended Attention

Freud describes that the therapist should meet the patient with 'evenly suspended attention', which 'consists simply in not directing one's notice to anything in particular and in maintaining the same "evenly-suspended attention"' (Freud 1958b[1912]:111). The therapist 'should simply listen, and not bother about whether he is keeping anything in mind' (Freud 1958b[1912]:112). The 'most successful cases are those in which one proceeds, as it were, without any purpose in view, allows oneself to be taken by surprise by any new turn in them, and always meets them with an open mind, free from any presuppositions' (Freud 1958b[1912]:114). In practice, this means that the therapist should remain as open as possible to what the patient consciously and unconsciously communicates in the therapeutic space, that he should (at times) simply go with the flow of the therapeutic and interpersonal process, and remain open to his own ideas, mental states and reactions in the interaction with the patient. Especially at the beginning of each session, it is often a good idea to allow oneself to be carried by the process that emerges, more or less spontaneously, in the therapeutic space; to let the patient's statements and acts—and what is initiated in the therapeutic relationship—unfold in order to develop a sense of 'where the patient is at', and what the patient is most focused on in the moment, on a conscious as well as an unconscious plane. Next, the therapist should be ready to alternate between structuring and focusing the conversation versus going with the flow of the therapeutic process, also referred to as the therapist's temporary regression in the service of the ego.

According to Freud, the therapist should hold back, resisting the urge to settle too quickly on what is the most important aspect and what to focus on in what the patient says and acts out in the therapeutic space; that requires patience and inner calm from the therapist as well as an ability to tolerate uncertainty. As much as possible, he should liberate himself from external and internal pressures that require him to act quickly in order to make a difference, give the patient something specific (in the form of goal-oriented interventions) and take control. This involves abandoning any illusions of omnipotence without, on the other hand, abandoning one's responsibility completely, thinking that 'anything goes'. He should also be able to tolerate the uncertainty of being in a situation where he does not immediately understand or know what to do, giving up any notion that the best way to help the patient is via targeted actions (showing agency, taking charge and so on). In order to help another human being one must first uncover 'what the issue is', the core of the other's difficulties, which takes patience, inner calm, empathy and the ability to listen. Only then can he offer a qualified opinion as to what can be done to help. In some cases, the most important and helpful approach is in fact to listen, take the necessary time and avoid immediately taking action, offering advice or initiating hasty and poorly timed interventions, which may, to varying degrees, be driven by his own needs to act and escape painful emotions or other overwhelming mental states. Over time, the patient gradually internalizes the tolerance, containment capacity and inner calm that the therapist displays in the therapeutic space.

Listening to the Unconscious—Manifestations in the Therapeutic Process

Evenly suspended attention is related to parts of what classical psychoanalysis refers to as the therapist's neutrality (see later). The purpose of evenly suspended attention is to promote a more creatively receptive approach to the patient that enhances the therapist's ability to see unconscious links and connections and recurring patterns in what the patient says and does in the therapeutic space. The therapist should devote part of his attention to noticing what the patient is not telling, or what she is saying between the lines, how it is said, and what the patient communicates by nonverbal means (in her nonverbal communication, what is activated in the therapist's countertransference, see Chap. 10) and avoid focusing exclusively on the specific and purely factual aspects of the patient's verbal narratives (cf. Mertens 2015:55). The therapist adopts a receptive position, where his primary task is to listen to, reflect on and process what is happening in the patient and in the therapeutic space—rather than taking action. As mentioned above, one could argue that the concept should be expanded to include an evenly suspended readiness to take on the roles one is assigned by the patient, temporarily and under certain conditions (Köhler-Weisker 1986:152). This further supports the rationale behind the evenly suspended attention: to provide a basis for the therapist's development of hypotheses on actualized unconscious dynamics in the patient in the present moment (Leuzinger-Bohleber 2007:975) and to enhance the therapist's awareness of important (relational) themes in the therapeutic space.

The therapist should hold back and remain open to the unknown, the surprising, the previously overlooked and repressed, rather than meeting the patient in a way that is aimed at quickly determining what it is the patient is trying to communicate, and what the patient's problem is. The latter approach would risk restricting the process through selective perceptions and specific expectations to what the patient intends to do, which might reduce the therapist's openness to other themes and issues in the patient's material. In the therapeutic space the therapist should be open to surprises and to meeting the unknown, the unfamiliar and the initially intimidating that challenges the established order and the therapist's initial understanding of the patient and her inner reality.

Meanwhile, the therapist should also remain alert to how his own impulses and needs may get in the way of the necessary openness and emotional neutrality in the meeting with the patient, where 'the feeling that is most dangerous' to the therapist, according to Freud (1958b[1912]:115), is 'the therapeutic ambition to achieve […] something that will produce a convincing effect upon other people.' The therapist's main task is to understand and help the patient, not to prove his own excellence to the patient by coming up with 'wise' interpretations of her material and difficulties, taking up room in the therapeutic space at the cost of the patient, let along being proven right in connection with disagreements (power struggles) with the patient. The evenly suspended attention should help the therapist, as Freud (1958b[1912]:115f) puts it, 'turn his own unconscious like a receptive organ towards the transmitting unconscious of the patient. He must adjust himself to the patient as a telephone receiver is adjusted to the transmitting microphone.' In this task, the therapist should be attentive to his own potential resistance to hearing or attending to certain themes in the patient's material that might touch upon his own unresolved issues. In order to remain as open as possible to what the patient communicates, consciously as well as unconsciously, the therapist should therefore have undergone therapy himself and 'have become aware of those complexes of his own which would be apt to interfere with his grasp of what the patient tells him' (Freud 1958b[1912]:116).

Listening Without Memory, Desire or Preconceived Comprehension

Generally, the more one feels the urge to act or rapidly initiate interventions, the more important it is to curb this desire. Such a powerful urge to act will often be driven by unconscious forces (countertransferences, projective identification, parts of the patient's material that one finds it difficult to contain, see Chap. 10), which must be made conscious and processed before they may, perhaps, be communicated to the patient or otherwise included in the therapy; they should never be allowed to direct the therapeutic work. Similarly, the therapist should register any strong urges in himself to say something in particular to the patient without really knowing why. Often, it will be well-advised to avoid saying it and perhaps remain silent, until one has considered what it would be helpful to say, and why. On a more practical level, one should not be preoccupied with elements outside the therapeutic space when one is with the patient. Experiences with other patients earlier in the day, incidents that have nothing to do with the current therapeutic space, personal problems and concerns that may interfere with one's ability to be fully present here and now should be put aside, as much as possible (although it is, of course, never fully attainable). It is thus often a good idea to set aside the necessary time to process what happened in the contact with a previous patient and prepare mentally in order to meet the next patient with a fairly well-ordered psyche. Exactly how much time one needs naturally varies from person to person and also depends on the patients and other factors, but based on experience, at least 15–30 min is advisable.

Reik (1948) writes that the therapist should use his 'third ear' to listen to the patient's material, and Bion (1967) recommends that the therapist should listen to the patient without a conscious intention of remembering anything in particular from previous sessions, identifying anything in particular in the patient's current material or quickly understanding the material ('without memory, desire or comprehension'); instead, one should let the patient's material unfold and wait for patterns to emerge. Bion recommends listening patiently and waiting for a more or less spontaneous—facilitated by the therapist's mainly unconscious psychological work ('reverie' in Bion's terminology)—crystallization of a focal point (a 'selected fact' in Bion's terminology) for understanding what the patient says and does in the individual session—an experience of meaningful coherence in the material (cf. Symington and Symington 1996:92f, 168f). The therapist should give the patient the necessary time and space to explain and display what is important and emotionally significant to her right now, without quickly guiding her in any particular direction through his interventions. The therapist should also give himself time and permission to be affected, via his inner resonance, by what the patient says and does. This may involve asking brief follow-up questions in order to understand the patient's perception of and emotional reactions to the material, without being controlled by particular prior assumptions or imposing a specific structure on what the patient presents. Spontaneous recollections (for example from previous sessions) or desires (for something specific to happen right now) are not included in Bion's recommendation for the therapist to meet the patient without memory or desire, but should rather be understood as reflections of or reactions to what happens in the therapeutic space and in the therapeutic relationship right now, which should be made the topic of reflection and decoded (Levine 2015:456).

When Bion recommends listening to the patient without memory, desire or preconceived comprehension, it is because the therapist's personal wishes ('desires') may impair his judgment, conscious memories do not necessarily provide an objective image of past events but are constructs coloured by unconscious forces, and the therapist's needs and preconceived understanding may impair his intuitive thinking and openness to processes in the therapeutic space and his ability to listen to the patient's unconscious (Ogden 2016a:71ff). Naturally, the call for the therapist to meet the patient without any personal wishes ('desires') does not involve denying or splitting off one's own wishes; rather, it encourages the therapist to remain consistently conscious of his own actualized wishes and inclinations in the therapeutic space in order to avoid, as much as possible, acting these out or allowing them to determine one's actions in the interaction with the patient (Thomä 2004). The therapist will always, to varying degrees, be influenced by his own desires and prior assumptions (countertransferences); the key is how that is handled. It should never be allowed to control his therapeutic work, nor should it be repressed or otherwise rejected as forbidden or non-existing; instead, it should be incorporated as a natural element in the effort to understand what plays out in oneself, in the therapeutic space and in the patient. Especially in some forms of psychoanalytic psychotherapy with a prominent focus on working in and with the transference, the dominant focus is on what is happening in the therapeutic space here and now—not on what happened (in the past) or what may happen (in the future). Similarly, the way we talk and think (process) is at least as important as what we talk and think about (content) (Ogden 2009:29). This focus on the present moment underscores the importance of the therapist's ability to be open and present in the moment. Arguably, evenly suspended attention contains a number of often overlooked meditative elements, in the sense that the therapist has to open himself up to pure observation, allow the process to unfold while observing it without normative judging and suspend his urge to control the process and to do anything in particular—all elements that can be used to cultivate the therapist's ability to be present, open himself up to the moment and listen to his own affective resonance (Zwiebel 2012:58).

Naturally, it may also be argued that it is often easier to understand why what is happening in the moment is happening, when we view it in light of what we know about the past (the patient's past life, previous sessions and, perhaps, one's own history) and about human psychology—compared to an understanding of events in the moment that is completely unframed by prior knowledge. In that sense, the therapist's suspension of memory and preconceived understanding will of course always be relative and temporary, and it will alternate with the activation of memories and scientifically validated knowledge. The psychotherapeutic stance thus implies that the therapist continuously maintains an appropriate balance between, on the one hand, observing the patient and what is happening in the therapeutic space through a lens of scientific knowledge and pre-established knowledge about the patient and, on the other hand, maintaining an unrestrained openness to the unknown and surprising (cf. Tubert-Oklander 2013:33). Moreover, the therapeutic context naturally also plays a role, and in short-term treatment of less severe disorders it may be helpful to define a treatment focus fairly early and stick to it.

Finally, it is worth noting that we are approaching two fundamentally different—but not necessarily irreconcilable—perceptions of what constitutes the core of psychotherapeutic work. One view is that the key process driving psychotherapeutic work is the only partially verbal (unconscious) communication between patient and therapist, which enables an understanding of the patient's non-articulated experiences and history (unconscious, procedural memory, implicit relational knowledge) combined with corrections or added nuance to the patient's (conscious or unconscious) interpretation of past events and their psychological consequences, that is, corrective experiences in the meeting with the therapist. An alternative view is that the core of psychotherapy lies in the more conscious interaction between patient and therapist here and now, including how they, on a more conscious level, perceive themselves and each other and play out certain roles or relational positions, and how patterns from the patient's other relationships are repeated in the therapeutic space and, not least, their common effort to verbalize, contextualize and understand these dynamics in the present moment, in part in light of the patient's history and the therapist's knowledge of the aetiology and manifestations of psychopathology.

9.3 Transference

The above-mentioned basic elements of Freud's psychoanalytic method point to the need for a therapeutic stance that aims to create optimal conditions for the patient's transferences to unfold and become the focus of the therapeutic work. With the introduction of the transference concept Freud, in a certain sense, transforms the therapeutic situation in a way that raises the demands on the therapist considerably. The patient's difficulties are no longer something that the therapist discusses with the patient with a certain detachment; it plays out in the therapeutic space here and now, and the therapist, to varying degrees, becomes emotionally involved. The therapist is not only managing a specific therapeutic method but becomes 'personally' involved and, to some extent, part of the process that drives the treatment, which requires very different and much more extensive training (cf. Heimann 1960:154).

According to Freud, the typical patient tends to repeat or re-enact core elements of her past relationships in the interaction with the therapist. Rather than recollecting and verbalizing key parts of her pathology, including interaction patterns, that originally led to and now perpetuate the patient's current difficulties, these are unconsciously repeated and acted out in the interaction with the therapist, in the transference. The patient does not recall what was forgotten or repressed; he acts it out. As Freud (1958c[1914]:150) puts it, the patient 'reproduces it not as a memory but as an action; he *repeats* it, without, of course, knowing that he is repeating it. For instance, the patient does not say that he remembers that he used to be defiant and critical towards his parents' authority; instead, he behaves in that way to the doctor.' At the same time, Freud believes that in a dynamic perspective we should view the transference as a manifestation of the patient's resistance to remembering important past experiences and acknowledge internal psychological conflicts.

From the perspective of a modern psychodynamic understanding, however, the transference must rather be seen as an indication that the patient is not conscious of, let alone able to verbalize, how certain patterns are repeated over and over again in his or her relationships. Instead, the patient unconsciously repeats key aspects of these patterns in the interaction with the therapist. The transference is associated with the activation of the patient's procedural rather than declarative memory (see Chap. 11), which opens a window to the patient's unconscious and internal (past) object relations and implicit relational knowledge via the patient's behaviour in the therapeutic space. Freud's view of the transference as being indicative of the patient's resistance to remembering reflects a classical one-person psychology. On the other hand, as mentioned earlier, his theory also contains the seeds to a two-person psychology, where the transference is viewed as something that plays out in the patient-therapist relationship, which they both contribute to and are involved in. From the perspective of a dynamic-relational understanding, the patient's transference and the therapist's reactions to this transference—in the countertransference—are what drives the therapeutic work. It should not be regarded primarily as an indication of the patient's resistance to remembering specific events or to the therapy as such, but rather as a different (unconscious) way to show or communicate to the therapist what is the core of her difficulties.

Essentially, the transference concept refers to the phenomenon that the patient perceives and behaves towards the therapist in ways that repeat important elements of her earlier relationships with significant others, thus also repeating and acting out key aspects of her interpersonally rooted difficulties in the therapeutic space. Hence, transference contains invaluable information about the background of the patient's pathology and makes this information accessible to therapeutic work in a context where it is emotionally activated and present in the here and now. 'What are transferences? They are new editions or facsimiles of the tendencies and phantasies which are aroused and made conscious during the progress of the analysis [...] they replace some earlier person by the person of the physician. [...] a whole series of psychological experiences are revived, not as belonging to the past, but as applying to the physician at the present moment' (Freud 1953[1905]:116). Core elements of a past relationship are repeated in the interaction with the therapist, which means that the patient's perception of the therapist is coloured or distorted by unresolved elements from the patient's past relationships.

Freud (1958a[1912]:101) describes transference as 'the most powerful resistance to the treatment', but also as 'the condition of success', if it is handled correctly. 'It cannot be disputed that controlling the phenomena of transference presents the psycho-analyst with the greatest difficulties. But it should not be forgotten that it is precisely they that do us the inestimable service of making the patient's hidden and forgotten erotic impulses immediate and manifest. For when all is said and done, it is impossible to destroy anyone in absentia or in effigie [sic]' (Freud 1958a[1912]:108). The correct and therapeutically optimal handling of the transference depends on the therapist's more personal qualities and, according to Freud, requires that the therapist successfully undergoes therapy himself with a view to learning about his own strengths, weaknesses and reaction tendencies; 'no psycho-analyst goes further than his own complexes and internal resistances permit; and we consequently require that he shall begin his activity with a self-analysis […] Anyone who fails to produce results in a self-analysis of this kind may at once give up any idea of being able to treat patients by analysis' (Freud 1957[1910]:141). In other words, the therapist's implicit relational knowledge, which is far from always conscious, and his (possibly inadequate) self-insight form the basis of his interactions with the patient and may therefore place limitations on his ability to meet, contain and understand certain patients.

Actualizing the Core of Pathology

According to Freud, the core of the patient's pathology is actualized and made accessible to intervention in the therapeutic space by virtue of the transference. We should therefore 'treat his illness not as an event of the past, but as a present-day force' (Freud 1958c[1914]:151). Thus, the psychotherapeutic task consists in elucidating and connecting what happens in the therapeutic relationship with the patient's history and general way of functioning in relationships. Freud attributes the persistent repetition of certain patterns in the patient's relationships to a drive-based compulsion to repeat that is part of human psychology, and which must be curbed through the therapeutic work. 'The main instrument, however, for curbing the patient's compulsion to repeat and for turning it into a motive for remembering lies in the handling of the transference. We render the compulsion harmless, and indeed useful, by giving it the right to assert itself in a definite field. We admit it into the transference as a playground in which it is allowed to expand in almost complete freedom and in which it is expected to display to us everything' (Freud 1958c[1914]:154). 'The transference thus creates an intermediate region between illness and life, through which the transition from the one to the other is made' (ibid.). The transference is, in a sense, both phantasy and reality; it creates a unique entity in the therapeutic space in the transition between phantasy and reality that should be treated as 'unreal' in the sense that the therapist should not act on it—he should not take part in re-enacting the patient's actualized interaction patterns; instead it should be used as a source of valuable information about recurring patterns and difficulties in the patient's relationships.

In this context, Freud also writes about the development of what he calls a transference neurosis, where most of the patient's difficulties are temporarily unfolded and concentrated in the patient's relationship with the therapist. Recovery may be attained by verbalizing and processing what happens in the therapeutic relationship here and now—focusing on and processing the transference neurosis. 'Provided only that the patient shows compliance enough to respect the necessary conditions of the analysis, we regularly succeed in giving all the symptoms of the illness a new transference meaning and in replacing his ordinary neurosis by a "transference-neurosis" of which he can be cured by the therapeutic work' (ibid.). Freud's theory on the transference neurosis and its role in the treatment is disputed. It is not meaningful to speak of the transference neurosis as a categorical entity that is either present or not. Instead, it is more apt to speak of degrees in the development of a transference neurosis, which will play out especially in long-term, in-depth psychotherapy, where the therapist and the therapeutic relationship may for a period become extraordinarily important to the patient. Here, it should be considered that Freud developed his transference theory before he fully realized that there are no decisive qualitative differences between normal and pathological psychology; rather, they exist on a continuum ranging from what we would perceive as 'normal' to what we define as 'pathological' (cf. Wallerstein 1993:59).

Positive and Negative Transference

Freud distinguishes between positive and negative transferences, where the former are, broadly speaking, dominated by positive experiences and emotions, while the latter have their roots in negative experiences (abandonment, violation of personal boundaries, lack of recognition/invalidation of the self) in earlier relationships with significant others, including parents and close caregivers, and cause the patient to view and treat the therapist with hostility, detachment and mistrust. 'Positive transference is then further divisible into transference of friendly or affectionate feelings which are admissible to consciousness and transference of prolongations of those feelings into the unconscious […] [which] invariably go back to erotic sources' (Freud 1958a[1912]:105). The former is also referred to as the positive inoffensive transference and forms an important part of the basis of what we now call the therapeutic alliance, while the latter is referred to as the positive, eroticized transference and may pose major challenges for the therapist and the therapist's ability to maintain a therapeutic stance towards the patient.

However, we should distinguish between what might be called 'transference love', which often occurs in long-term therapy, and actual eroticized transference, where the patient's sexual attraction to the therapist moves into the foreground, and the transference is more at risk of losing its important 'make-believe' quality and may become more difficult for the therapist to handle. In practice, however, these are rarely clear-cut categories but should rather be seen as existing on a continuum, and in some cases it can be difficult to distinguish clearly between the positive inoffensive transference and transference love, both of which may promote the therapeutic alliance, and between transference love and the eroticized transference. A thorough treatment of the nuances in the transferences dynamics lies outside the scope of the present book. It can be said, however, that part of the reason why it can be difficult to draw a sharp distinction between the positive inoffensive transference and transference love is that the intense emotional contact and psychological closeness that is pursued within the therapeutic space is not unrelated to human sexuality and may also activate it. Finally, the positive transference may also become unrealistic and potentially problematic to the therapeutic process for other reasons besides its eroticized character. For example, a strong positive transference may lead to an excessive idealization of the therapist, with related phantasies about the therapist's ability to meet all the patient's needs and solve all her problems—an idealization that may naturally also stem from other dynamics, including the patient's more or less unconscious hopes (of being rescued by the therapist) or fears (of being abandoned, left to fend for herself and so on).

What we now refer to as the therapeutic alliance could in fact, with reference to Freud's writings, be viewed as an alliance between the therapist's ego and a rational core or rational aspects of the patient's ego, driven by positive inoffensive transferences—positive transferences that promote the formation of a trust-based relationship. As Freud wrote, 'the essence of the analytic situation is that the analyst enters into an alliance with the ego of the analysand', and 'If we want to make a compact with the patient's ego, that ego must be normal' (Freud 1937:389f). This also means that persons with severe ego disorders—what we would now describe as patients with psychosis or severe personality disorder, deficiency pathology and severe attachment disorders—may be more poorly equipped to enter into a sustainable therapeutic alliance (Küchenhoff et al. 2017), although it is far from impossible.

If negative transferences dominate, according to Freud, the psychotherapeutic space collapses, or, as he puts it, 'the whole analytic situation is broken up'. The 'patient now regards the analyst simply as an alien personality who makes disagreeable demands upon him [the patient] and he [the patient] behaves towards him [the therapist] exactly like a child who does not like a stranger and has no confidence in him' (Freud 1937:394). This sort of situation places different and greater demands on the therapist. When the positive inoffensive transference is very fragile or near-absent (it is rarely, if ever, fully and permanently absent), and the patient only has limited past experiences with positive relationships that may serve as a basis for trusting the therapist, it takes a bigger and more prolonged effort by the therapist to form a sustainable therapeutic alliance, which may thus become the primary treatment goal for much of the duration of the therapy. When the patient has developed enough—and sufficiently stable—trust in the therapist to be able to enter into a lasting alliance with the therapist, the patient who initially had a severe attachment disorder is well on her way to recovery. The positive transference also lends the therapist an air of authority in the eyes of the patient that makes the patient more receptive to the therapist's interventions and to the therapeutic work by strengthening the patient's positive expectations and epistemic trust in the therapist (see Chap. 3). The determining factor for the treatment outcome, in Freud's words (1963[1917]:445f), is not the patient's intellectual insight, 'but simply and solely his [the patient's] relation to the doctor. In so far as his [the patient's] transference bears a "plus" sign, it clothes the doctor with authority and is transformed into belief in his communications and explanations. In the absence of such a transference, or if it is a negative one, he would never even give a hearing to the doctor and his arguments'.

9.4 Transference Love and Eroticized Transference

Less experienced therapists in particular may become overwhelmed and struggle to handle a highly eroticized transference, but experienced therapists too may get caught up in taking part in acting out—or failing to set sufficiently clear boundaries for and deal therapeutically with—an eroticized transference. Freud's treatment of this theme focuses solely on female patients' eroticized transference and transference love in the interaction with male therapists, which is explained in part by the gender distribution among patients and therapists in Freud's time and the fact that this part of Freud's theory is based on his own experiences in the therapeutic space and in part by the prevalence of cultural themes at the time, when prominent authors and playwrights, including Ibsen, Strindberg and Schnitzler, presented the female as a dangerous, drive-motivated being who might threaten the man and his defence of spiritual and social order (cf. Cremerius 1984:774).

From a contemporary perspective, it is of course remarkable that Freud never explicitly addresses the possibility of an eroticized transference between the female therapist and the male patient or of a homosexual eroticized transference. He also only indirectly addresses the risk that an inexperienced and impulse-driven (male or female) therapist might exploit (and actively contribute to fostering) an eroticized transference in order to satisfy his or her own sexual and emotional needs in a way that is completely unacceptable within the therapeutic context. Nevertheless, elements of his descriptions and attempts to understand what might play out in the therapeutic relationship in connection with an eroticized transference—and how the therapist should deal with this—still has validity today, beyond Freud's own time and beyond the therapeutic relationship between the younger female patient and the older male therapist. Hence, it is still worthwhile to consult Freud's reflections on this issue, with the awareness that his writings are in some regards in need of updating and contextualization. As mentioned earlier, some of Freud's technical recommendations should be seen as part of an efforts to protect psychoanalysis and its legitimacy against therapists who lack a proper understanding of personal boundaries, so in some regards they are a little simplistic and rigid, just as today's understanding of psychotherapeutic practice is, in many regards, much more sophisticated than it was in Freud's day. On the other hand, Freud's descriptions of the eroticized transference does capture certain universal and timeless aspects of human psychology.

When the therapeutic relationship is dominated by an eroticized transference or, in less radical situations, by transference love, it may seem, as Freud (1963[1917]:291) puts it, as if the patient is in love with the therapist, and all her 'interest in the immediate situation in the treatment and all the obligations they undertook at its commencement vanish'. The patient's approach to the therapist, the therapeutic relationship and the therapeutic work changes radically, and the therapeutic space may collapse unless the therapist manages to handle the situation and is seduced into taking part in a form of acting out of the patient's transference phantasies. 'There is a complete change of scene; it is as though some piece of make-believe had been stopped by the sudden irruption of reality—as when, for instance, a cry of fire is raised during a theatrical performance' (Freud 1958d[1915]:162). A situation may arise where the patient 'suddenly loses all understanding of the treatment and all interest in it, and will not speak or hear about anything but her love, which she demands to have returned' (Freud 1958d[1915]:162). What plays out in the transference and the therapeutic relationship may lose its important 'make-believe' character, and the therapeutic relationship may change from a relationship where all activity is directed at understanding the patient to an 'ordinary' interpersonal relationship, where impulses are not used as material for new understanding but are acted out.

As is the case with transference in general, Freud perceives eroticized transferences as manifestations of the patient's resistance to the treatment, but he also points out that they include 'so much of the most important material from the patient's past and bring it back in so convincing a fashion that they become some of the best supports of the analysis if a skilful technique knows how to give them the right turn' (Freud 1963[1917]:291). Again, the key is how the therapist meets and deals with the patient's transference and its concrete manifestations in the therapeutic space. The therapeutic stance towards the patient, towards the manifestations of the patient's pathology and towards the therapist's own experiences in the interaction with the patient becomes the driver of the process.

Freud warns against the countertransferences that eroticized transference can activate in the therapist. The therapist 'must recognize that the patient's falling in love is induced by the analytic situation and is not to be attributed to the charms of his own person; so that he has no grounds whatever for being proud of such a "conquest"' (Freud 1958d[1915]:160f). The patient's love may be genuine in a sense, as any love, according to Freud (1958d[1915]:168), repeats 'infantile reactions', but is also induced and intensified by the psychotherapeutic situation, including the often asymmetrical relationship between the vulnerable patient and the idealized therapist (perceived authority), and 'it is lacking to a high degree in a regard for reality, is less sensible, less concerned about its consequences and more blind in its valuation of the loved person [the therapist]' (Freud 1958d[1915]:168f). Today, more than a century after Freud presented his recommendations, we may ask whether it is really essential to evaluate and, in a sense, reach a normative judgment on whether the patient's feelings in the therapeutic space are real, mature and appropriate or unreal (because they are determined by transferences), immature and inappropriate. The therapist's task is to examine the patient's inner psychological (subjective) reality, not to determine to what extent it matches any imagined objective reality (Hoffer 1993:1031).

Handling Ambivalence

The eroticized transference may cause the therapist 'to come to grief', as Freud (1958d[1915]:163) puts it. Freud also emphasizes that it is the therapist's responsibility to meet the eroticized transference or transference love in a balanced and therapeutic manner by not explicitly rejecting the patient's feelings, with reference to norms and rules, or pretending to reciprocate the patient's tender feelings, while 'at the same time avoiding any physical implementation of this fondness' (Freud 1958d[1915]:164). Freud warns explicitly that the 'experiment of letting oneself go a little way in tender feelings for the patient is not altogether without danger. Our control over ourselves is not so complete that we may not suddenly one day go further than we had intended.' (ibid.). The patient who is overwhelmed by the eroticized transference seeks to act out the activated feelings rather than examine and process them, and if 'the patient's advances were returned it would be a great triumph for her, but a complete defeat for the treatment' (Freud 1958d[1915]:166).

Freud (ibid) points out that the therapist 'must take care not to steer away from the transference-love, or to repulse it or to make it distasteful to the patient; but he must just as resolutely withhold any response to it. He must keep firm hold of the transference-love, but treat it as something unreal.' 'It is, therefore, just as disastrous for the analysis if the patient's craving for love is gratified as if it is suppressed' (bid.). The therapist must avoid becoming personally and emotionally entangled in the patient's eroticized transference; the more plainly the therapist lets 'it be seen that he is proof against every temptation,' the more likely, according to Freud (ibid.), it is that the patient will 'feel safe enough to allow all her preconditions for loving, all the phantasies springing from her sexual desires, all the detailed characteristics of her state of being in love, to come to light,' which allows for working therapeutically with the elements and dynamic background of the transference. This requires the therapist to maintain the therapeutic stance in the meeting with the patient's at times insistent eroticized transference. The therapist must also bear in mind that the eroticized transference may contain other relational dynamics as well. For example, it may reflect the patient's more or less unconscious attempts at achieving a sense of control in/over the therapeutic relationship or it may be related to her efforts to gratify other, non-sexual needs (for attention, nurture, contact). The former situation may be related to having learned, in previous relationships, that it is possible to attain a sense of control over a relationship by sexualizing it, while the latter may stem from having learned that she has to 'pay' with her sexuality for contact and the gratification of basic emotional needs.

A brief example from clinical practice may illustrate this complicated dynamic. A patient has for some time explicitly expressed her interest in some form of personal and sexual relationship with the therapist. At the outset of the therapy, the therapist clearly communicated the conditions for the treatment, including that needs and urges that come up in the therapeutic space should be used as a basis for understanding the patient and her difficulties, rather than being acted out, and that any form of physical contact or more personal contact between patient and therapist outside the therapeutic space is ruled out, as it would ruin the possibilities of therapeutic work, and besides, the therapist is bound by a set of professional ethical guidelines. Over some time the therapist refers, in various ways, to the conditions of the treatment when the patient expresses her desire to change the character of the therapeutic relationship, and the therapist consistently invites the development of a common understanding of what it is that is played out and repeated when the patient feels the urge to change the character of the therapeutic relationship.

This is done in ways where the therapist acknowledges and respects the patient's desire but also avoids explicitly addressing how he might have hypothetically responded, had the patient expressed the same interest in a normal, non-therapeutic relationship (to prevent the patient from feeling rejected or, conversely, encouraged to push further to change the character of the relationship). Meanwhile, he maintains focus on the task: to uphold the therapeutic context and the therapeutic space, and to use everything that happens in the space and in the therapeutic relationship as a basis for understanding and helping the patient—while avoiding to act on what happens as if it were a normal non-professional relationship. It gradually becomes clear that the patient has a history where emotional and sexual contact are fused. She has difficulty distinguishing between, on the one hand, being in emotional contact (something that, in a sense, she has never experienced before in her life), experiencing psychological closeness and feeling seen and contained and, on the other hand, having physical sexual contact. In her experience, if she wanted to establish or maintain any form of emotional contact, which she so desperately needs, she had to 'pay' in the form of sexual contact. Later in the treatment the patient explicitly expresses that although she did at one point have a strong desire for personal and sexual contact with the therapist, she would also have been furious if he 'had played along', because 'then you would have ruined all the trust and intimacy we have established,' as she put it.

The patient's sense of security would have been breached, and she would have been trapped in another repetition of a far-too-familiar pattern of constantly devoting a large share of her mental energy to reading the other's (sexual and other) needs and doing everything she can to gratify them. Thus, although the patient on a conscious, manifest level expresses a desire for sexual contact with the therapist and for changing the therapeutic relationship into a personal one, had the therapist met this need, that would have constituted a repetition of a maladaptive pattern from her earlier life that would have been destructive to her and to the therapeutic relationship, and it would have caused the therapeutic space to collapse. Arguably, another part of her—unconsciously—wanted the therapist to meet her in a way that was different from what she was used to and which she invited—a meeting that would break her earlier pattern and help her understand herself and her way of handling contact.

She wanted contact—emotional contact, psychological closeness and attachment, not sexual contact. Her transference was not primarily, as claimed by classical psychoanalysis, motivated by sexual drives but rather by a yearning for contact and closeness. The therapist's way of handling the patient's communicated need helps her realize that she can achieve emotional contact with others without this resulting in her (and the relationship) being flooded by (her own or others') uncontrollable sexual needs or having to 'pay' the other in some way for the contact. One might also consider whether the patient—consciously or unconsciously—was testing the therapist to see whether she might trust him enough to allow him to get closer emotionally, with the heightened vulnerability and exposure that this involves, or whether he was 'like all the other men' in her life, who, in her experience, expected sexual favours as payment for contact and acceptance.

Towards the end of the treatment, when the transference has taken on a different and much more mature character, the patient says to the therapist (note the interesting shifts in grammar): 'I have had great admiration for you in my therapy, almost like being in love. But I have always known, in some sense, that it wasn't you as a person I was in love with. The many warm feelings and the enchantment isn't about you as a person, because I don't know who you are, other than the little glimpses I've seen—so I can't be in love with who you are as a whole, because I don't know … I don't know what you're like when you are angry, crazy, loving […] but I have been in love with the feelings you gave me, the feelings of acceptance and containment that you have shown me, I was enchanted by that, and I still am.'

9.5 Neutrality

> 'General emotional withdrawal and uninvolvement with the patient are […] ominous signs and make for an inability to perform psychoanalysis except as a caricature of the true procedure.' (Greenson 1967:400)

Historically, the neutrality of the psychoanalytic therapist has been associated with at least five kinds of neutrality (Mertens 1993:15f), where the first and, to some extent, the second are particularly firmly rooted in classical (one-person) psychoanalytic theory and today appear both obsolete and impracticable, even if one might think they were worth pursing. On the other hand, a moderate version of the other three (especially the latter two) are relevant elements of the psychotherapeutic stance:

1. *Behavioural neutrality*, linked to the therapist's relative anonymity in relation to the patient.
2. *Neutrality in the attitude towards the patient's material*, where the therapist avoids normative, value-based judgments and avoids taking part in internal conflicts between the patient's id, ego and superego (drives/needs; self; conscience, values and ideals).
3. *Interpersonal neutrality*, where the therapist avoids taking sides in connection with conflicts in the patient's actual relationship, for example by uncritically siding with the patient in her presented conflicts with her 'mean parents' instead of inviting shared reflection on them.
4. *Interactional neutrality*, associated with a flexibility in the therapist's attitude to the patient's actualized internal object relations and interaction patterns, when these are played out in the therapeutic relationship (see section on evenly suspended role-responsiveness).

5. *Essential neutrality*, which implies that the therapist is open to the fact that there are multiple possible understandings of reality and that his or her interpretations merely represent one among several possible perspectives on reality.

As mentioned, the demand for neutrality on the part of the psychoanalytic therapist springs from elements of Freud's theory, including his drive theory, which must now be considered outdated. Generally, the notion of therapist neutrality can be traced back to Freud and the roots of early psychoanalysis in the natural and medical sciences, including the image of the neutral physician/surgeon or scientist. Earlier, for example, the ideal analyst was supposed to remain relatively anonymous and act as an opaque mirror to the patient in order to avoid gratifying what was perceived as the patient's primitive or infantile needs (cf. the rule of abstinence, see above), so that split-off drives and repressed (unconscious) ideas could surface, become conscious and thus become accessible to analytic interpretation. One should, however, be cautious to compare neutrality and abstinence, since neutrality, as mentioned, can be defined in different ways and include a range of elements, including the therapist's handling of the patient's transferences, while abstinence primarily refers to the need for the therapist to refrain from gratifying (especially the more primitive) needs in the patient.

According to Freud (1958b[1912]:118), the therapist should only have a limited explicit emotional and personal presence in the treatment; he refers to this as the therapist's 'intimate attitude' towards the patient and recommends that the therapist should 'be opaque to his patients and, like a mirror, should show them nothing but what is shown to him.' Moreover, it was imagined that the analyst's neutrality—where the therapist only reveals himself to a limited degree with his individuality and subjectivity—affords optimal conditions for the patient's transferences to unfold and be made the object of therapeutic work. There is nothing to suggest, however, that Freud fully adhered to his own strict requirements of neutrality in his own therapeutic work.

The Surgeon as a Model

In line with the one-person psychology underlying classical psychoanalysis, Freud largely considered the patient's transferences as a manifestation of resistance (to remembering and insight), and one of the analyst's most primary tasks, according to Freud, is to analyse and interpret, among other things, the patient's defences and manifestations of internal conflicts in the analytical space. He therefore recommends that the therapist should model himself on the surgeon 'who puts aside all his feelings, even his human sympathy, and concentrates his mental forces on the single aim of performing the operation as skilfully as possible' (Freud 1958b[1912]:115).

Interpreting Freud's surgeon metaphor to mean that the therapist should repress, deny or shut off the feelings activated in the therapeutic work carries a considerable risk of impairing one's emotional sensitivity and ability to be present as a person—factors that are crucial to a successful outcome (Heimann 1960:151). Moreover, the therapist will always inevitably influence the patient's experiences and behaviour with his personality and behaviour in the therapeutic space, so the so-called neutral therapist will only invite the patient to demonstrate how he or she reacts to a person who appears and acts in this specific manner (Wachtel 2008:17). In that sense, the neutral therapist (the objective observer who does not influence the observed with his or her subjectivity) is a problematic illusion in several regards. Similarly, it can be problematic to apply Freud's mirror metaphor to the therapist's attitude and stance towards the patient.

Over time, the prevailing psychoanalytic understanding of the therapeutic stance has changed considerably, from the notion of a largely dispassionate, neutral therapist to that of a more supportive and explicit approving therapist who, to varying degrees, is flexible and patient and tries to build trust with the patient. Here, it is naturally important to note that what it takes for the therapist to build trust will differ greatly across different patients, depending on the individual patient's psychological constitution and relational history. This historical shift in the perception of certain aspects of the psychotherapeutic stance is reflected in and, to some extent partially connected to, changes in late modern Western societies towards more democratic relations, an ability to challenge (previously largely unassailable) authority figures and a critical detachment from objective truths (which have arguably gone too far in recent years, cf. social constructivism and other developments).

In the early 1960s Leo Stone presents a study of the psychoanalytic situation (Stone 1961), which represents one of the first major breaks with the traditional notion of the therapist's neutrality. Today, most would argue that an anonymous and, in that sense neutral, therapist (cf. point 1 and, in part, point 2 above) presents more of an obstacle to the therapeutic work with inner conflicts and could be harmful in the work with patients with more severe psychological disorders, such as personality disorders (deficiency pathology, Killingmo 1989), where the therapist ability to be authentically present and 'hold' the patient is a crucial factor (cf. Kutter 1988:20f), while pronounced neutrality may be perceived as indifference or as a sign that the therapist 'is siding with the others' against the patient in her interpersonal conflicts. These patients often need a therapist who is more emotionally involved and present in the therapeutic space, not another alienating relationship without real relatedness, where the patient feels abandoned, insignificant and without contact.

The therapist's neutrality and absent or very controlled emotional responsiveness can add unnecessarily to the emotional burden on the patient and hamper the psychological and emotional contact the patient needs to develop her capacity for contact and self-regulation (Hansel 2008). The classical Still Face experiment (see https://www.youtube.com/watch?v=apzXGEbZht0), which shows how children react with clear signs of escalating emotional discomfort (dysregulation) and attempts at making contact when an attachment figure meets them with an inexpressive and non-responsive facial expression, offers a good illustration of how it affects a person to be in a relationship where the other is absent as a subject and fails to respond to invitations to interpersonal and emotional contact (Ham and Tronick 2009).

The fact that the requirement of therapist neutrality and personal anonymity has persisted as long as it has stems in part from a fear that abandoning it would throw the door wide open to mercurial approaches and 'anything goes', where irresponsible, transgressive and incompetent therapists would be wreak havoc to the reputation of psychoanalysis. That fear is understandable, to some degree, but it should not result in a rigid insistence on obviously inappropriate guidelines for therapeutic work

(Mitchell 1997:xi). The experience of intersubjective recognition (from the therapist) and (marked and congruent) mirroring of the self in the other (the therapist), who does not (as an opaque mirror) offer 'objective' mirroring but mirroring coloured by his or her own subjectivity, contributes to a better and more grounded sense of self in the patient. In addition, a therapist who is clear in his or her reactions to what the patient does in the therapeutic relationship, demonstrating and verbalizing the interpersonal consequences of the patient's way of relating to others, can help the patient understand and change her implicit (procedural) relational knowledge, including understanding how her behaviour affects others and may evoke certain (often painful to the patient) reactions in others (Streeck 2017:249).

Contemporary Concept of Neutrality

A contemporary, yet still psychoanalytically informed, understanding of the therapist's neutrality could be that the therapist should avoid intruding on the patient or otherwise imposing his or her own wishes, ideas, values and private experiences or concerns, which far from precludes the possibility of also being friendly, authentically present and accommodating (cf. Sandell et al. 2006:640) and at times gratifying the patient's needs, especially the more mature and relational ones, by inviting emotional contact and psychological closeness. Therapeutic neutrality thus represents respecting the patient's autonomy and fundamental otherness while also inviting the patient into a form of contact where the therapist is present on a personal level. On the other hand, it should be remembered that psychotherapy, as mentioned earlier, can also contain an element of (re)socialization to contemporary culture. This implies that some patients may, to varying degrees, need for the therapist to represent a reflected verbalization of what could, for want of a better term, be called common human (and social) norms and values (related to basic self-nurture, basic conditions for establishing well-functioning and mature relations with others and so on), which the patient needs to know and, in part, internalize to achieve a basic psychological and interpersonal level of functioning. Similarly, some patients may, for shorter or longer periods, need a therapist who appears as a competent authority figure that they can lean on, identify with or challenge—and who can help them form a better and more nuanced self-perception.

Naturally, this raises a number of questions and requires that the therapist has good judgment and is able to balance different concerns in the given situation: when does a sexual practice that the patient engages in go from being experimental in relation to prevailing norms (and perhaps the therapist's own narrow views of human sexuality) to being destructive to the patient? When does the patient's insistence on being spontaneous and avoiding making plans become a sign of pathological impulsivity and a (painful) inability to plan and hold on to long-term goals that leads to a painful chaos and in practice blocks the patient's development? Exactly when do alcohol and drug use tip over into abuse, where the therapist needs to confront the patient with the self-destructive consequences? When are the symptoms of a medical condition or somatic illness in the patient so severe that the therapist has to insist that the patient is seen by a medical doctor, even if the patient refuses and denies that she needs medical help? Questions such as these may be further complicated when the therapist belongs to and represents a different (sub)culture than the one the patient knows and grew up in—an issue that it may be helpful to address with the patient. A brief example may serve to illustrate this point: a patient with a history of countless violations of her personal boundaries begins a session by describing a recent incident where a men she had met not long ago 'suddenly' violates her boundaries by holding her firmly and kissing her against her will. Even though the patient initially trivializes the experience (despite the fact that it re-actualized self-loathing and suicidal ideation), saying that she has experienced similar incidents many times before, the therapist insists that they work on what happened prior to the violation, including whether the patient had noticed previously that this man behaved in ways that overstepped her boundaries (which it quickly turns out he had, although the patient trivialized it)—and, not least, the patient's perception of and emotional reaction to the transgressive behaviour. Suddenly the patient says to the therapist: But I've never learned that it's okay to set boundaries, especially not with men, so it's very novel to me when you say that I need to sense my own boundaries and uphold them. It is as if I come from one culture, and you're showing me that there's a different culture, where it's okay to set boundaries with other people, but I don't know if I'll know how to be in that other culture.' In this sort of situation the therapist has to strike a balance between, on the one hand, avoiding imposing certain norms and values from his own culture on the patient and, on the other hand, sticking to his professional knowledge about what is good and bad for human psychological well-being.

Generally, it is a part of the psychotherapeutic stance that the therapist adopts a curious explorative, rather than a moral-normative, attitude to what the patient says and does in the therapeutic space. On the other hand, there are certain situations, where the therapist would de facto fail the patient and his therapeutic responsibility if he did not, at least, explicitly express his concern for the patient's situation and behaviour, including pointing out the need to act. It is neither possible nor meaningful to articulate specific guidelines stating exactly when it may be necessary for the therapist to step away, temporarily, from the more curious and explorative position that is part of the psychotherapeutic stance, nor exactly what form it should take in the given situation. Here too, the therapist's good judgment and more personal qualities (including experience and maturity) serve as an important compass in determining what is the most appropriate way to act in the situation.

Therapy has little chance of success if the therapist acts in an unnatural way, suppresses his own feelings and countertransferences or pretends to be neutral. The line between being neutral in a positive sense and being a bland, featureless, inauthentic therapist who simply performs the role of 'the neutral therapist' can be razor-thin (Heimann 1978:313). The key is that the therapist is aware of his influence on the patient and thus what is observed in the therapeutic space and understands that it is neither possible nor desirable to be a fully objective (cf. the surgeon) and uninvolved therapist (Renik 1993). Of course, this awareness does not eliminate the influence, but it does help to initiate helpful reflections on how one might have influenced what the patient says and does, that is, on one's own active role in what happens in the therapeutic space.

The therapist's subjective involvement in the interaction with the patient cannot—and should not—be eliminated; at most it can be repressed or denied, which hardly makes it less important or problematic, on the contrary (Mitchell 1997:13). Listening to and interacting with the patient and the specific use of various therapeutic methods will always involve the therapist's own subjectivity and psychology (Renik 1993:560). Here it is worth remembering that our patients typically know much more about us than we might think—a knowledge they gain, in part, via our countertransference reactions, our appearance as persons in the therapeutic space and, perhaps, our appearance in public settings outside the therapeutic space. A rigid insistence on traditional concepts of neutrality may be driven by our own defences and our own urge to maintain an emotional distance to what plays out in the therapeutic space (Treurniet 1997:600f).

A contemporary two/multiple-person psychology calls for a more personal and human approach, where the therapist meets the patient in a subject-subject relationship, and where the therapist's person and way of relating to the patient is in itself seen as an important part of the treatment (cf. Köhler-Weisker 1986:148f). The main focus is shifted from internal psychological conflicts in a patient, who is inherently seen as being trapped in his or her own inner universe, to what plays out between patient and therapist in transference and countertransference, where the therapist both participates in and is able to take a step back from what is happening in the therapeutic relationship (Gullestad and Killingmo 2013:168). In a parallel development, the attention to the specific (cognitive) content of the verbal communication is toned down somewhat in favour of an increased interest in the affective and relational context of the patient's stories in the therapeutic space (Bromberg 2012:5).

The German psychoanalyst Zwiebel (2004) speaks of a shift from the classical psychoanalytic method, where the therapist as a person was largely required to stay in the background, to a postclassical approach where the therapist is far more open to his or her own subjectivity and the impact of his or her own countertransferences om what happens in the therapeutic space. The emphasis is on the emotional contact with the patient, from a stance that is non-intrusive and expresses recognition, and on the need to alternate, as one inevitably will, between acting out/with the patient and taking a step back and relating analytically to this process. Finally, the therapist has to acknowledge and accept his or her own inevitable personal limitations as a therapist, including the unavoidability of missteps and incidents of unhelpful acting out countertransferences, rather than holding on to unrealistic heroic ideals and demands. No therapist is perfect or infallible. The therapist who thinks he is—or who requires himself (and perhaps others) to be—infallible is unlikely to be a particularly competent therapist, a supposition that is supported by empirical studies (see Chap. 7; Nissen-Lie et al. 2016).

References

Balint, M. (1968[1994]). *Grundbristen* [The basic flaw]. Copenhagen, Denmark: Hans Reitzels Forlag.

Bion, W. (1967). Notes on memory and desire. In E. B. Spillius (Ed.), *Melanie Klein today, Vol 2: Mainly practice* (pp. 17–22). London, England: Routledge.

Bromberg, P. M. (2012). Stumbling along and hanging in: If this be technique, make the most of it! *Psychoanalytic Inquiry, 32*, 3–17.

Cremerius, J. (1984). Die psychoanalytische Abstinenzregel. Vom regelhaften zum operationellen Gebrauch [The psychoanalytic rule of abstinence: From rule-bound to operational use]. *Psyche, 38,* 769–800.

Freud, S. (1937). Analysis terminable and interminable. *International Journal of Psychoanalysis, 18,* 373–405.

Freud, S. (1953). Fragment of an analysis of a case of Hysteria. In J. Strachey (Ed. and Trans.), *The standard edition of the complete psychological works of Sigmund Freud* (Vol. 7, pp. 1–122). (Original work published 1905).

Freud, S. (1955). Lines of advance in psycho-analytic therapy. In J. Strachey (Ed. and Trans.), *The standard edition of the complete psychological works of Sigmund Freud* (Vol. 17, pp. 157–168). London, England: Hogarth (Original work published 1919).

Freud, S. (1957). The future prospects of psychoanalytic therapy. In J. Strachey (Ed. and Trans.), *The standard edition of the complete psychological works of Sigmund Freud* (Vol. 11, pp. 139–152). London, England: Hogarth (Original work published 1910).

Freud, S. (1958a). The dynamics of transference. In J. Strachey (Ed. and Trans.), *The Standard edition of the complete psychological works of Sigmund Freud* (Vol. 12, pp. 97–108). London, England: Hogarth (Original work published 1912).

Freud, S. (1958b). Recommendations to physicians practising psycho-analysis. In J. Strachey (Ed. and Trans.), *The standard edition of the complete psychological works of Sigmund Freud* (Vol. 12, pp. 109–120). London, England: Hogarth (Original work published 1912).

Freud, S. (1958c). Remembering, repeating and working-through. (Further recommendations on the technique of psycho-analysis II). In J. Strachey (Ed. and Trans.), *The standard edition of the complete psychological works of Sigmund Freud* (Vol. 12, pp. 145–156). London, England: Hogarth (Original work published 1914).

Freud, S. (1958d). Observations on transference-love (Further recommendations on the technique of psycho-analysis III). In J. Strachey (Ed. and Trans.), *The standard edition of the complete psychological works of Sigmund Freud* (Vol. 12, pp. 157–171). London, England: Hogarth (Original work published 1915).

Freud, S. (1963). Introductory lectures on psycho-analysis (Part III). In J. Strachey (Ed. and Trans.), *The standard edition of the complete psychological works of Sigmund Freud* (Vol. 16). London, England: Hogarth (Original work published 1917).

Friedman, L. (1991). A reading of Freud's papers on technique. *Psychoanalytic Quarterly, 60,* 564–595.

Greenson, R. R. (1967). *The technique and practice of psychoanalysis*. London, England: Hogarth Press.

Gullestad, S. E., & Killingmo, B. (2013). *Underteksten. Psykoanalytisk terapi i praksis* [Subtext. Psychoanalytic therapy in practice] (2nd ed.). Oslo, Norway: Universitetsforlaget.

Ham, J., & Tronick, E. (2009). Relational psychophysiology: Lessons from mother-infant physiology research and dyadically expanded states of consciousness. *Psychotherapy Research, 19,* 619–632.

Hansel, J. (2008). Psychoanalytic aims and attitudes. *The Psychoanalytic Quarterly, 77,* 1179–1192.

Heimann, P. (1960). Countertransference. In P. Heimann (Ed.), *About children and children-no-longer* (pp. 151–160). London, England: Routledge.

Heimann, P. (1978). On the necessity for the analyst to be natural with his patient. In P. Heimann (Ed.), *About children and children-no-longer* (pp. 311–323). London, England: Routledge.

Hoffer, A. (1993). Asymmetrie und Gegenseitigkeit in der analytischen Beziehung: Lektionen für heute aus der Beziehung zwischen Freud und Ferenczi [Asymmetry and mutuality in the analytic relationship. Lessons to be learned from the relationship between Freud and Ferenczi]. *Psyche, 47,* 1027–1040.

Jørgensen, C. R. (2002). *Psykologien i senmoderniteten* [Psychology in late modernity]. Copenhagen, Denmark: Hans Reitzels Forlag.

Jørgensen, C. R. (2009). *Personlighedsforstyrrelser. Moderne relationel forståelse og behandling af borderlinelidelse* [Personality disorders. Modern relational understanding and treatment of borderline disorder] (2nd ed.). Copenhagen, Denmark: Hans Reitzels Forlag.

Jørgensen, C. R. (2012). *Danmark på briksen. Et psykologisk perspektiv på Danmark og danskerne i det senmoderne* [Denmark on the therapist's couch. A psychological perspective on Denmark and Danes in later modernity]. Copenhagen, Denmark: Hans Reitzels Forlag.

Jørgensen, C. R. (2014). *ADHD. Bidrag til en kritisk psykologisk forståelse* [ADHD. Contributions to a critical psychological understanding]. Copenhagen, Denmark: Hans Reitzels Forlag.

Killingmo, B. (1989). Conflict and deficit: Implications for technique. *International Journal of Psychoanalysis, 70,* 65–79.

Killingmo, B. (1997). The so-called rule of abstinence revisited. *Scandinavian Psychoanalytic Review, 20,* 144–159.

Klüver, R. (1983). Agieren und mitagieren [Acting-out and counter-acting-out]. In S. Hoffmann (Ed.), *Deutung und Beziehung. Kritische Beiträge zur Behandlungskonzeption und Technik in der Psychoanalyse* (pp. 132–45). Frankfurt am Main, Germany: Fischer Verlag.

Köhler-Weisker, A. (1986). Zum Begriff der Haltung des Psychoanalytikers am Beispiel einer Fokaltherapie [On the concept of the psychotherapist's stance as an example of focal therapy]. *Jahrbuch der Psychoanalyse, 18,* 143–173.

Körner, J. (2002). The didactics of psychoanalytic education. *International Journal of Psychoanalysis, 83,* 1395–1405.

Küchenhoff, J., Prause, K., & Schulz, G. (2017). Engagement und Respekt. Psychotherapeutische Haltung und Bezieungsarbeit in der Psychotherapie mit psychotisch erlebenden Menschen [Commitment and respect: Psychotherapeutic attitude and work on analyst-patient relationships in psychotherapy for individuals with psychotic experience]. *Psyche, 71,* 60–81.

Kutter, P. (1988). Grundhaltung, professionelle Einstellungen und psychoanalytische Methode. In P. Kutter, R. Paramo-Ortega, & P. Zagermann (Eds.), *Die psychoanalytische Haltung* (pp. 17–29). Munich, Germany: Verlag Internationale Psychoanalyse.

Leuzinger-Bohleber, M. (2007). Forschende Grundhaltung als abgewehrter „common ground" von psychoanalytischen Praktikern und Forschern? [The explorative attitude as repelled 'common ground' of psychoanalytic practitioners and researchers?] *Psyche*, *61*, 966–994.

Levine, H. B. (2015). The transformational vision of Antonio Ferro. *Psychoanalytic Inquiry, 35,* 451–564.

Mertens, W. (1993). Die psychoanalytische Haltung [The psychoanalytic stance]. In M. Ermann (Ed.), *Die hilfreiche Beziehung in der Psychoanalyse* (pp. 11–34). Göttingen, Germany: Vandenhoeck & Ruprecht.

Mertens, W. (2015). *Psychoanalytische Behandlungstechnik. Konzepte und Themen psychoanalytisch begründeter Behandlungsverfahren* [Psychoanalytic treatment technique. Concepts and themes of psychoanalytically motivated treatment methods]. Stuttgart, Germany: Kohlhammer.

Mitchell, S. A. (1997). *Influence and autonomy in psychoanalysis.* Hillsdale, MI: Analytic Press.

Nissen-Lie, H.A., Goldberg, S.B., Hoyt, W.T., Falkenström, F., Holmqvist, R., Nielsen, S.L. & Wampold, B.E. (2016). Are therapists uniformly effective across patient outcome domains? A study on therapist effectiveness in two different treatment contexts. *Journal of counseling psychology, 64*(4), 367–78

Ogden, T. H. (2009). *Rediscovering psychoanalysis. Thinking and dreaming, learning and forgetting.* London, England: Routledge.

Ogden, T. H. (2016). *Reclaiming unlived life: Experiences in psychoanalysis.* London, England: Routledge.

Pflichthofer, D. (2010). Zwischen Gesetz und Freiheit. Die Suche nach dem Rahmen und dem Objekt [Between law and freedom: The search for setting and object]. *Psyche, 65,* 30–62.
Reik, T. (1948). *Listening with the third ear: The inner experience of a psychoanalyst.* New York, NY: Grove Press.
Renik, O. (1993). Analytic interaction: Conceptualizing technique in light of the analyst's irreducible subjectivity. *Psychoanalytic Quarterly, 62,* 553–571.
Sandell, R., Lazar, A., Grant, J., Carlsson, J., Schubert, J., & Broberg, J. (2006). Therapist attitudes and patient outcomes: III. A latent class analysis of therapists. *Psychology and Psychotherapy: Theory, Research and Practice, 79,* 629–647.
Sandler, J. (1976). Countertransference and role-responsiveness. *International Review of Psychoanalysis, 3,* 43–47.
Stone, L. (1961). *The Psychoanalytic Situation: An examination of its development and essential nature.* New York, NY: International Universities Press.
Streeck, U. (2017). Denn sie wissen nicht, was sie tun. Über unbewußte Beziehungsregulierung [For they know not what they do. About unconscious relational regulation]. *Forum Psychoanalyse, 33,* 235–250.
Strenger, C. (1989). The classic and romantic vision in psychoanalysis. *International Journal of Psychoanalysis, 70,* 593–610.
Symington, J., & Symington, N. (1996). *The clinical thinking of Wilfred Bion.* London, England: Routledge.
Thomä, H. (2004). Ist es utopisch, sich zukünftige Psychoanalytiker ohne besondere berufliche Identität vorzustellen? [Is it utopian to imagine a future psychoanalyst without any particular professional identity?] *Forum der Psychoanalyse, 20*(2), 133–157.
Treurniet, N. (1997). On an ethic of psychoanalytic technique. *Psychoanalytic Quarterly, 66,* 596–627.
Tubert-Oklander, J. (2013). *Theory of psychoanalytical practice. A relational process approach.* London, England: Karnac.
Wachtel, P. L. (2008). *Relational theory and the practice of psychotherapy.* New York, NY: Guilford.
Wallerstein, R. S. (1993). On transference love: Revisiting Freud. In E. S. Person, A. Hagelin, & P. Fonagy (Eds.), *On Freud's 'Observations on transference-love'* (pp. 57–75). New Haven, CT: Yale University Press.
Zwiebel, R. (2004). Der Analytiker als Anderer: Überlegungen zum Einfluß der Person des Analytikers in der analytischen Praxis [The analyst as 'other': Thoughts on the influence of the analyst's personality in the analytical practice]. *Psyche, Zeitschrift für Psychoanalyse, 58,* 836–868.
Zwiebel, R. (2012). Von der Schwierigkeit Psychoanalytiker zu werden und zu bleiben [On the difficulty of being and remaining a psychoanalyst]. In C. E. Walker, H. Blass, R. Paul, & M. Teising (Eds.), *Die Psychoanalytische Haltung* (pp. 53–69). Frankfurt am Main, Germany: Congress-Organisation Geber & Reusch.
Zwiebel, R. (2013). *Was macht einen guten Psychoanalytiker aus? Grundelemente professioneller Psychotherapie* [What makes a good psychoanalyst? Basic elements of professional psychotherapy]. Stuttgart, Germany: Klett-Cotta.

Chapter 10
What Characterizes the Psychotherapeutic Stance?

The content of the psychotherapeutic stance is not defined in the sense that it can be reduced to a collection of techniques or methods that can be standardized; instead, it reflects a certain attitude to or way of experiencing, interpreting and relating to the patient and his or her issues and what happens in the therapeutic space, including the therapist's own subjective experiences and reactions in the interaction with the patient. The psychotherapeutic stance creates a unique therapeutic space and interpersonal field that do not in themselves dictate any specific topic or focus but serve as a platform for the psychotherapeutic work. Patient and therapist can work with virtually any topic (Küchenhoff 2013:369); the key is how it is handled and addressed, that is, how the therapist meets and relates to the patient, her material and himself. The psychotherapeutic stance reflects a certain view of humanity, mainly informed by humanistic values (see Jørgensen 2012:263ff). It is associated with a way of meeting the patient as an equal subject with the goal of cooperating with the patient on the shared task of enabling the patient to achieve a better understanding of herself, change the way she relates to others and, as much as possible, break free from the difficulties that caused her to seek treatment. The psychotherapeutic stance contains both predominantly intentional elements, which are central elements of the therapeutic method, and more subjective elements related to the individual therapist's basic approach to the world and his patients. It depends, to varying degrees, on the therapist's personality, implicit relational knowledge (see this chapter) and internalization of other therapists' work based on his own therapy, therapeutic training and supervision. Over time, this internalization gradually becomes second nature for the therapist, an almost natural (reflexive, nearly automatic) way of meeting the world and others, of course primarily (but rarely exclusively) in the therapeutic space.

Perhaps the most important and complex tasks, especially in long-term and more intensive psychotherapy, is to establish and remain in prolonged emotional contact with the patient while adopting and maintaining a basic psychotherapeutic stance to him or her, oneself (own subjective experiences and reactions) and everything that happens in the therapeutic space. Psychotherapists need to focus not only on specific and factual aspects, the patient's observable behaviour and the search for specific solutions to specific problems; they must also direct the shared attention at

C. R. Jørgensen, *The Psychotherapeutic Stance*,
https://doi.org/10.1007/978-3-030-20437-2_10

subjective experiences, mental states, interpersonal processes, (dynamic-relational) psychological dynamics underlying the patient's specific problems and, not least, what plays out in the therapeutic space here and now, including how key elements of the patient's difficulties are actualized in the interaction with the therapist (and with others outside the therapeutic space). Moreover, they have to make sure the work is driven by the long-term goals of the therapy, holding on to these goals throughout, also in situations with intense emotional drama or states of alarm, where a therapist might be tempted to focus solely on the specifics of the moment and thus lose sight of the patient's more basic problems thus the long-term therapy goals.

A patient who recently experienced a break-up (again) or who just had an intense conflict with her mother may seem very convincing in her insistence that the current situation is the most important issue in the world and should be the theme of the entire session. Although it is, of course, important to listen to the patient's current experience, the main therapeutic task will often be to explore, with the patient, how it contains repetitions of recurring experiences and patterns from the patient's life and to examine how these repetitions may be understood. Naturally, that also includes examining how the experience affects the patient, how she feels, here and now, as she describes it, and how that may re-enact certain mental states, difficulties with regulating certain affects, the activation of certain defensive strategies and so on. Why does the patient keep being abandoned, why is she involved in intense conflicts with others over and over again, and what happens in and to her in these situations?

10.1 The Main Elements of the Psychotherapeutic Stance

Fundamentally, the psychotherapeutic stance invites an equal subject-subject relationship, rather than a potentially more instrumental subject-object relationship, between patient and therapist. The therapist's psychotherapeutic stance is characterized by the following main elements:

(1) *Seeing and meeting the patient as an intentional subject.* A certain way of meeting and entering into a relationship with the patient, where the primary attention and focus are on the patient as a perceiving, experiencing and actively acting (intentional) subject, not on any quantifiable symptoms, deviant behaviour (specific diagnostic criteria) or biochemical brain processes (which should primarily be treated medically). The main task is to understand the patient's subjective experience and inner universe on the patient's own terms.

(2) *Seeing symptoms as meaningful.* The therapist receives, experiences, considers and understands what the patient says and does in the therapeutic space based on contemporary dynamic relational theory and a contemporary model of pathology (see Chap. 7), possibly a different psychological theory, provided it does not reflect an obvious reduction of the complexity of reality. The therapist meets the patient with the basic assumption that her presented difficulties—symptoms and, to an initial observation, dysfunctional behaviours, as

they are reported and demonstrated in the therapeutic space—are meaningful and potentially understandable manifestations of psychological (including interpersonal) dynamics in her past and present life and of her subjective experiences and mental states; that is, symptoms and seemingly dysfunctional, pointless or irrational behaviours have and/or have had a function in the patient's psychology (that is, they spring from meaningful reasons), which the patient and therapist can uncover in a shared effort.

(3) *Focusing on the borderland in between internal psychological and external reality.* The therapist must acknowledge that the patient has perceptions of self, others (including the therapist) and reality, while insisting that these ideas about reality—the internal psychological reality—are not necessarily objective reflections of, let alone identical with, actual (external) reality but may, to varying degrees, be generated or profoundly coloured by psychological factors, including anxiety and other mental states. Their shared attention is therefore directed at both the relationship between the patient's perceptions of self, others and the world in general (internal psychological reality) and the actual external reality and at the possible underlying reasons or motivations behind the patient's perceptions (internal psychological reality). The goal of the therapeutic work is not primarily to arrive at an 'objective' version of reality but, in part, to challenge and explore the relationship between the patient's (and the therapist's) internal psychological reality and the external reality. This also helps the patient take a step back from her (often pathologically distorted) perceptions of self, others (typically based on emotionally intense experiences with individual significant others) and reality and to take a fresh look at them from outside.

(4) *Containing and inviting reflection.* The therapist receives, contains and mirrors (verbalizes) the affects and other, at times intense, painful or frightening mental states that the patient comes into contact with and communicates in the therapeutic space. These are made the object of (eventually shared) reflection rather than being acted out in the form of exaggerated attempts to calm or comfort the patient or correct her perception of reality, perhaps driven by self-interest (for example, the therapist may comfort the patient because he cannot bear seeing her upset). Affects and other mental states in the therapeutic space are used as an entrance to understanding the patient's inner universe, difficulties, self-regulation strategies and relational patterns (cf. Kernberg 2016:216). As much as possible, the therapist's mirroring of the patient and her mental states should be congruent (consistent with what is mirrored) and marked (clearly distinct from and signalling the ability to contain and handle what is mirrored), as that in itself enhances the patient's ability to distinguish self from others, her sense of self or identity ('who am I?') and her perceived agency/autonomy.

(5) *Curiosity and genuine interest.* The patient is met with basic curiosity and interest in understanding who she is and the difficulties that made her seek treatment ('This is important. How can we understand this together?')—a curiosity and an interested wondering that opens the world and invites an explorative approach to the world, the unknown and the unexpected, rather than an approach driven by anxiety that closes off and looks for quick

(illusorily) clear-cut answers, and which rigidly holds on to a certain, often simplistic understanding of the world (Buechler 2004:27ff). The therapist's meeting with the patient in each session is not based on knowing ahead of time what is the patient's most urgent problem right now, or what the background is—a knowledge that simply needs to be conveyed to the patient—but on the notion that they can discover this together. The therapist seeks to establish a contact with the patient as a person, where the patient can feel seen and understood as a person, in contrast to an experience of being seen as an object, a diagnosis, a disorder.

(6) *Introducing new perspectives on the patient's reality.* The therapist makes himself available to the patient with his ability to observe her subjective experiences and difficulties from different perspectives, handling (tolerating and processing) conflicts between different, apparently incompatible, perspectives on reality and engaging in nuanced thoughts about her psychology, including what might be the dynamic psychological background of her presented symptoms, painful subjective experiences and maladaptive behaviour. Patiently, the therapist insists that reality, including the patient's difficulties and significant events in her past and current life, can be viewed from several equally valid perspectives—and he insists on exploring these different perspectives on reality together with the patient (see also Bateman and Fonagy 2016:183)—also when the patient initially maintains that there is only one way to understand a given experience or event (one—and only one—possible perspective). The therapist thus helps the patient recognize recurring patterns in her life and verbalize significant past and present experiences from different angles. This all takes place in an ongoing dialogue with the patient, where the therapist also seeks to arouse the patient's own curiosity to understand reality, with its complexity, and to have nuanced thoughts rather than resorting to impulsive acts or her existing (typically simplistic and rigid) interpretations of reality. For the therapist, this involves seeing, focusing on and perhaps insisting on working with what happens in the therapeutic relationship in the here-and-now, including repetitions of patterns from the patient's life (transferences) and any complications that arise in the therapeutic relationship (ruptures in the alliance). The therapist has to be prepared that the patient may sometimes be annoyed with this insistence on the complexity of reality and may find it much easier to hold on to her existing (simplified) interpretation of the world. Here, it is the therapist's responsibility, in a friendly but firm manner, despite the patient's resistance, to maintain the effort to arrive at a more nuanced understanding of the complexity of reality.

(7) *Listening to multiple channels of communication from a position of not knowing.* The therapist not only listens to what the patient communicates through verbal communication but also listens for nonverbal communication, including what may not be communicated, because it has, for various reasons, been excommunicated from the patient's conscious, perhaps due to anxiety, shame or fear about how it might be received by the therapist and others. In this process, the therapist has to remain aware that explicit verbal communication can in some cases act as a diversion or a defence against coming into contact

with and becoming aware of painful, unrepresented, dissociated and possibly unbearable experiences. What the therapist believes to hear and notice is verbalized (with consideration for the patient's current functioning level) and is made the object of common reflection and processing. With a view to maximizing his openness to the patient's unconscious and his ability to listen, the therapist should at times, as proposed by Wilfred Bion, strive to meet the patient from a position without memory (focus on previous events and statements), desire (own wishes, needs or goals) and (pre-conceived) comprehension (Symington and Symington 1996:166ff, see Chap. 9). Although this ideal can never—and never should—be fully achieved, it is an excellent reminder in the ongoing effort to remain open and receptive in the meeting with the patient and (at times) allow the spontaneous therapeutic process to unfold, also at the later stages of the therapy where it may be tempting to think that one has already grasped the full story—a notion that may diminish the therapist's openness and curiosity in the meeting with the patient. This may be described as a professional not-knowing stance characterized by openness, curiosity and a fundamental scepticism towards the perceived certainty, relief and sense of security that typically accompanies a seemingly quick ability to understand and explain complex clinical challenges (Leuzinger-Bohleber 2007:968); moreover, it reflects the therapist's faith in the therapeutic process—a belief that the process will take us to a place where we will work on something that is important to the patient, and that we can find meaning and understanding together, even if it may look difficult at times and may take time. This is not a specific technique but a certain way of being in the therapeutic space and of listening to and meeting the patient (Bonaminio 2008:1111). To assume this not-knowing position in the meeting with the patient sometimes, the therapist has to be able to tolerate being in such a position, with the risk it entails of (temporary) perceived confusion, disorientation and powerlessness, without resorting to acting or being overwhelmed by expectations of knowing exactly what to do that most people (in a sense, justifiably; but only in a sense, when it comes to some aspects of the psychotherapeutic work) associate with the position of a treatment professional and expert.

(8) *Attending to underlying and recurring themes.* The therapist listens to and is continuously attentive to possible underlying or recurring themes in what the patient says and in what plays out in the therapeutic space (including transferences and countertransferences) in the individual session, possibly across sessions, with a view to piecing together (creating links) and generating a coherent and meaningful understanding of what may be the dynamic-relational core of the patient's difficulties. This includes attending to what are the most emotionally important or urgent aspects in the patient's material (see below). Based on an assessment of the patient's current functioning level (are the patient's emotional arousal and anxiety levels so high that it is wise to postpone?) the therapist determines if, or rather when, this should be made the topic of their shared attention. For example, the patient may bring up that she misses having a boyfriend, and gradually a picture seems to emerge that it is fear about the powerful feelings and the desire she comes into contact with

when she gets close to a man (and, to some extent, people in general) that makes her run away. Thus, she moves in and out of situations with emotional closeness—a pattern that also plays out in the therapeutic space, where the patient, on the one hand, says that she needs to talk about emotionally intense experiences she has had in the contact with others and then, on the other hand, soon 'runs off' (tries to change the topic, dismisses it as unimportant, says 'I don't know,' 'I don't remember' and so on) when the conversation turns to these experiences. When that happens, it is an important therapeutic task to verbalize the underlying theme and how it also appears to play out in the therapeutic space. The patient's verbal self-narratives, descriptions of specific events and explicit messages about what is the core content of her material are not taken at face value as objective descriptions of reality but as expressions of the patient's perspective on and subjective experience of the described issues in the present moment, which may be coloured by her need for reality to be or appear in a certain way. Similarly, the patient's desire for certain reactions from the therapist or for the therapist to have a certain image of her may influence what she says and brings up, and how she addresses it. As a way of handling this, it may in some cases be helpful to explore key aspects of the patient's narratives with a focus on what happened specifically and in detail in the situations the patient brings into the therapy, that is, what the involved parties specifically said and did and, not least, what emotions and other mental states and interpersonal processes were at play in these specific situations.

(9) *Focusing on emotionally central elements of the narrative and the here-and-now.* When the patient talks about her experiences, the therapist's focus is not only on the specific content but also on what is most emotionally important, how the patient feels as she is talking, and what it does to her to tell the therapist about certain experiences; the patient's subjective experiences and mental states take centre stage. Thus, the therapist's interest is far from limited to what the patient is saying but also includes what the patient is experiencing—what is 'happening' in the patient here and now—while she talks, and how she speaks and tells her story. Talking about significant experiences can thus initiate processes on several levels. The patient may get into renewed contact with the described experiences, and she is opening up and may thus make herself vulnerable to another person, which might activate themes related to trust, fear of being seen as 'wrong' or weak and so on. The focus is more on emotionally central aspects and mental states than on specific behaviour in the patient's descriptions and narratives (see also Bateman and Fonagy 2016:182f). Also, the therapist continuously looks for links between any descriptions of past events and the patient's current life and processes in the therapeutic space (cf. above). However, the therapist should strive to avoid getting lost in general or very detailed narratives about the patient's distant past. The primary focus is on the patient's current relationships, mental states, symptoms and difficulties—not their possible roots in a distant past that we can only, at best, have access to (re)constructed images of, which may be coloured by both subsequent experiences and current needs. On the other hand, of course, that does

not mean that it is impossible to work with any traumatic experiences in the patient's history and their potential impact on her current life. This may include, for example, the patient's difficulties with developing trust and engaging in more intimate relationships (as a consequence of past abuse, betrayal and so on), severe dependence on others (related to experiences with powerlessness, loneliness) or urge for control (related to frightening experiences involving loss of control and so on). In the work with past traumatic experiences, the key focus is on how they influence the patient's current life and functioning. Finally, as mentioned earlier, one should notices whether any parts of the patient's self might have been split off and are therefore excluded from her narratives.

(10) *Continuously attuning interventions to the patient here and now.* The therapist intervenes with a sense of timing and attunes interventions to the patient's current functioning level and needs. The therapist applies well-developed responsiveness in his work with the patient (see below). Among other things, this implies that the psychotherapeutic stance cannot be standardized or reduced to a set of specific guidelines for 'correct' therapist behaviour, as the actual manifestation of the psychotherapeutic stance must always be attuned to the individual patient and her current state. What is the optimal actual realization of the psychotherapeutic stance right now always depends on a wide range of factors in the given situation, and it is the responsibility of the therapist (based on his professional and personal judgment) to capture, assess and accommodate this in his interventions and ways of relating to the patient (see the section below on good judgment).

(11) *Incorporating own mental states and reactions in his understanding of the patient.* The therapist relies on his own (internal) subjective experiences, emotional fluctuations (mental states) and reactions (countertransferences) in the therapeutic space as an important way to understand the patient. This is done with the awareness that these may also, to varying degrees, spring from strictly personal factors, and that it is therefore important to pay attention to the borderland between objective and subjective countertransferences (see Chap. 11). Thus, the therapist has to notice which aspects of his own experiences and reactions in the interaction primarily offer insight into the patient (current mental states and so on) and her interpersonal style (recurring patterns in interpersonal interactions), and which relate primarily to his own internal dynamics and personal issues. When the therapist is emotionally affected by what the patient says and does in the therapeutic space, he should not try to suppress or dismiss the reaction but use it as a valuable therapeutic tool. This involves using one's own immediate thoughts, urges, emotions and other mental states in the therapeutic space as therapeutic material, that is, as indications that one's own psychology and inner life resonates with the patient and thus may contain valuable information about the patient's inner life and difficulties and about current themes in the therapeutic work. The psychotherapeutic stance thus not only describes how the therapist relates to the patient but also how he relates to his own thoughts and reactions, which should not be viewed as neutral or

objective interpretations of or reactions to reality but as subjective objects in the transitional space (or 'the potential space', cf. Winnicott 1971:50ff) between the internal psychological reality and the concrete external reality, which may be viewed from different perspectives and made the object of shared reflection (can be 'played with', ibid.) in the therapeutic work (Bollas 1987:206). See also Chap. 11 about the use of the countertransference.

(12) *Considering own actions and reactions as efficacy factors.* The psychotherapist (consciously and unconsciously) uses his own (external, manifested) reactions—his own behaviour and way of being—in the interaction with the patient as part of the therapeutic intervention and strategy, which may enable emotionally intense corrective experiences for the patient in the therapeutic space—experiences that disprove the patient's negative perceptions of self, others, interpersonal relations and the world in general. This means disproving the patient's existing (typically negative) perceptions and providing experiences that may, over time, alter the patient's object relations, internal working models and implicit relational knowledge for handling relationships (see Chap. 4) and 'detox' the patient's often painful self-criticism. More specifically, this means that the therapist seeks, to varying degrees, to attune his way of relating to and acting in the interaction with his patients to the diverse patterns that have shaped the patients' past life and to the individual patient's needs for certain types of corrective experiences in the therapeutic relationship. Based on an understanding of the interpersonal patterns that dominated and played a maladaptive role in the individual patient's life—developed through exploration in connection with assessment and the therapeutic work—the therapist strives to engage in the interaction with the patient in a way where he avoids participating in a repetition of these patterns in the therapeutic relationship and instead offers a corrective to the patient—and over time helps the patient recognize those aspects of her perceptions of and emotional reactions to the therapist and others that are irrational and not adapted to the current reality. This should happen in a way where the therapist remains authentic and does not seek to convey any particular emotions (that he does not have) or play a certain role in the contact with his patients (that he cannot identify with). The latter naturally limits what types of patients one will be able to help (see also corrective emotional experience as an efficacy factor, Chap. 4). Through the way he relates to the patient the therapist becomes a model for changes in the patient's (internalized) perceptions of and way of treating oneself. Thus, over time, for example, the open-minded and tolerant therapist who meets the patient as an equal, intentional subject can help the patient become more open-minded, tolerant and accepting of herself and to begin to see herself as an intentional subject rather than a worthless object. Similarly, showing nurturing interest in the patient's body (cf. the patient's often inadequate self-care or objectifying treatment of herself and her body) can help change the patient's perception of and way of treating her body. That

may be of particular relevance and importance when working with patients with eating disorders and other types of self-harm. The therapist appears as a clearly defined person who thinks out loud and communicates clearly about psychological processes and mental states. The therapist's more personal qualities (way of being in the therapeutic space and in the interaction with the patient) are important for this element of the psychotherapeutic stance.

(13) *Recognizing and validating the patient's subjective experiences and perceptions.* The therapist meets the patient in a way that recognizes and validates his or her subjective experiences and perceptions, psychological reality and perspective on reality as true to him or her. He avoids entering into a position where he confirms or disproves the patient's perceptions or subjective experiences from a normative perspective. The main task is to help the patient attain a richer and more nuanced perception of self, others and reality (Mitchell 1997:96). The primary mechanism of change in this context is not that the therapist addresses the validity of the specific content of the patient's subjective experience or begins to offer reality correction; instead, it is that the patient encounters a significant person who recognizes her legitimate right to exist and have her own perception of reality. Generally, thus, the therapist should strive to suspend any urge to normative-moral evaluations of what the patient says and instead communicate his empathic understanding of what it is like to be the patient and seek to see reality from his or her perspective. This understanding should ideally be backed up with reference to specific events and mental states in the patient rather than merely taking the form of general and abstract declarations of the type 'I understand'—an understanding and a validation that may also introduce possible cause-and-effect chains, link mental states and behaviour and different experiences together and thus enhance the patient's internal integration. 'If you perceived your boyfriend's silence as a sign that he was going to leave you, as I see it, it makes sense that you became so scared and desperate that you went into the kitchen and cut yourself.' Later, perhaps, one may invite the patient to consider other possible ways of understanding the specific situation: 'I know it's hard for you to handle when your boyfriend is silent, because it reminds you of unpleasant experiences earlier in your life. But I wonder if his silence might be understood in other ways than as a sign that he is going to leave you?' (With reservation for the possibility that some patients may, for example, experience silence as an unbearable expression of a lack of contact and thus a sense of abandonment, of ceasing to exist, where it is not therapeutic to shift the focus to the other's possible intentions). Perhaps supplemented with, 'Sometimes it also makes you nervous when we are silent here; I wonder if there might be a connection?' The patient's feeling of being understood by the therapist strengthens the therapist's perceived authority and the patient's general epistemic trust in what (see Chap. 4) the therapist communicates (Allison and Fonagy 2016:290); this in turn improves the chance of positive transferences and thus strengthens the therapeutic alliance. Although

the therapist should generally avoid moral or normative evaluations of what the patient says, there may be situations where he should deviate from that approach—for example when the patient is severely self-harming, poses a risk to herself/others or is involved in a profoundly destructive relationship, and the patient, for various reasons, is unable to protect or even show a minimum of nurture for herself (or any children she may have). Here, it should be remembered that 'good parents' (and the more mature superego) are not just moralistic, oppressive and restrictive but also contain elements of loving care for and protection of the self in situations when the self has trouble protecting and looking after itself—a position and a task that the therapist should, in some situations, temporarily take on or represent in the therapeutic space.

(14) *Being a participant observer.* The therapist should continuously alternate between (I) participating in and experiencing how parts of the patient's inner life, object relations and implicit relational knowledge are actualized in the therapeutic relationship and (II) apply an analytical gaze on this, including exploring his own experiences, emotional reactions and mental states (countertransferences) in the interaction with the patient. The therapist lets the patient's behaviour, projections, transferences and perceptions influence his own self and emotions while simultaneously taking a step back to register and reflect on the fact that this is happening. The therapist adopts the position of a participant observer, where (a) the experiencing, receiving and (b) the analytical, structuring and meaning-making perspective on what plays out in the therapeutic space are both kept distinctly separate and continuously integrated. This requires the therapist to strike a balance between, on the one hand, being authentically present as a fellow human subject and, on the other hand, exercising professional self-discipline. When the therapist takes a step back to observe and analyse, he must always do so within a framework where the patient feels seen and recognized as an equal subject, which helps protect the patient against an experience where the therapist is perceived as not only observing and analysing but also judging the patient for her self-perceived flaws, shortcomings and inadequacies, especially in comparison with the temporarily idealized therapist. In particular, patients with attachment disorders can be vulnerable in a situation where the therapist takes a step back and marks a form of separateness from the patient.

(15) *Being present and accessible as a person in the contact with the patient.* The therapist must be authentically present as a person, a subject, and invite the patient into psychological closeness and emotional contact. The therapist should strive to be open to and ready to seize the openings for emotional contact and the authentic intersubjective or interpersonal meeting ('moments of meeting', see Chap. 11) that arise spontaneously in the therapeutic space, instead of rigidly adhering to a more formal contact and standardized guidelines. Meanwhile, the therapist has to stay within

the boundaries of what characterizes a professional contact (see Chap. 1) and essentially maintain the other elements of the psychotherapeutic stance. This involves remaining open to—and continuously aware of developments in—one's own emotional and bodily sensations and reactions in the therapeutic space. They often reflect one's affective resonance in the interaction with the patient and may thus enable a new and deeper understanding of the patient (Stern 2004:223). Important elements of this contact and mental resonance may play out in the nonverbal communication, including facial expressions, breathing, posture, self-touching (stroking one's hair, picking at fingernails, touching wounds/scars after self-injury and so on), shifting in the chair, eye contact and others types of nonverbal contact. In the therapeutic space, a similar continuous (implicit) procedural dialogue, which relates in part to—and may teach the patient—what it means to be in psychological and emotional contact with another person (and oneself), including how to act in such a contact (Beebe and Lachmann 2014:71f). Hence, the therapist should be aware what is playing out in these aspects of the interaction with the patient, without necessarily verbalizing it in the moment (as verbalization may shift the focus to the verbal communication and thus contribute to closing down the procedural dialogue). Similarly, the therapist has to remain aware that especially more fragile patients may experience these moments of intense emotional contact and psychological closeness as quite overwhelming and may thus subsequently need help to organize, process and understand what is happening, and what they experience in this contact.

Precisely because the psychotherapeutic stance cannot be standardized but can only be articulated as a general approach to and way of thinking about and understanding the psychotherapeutic work, and because the individual therapist's person inevitably has a significant influence on what plays out in the therapeutic space, each therapist must find his only personal style and 'voice' in the specific manifestation of the psychotherapeutic stance—a style that in some regards will vary from patient to patient and over time, as the individual patient inevitably influences the therapist and sets the conditions for his contributions.

The Therapist Makes Himself Available as a Subject and 'Is Used'

The ability to establish and maintain a psychotherapeutic stance—also in long-term psychotherapy with more severely disturbed patients, where it may at times come under heavy pressure—is a fundamental psychotherapeutic meta-competence that frames and is a condition for the intended effect of more specific interventions. On an emotional level, it requires the therapist to be able to tolerate conflicts, silence, anger, loneliness, emptiness, anxiety, grief, mental anguish, lack of appreciation and, at times, very personal attacks from the patient as well as other burdensome or painful mental states in the therapeutic space without fundamentally abandoning the psychotherapeutic stance in favour of a different role or a different type of relationship with the patient. The therapist should strive to contain and hold the patient, make himself available to the her, show patience and remain calm—also when the therapeutic work involves contact with intense emotions and experiences. He has to be ready to 'show his own mind': in his efforts to understand the patient he should strive to make his own subjective experiences, emotions and other mental states clear to the patient, including his doubts and thoughts (cf. Bateman and Fonagy 2016:190). That requires honesty, authenticity and taking ownership of one's own experiences but also having a 'mature character' and a firm ethical foundation, just as one should have a fairly good psychological functioning level. Here too, there is reason to point out that the therapist's more personal qualities are crucial for the psychotherapeutic work and for his ability to adopt and maintain the psychotherapeutic stance, as it is outlined above—although this should not, on the other hand, be understood as a superhuman demand for perfection that no one, or very few people, could ever live up to. Everyone inevitably makes mistakes and at times find it difficult to maintain the psychotherapeutic stance, which is not normally a serious problem in itself, provided one acknowledges and subsequently takes it in hand. Someone who is far from having the personal qualities that are a condition for practicing intensive psychotherapy should not be in charge of psychotherapeutic work.

Winnicott (1971:102ff) writes that the therapist should allow himself to be used and 'destroyed' as an object by the patient. According to Winnicott, the act of making oneself available for the patient and 'surviving' any attacks from her on one's person, professional capacity and the therapeutic stance (framework and technique) is crucial for the patient's development process, especially in the work with patients with more severe pathology. Attacks may take on many different forms, including being ignored by the patient, devalued, cut off from emotional contact or perceived as irrelevant or incompetent. Alternatively, the patient may test whether the therapist is able to contain and survive her anger, desperation, instability or impulsivity ('Can I trust you to handle me, can you stand your ground, and will you stay with me when I freak out or show you how damaged I am?').

Patients who for much of their lives have learned that emotional contact is associated with betrayal, abandonment and violation of their boundaries, and who gradually feel a growing trust and a hope that emotional contact may lead to something other than betrayal, abandonment, boundary violations and mental anguish may find themselves in a difficult situation. Should they give up their previous self-protection strategies (keeping their distance, attack or break off contact in the face of growing emotional closeness) and revise their previous perception of others, or is that too risky? Will they need to hold on to the defence mechanisms they know and rely on, even if they cause them to be lonely and yearn for contact? As an element in attempting to handle this difficult situation they may test the therapist in a variety of ways in order to discover whether relationships may actually be so very different than they thought. Are there really others who can contain her, like her and show her kindness, even when she is herself and reveals sides that she herself does not like?

This may be seen as an opening to corrective experiences, where it is important that the therapist passes the tests. In this process, the therapist may doubt whether he is, indeed, a good-enough therapist. He may doubt his ability to contain and help the patient, where the very fact of 'surviving', containing or overcoming this doubt sets the patient free to use the therapist and the therapy as a basis for developing (Ogden 2016:1250), exploring and unfolding her individuality, her 'true self' and her own psychological reality, the way a child uses the parents in his or her development process.

The therapist must refrain from acting out any, perhaps, superficially interpreted, understandable, urge to counterattack or become defensive in the face of perceived attacks from the patient, perhaps via seemingly correct but poorly attuned (subtly devaluing, attacking, controlling, defensive and so on) interventions. For the patient to be able to use the therapist as an object, the therapist has to be present and visible as a subject who is emotionally affected by the patient and their interaction but who still remains clearly separate from her and maintains his personal and professional integrity (cf. Greenberg and Mitchell 1983:196f) as well as the psychotherapeutic stance. There has to be emotional contact between patient and therapist, and the patient has to experience that she matters to the therapist, without the therapist becoming overwhelmed, emotionally destabilized or regressive in his psychological functioning level for long. The therapist must not appear as a subjectless 'technician', let alone an unaffected container to the patient's (projected) perceptions and thus an extension of the patient's self; he must remain clearly identifiable as a reel external other, a human subject (person) that the patient can use, spar with and generate new experiences in interaction with (Ogden 2016:1245). This also implies that the therapist may at times become 'situationally disturbed' (knocked off balance) by what plays out in the therapeutic relationship (Gorkin 1987:74).

The very fact that the therapist is visibly affected and survives the patient's attacks constitutes him as an external object that is separate from the patient and her perceptions of the therapist and outside the patient's omnipotent control. The therapist emerges as a separate and real person in his reactions and his ability to survive as a separate subject when the patient attacks and uses him to satisfy her own needs or (unconsciously) tests her own perceptions of reality and others (Winnicott 1971:106f). As part of this, it may in itself be educational for the patient to observe how the therapist reacts to and processes what happens in the therapeutic space. This may also include interactions where the patient experiences that the therapist survives her dependency, greed and (in the patient's own experience) destructive and harmful influence on anyone who gets close to her—an experience that may help to revise her maladaptive self-perception, founded in earlier relationships.

Respecting and recognizing the patient's subjectivity, uniqueness (unlike reducing the patient to a psychiatric diagnosis), autonomy and dignity are among the core values underlying the psychotherapeutic stance. The therapist meets the patient, takes an interest in and empathizes with her experiences and universe without trying to impose his own norms, values and ideals on her, where symptoms and deviant behaviour are not simply reduced to a disorder or dysfunction, but are also seen as potential expressions of the patient's subjectivity and attempts to protect the self. This approach enables her to use the therapist to experience and explore her own individuality, her true self; she is able to experience her psychological reality on her own terms and at her own pace (Treurniet 1997:603). In the therapeutic space, the patient ideally has the opportunity—perhaps for the first time in her life—to be in a relationship where she does not have to sacrifice or hide her true self to preserve the relationship but is free to discover what it means to be oneself in a relationship, without having to pay a price in form of consistently satisfying the other's needs or being afraid to lose herself, alternatively lose the other and go back to being alone (feeling lonely and so on). As a former borderline patient described what she experienced in the relationship with her therapist (slightly abbreviated): 'I've been able to be myself and show you every side of myself, even the ugly ones. You have accepted me without me having to give you a lot back or constantly needing to devote all my energy to "go inside you" and read your needs. So now it's much easier for me to accept myself.' Maybe what she is saying here is that she experienced being able to connect with another person without having to give up herself or her identity and separateness.

As human beings we develop our subjectivity—'we become human'—by being seen and treated as subjects, as unique individuals, by significant others—an experience that the patient should have in the therapeutic space. Similarly, the patient should be able to see the therapist as a subject, a person, which enables the development of the patient's capacity to empathize with and understand other subjects and their inner life, motivations, affects and other mental states; conditions for engaging in mature subject-subject relationships. The therapist's coherent and stable psychotherapeutic stance helps create a therapeutic atmosphere and a secure base in the therapeutic space, where the patient, together with the therapist, can explore herself, her own internal and relational life, others' mental states and acts and recurring maladaptive patterns in the way she relates to the world. The psychotherapeutic stance contributes to a secure atmosphere in the therapeutic space that gives the patient optimal conditions for experiencing and talking about her difficulties (and resources) and addresses them psychotherapeutically, in part by taking a step back from her difficulties, with the therapist's help, and trying to understand and think nuanced thoughts about her difficulties (and resources), in contrast to merely talking about her problems and release pent-up emotions (achieving brief catharsis), as it is often possible in a good and close (but not psychotherapeutic) interpersonal relationship.

The Therapist as a Participant Observer

The authors of classical psychoanalytic works in particular imagined that the therapist would be able to occupy a neutral position outside the interpersonal field of the psychotherapeutic space, from whence he would observe the patient, including the way she interacts with the therapist, and intervene from a sort of objective, uninvolved position. That is neither possible nor desirable, however. As described in contemporary (two-person) relational psychology (see Table 8.2) the therapist is inevitably involved in what happens in the therapeutic relationship, which opens unique opportunities for understanding the patient and her way of engaging in interpersonal interactions. Before we can verbalize and begin to consider the patient's relational and other difficulties (mainly related to the procedural rather than the declarative memory), these have to be enacted, that is, repeated in the therapeutic relationship, where the therapist strives to contain, digest and begin to verbalize what he or she sees in the therapeutic space. The psychotherapeutic stance thus helps bridge the gap between these two 'realities'—between the internal reality in the form of non-conscious interaction patterns (implicit relational knowledge), perceptions of self and others (ego-identity, Jørgensen 2008, 2009), self-regulation strategies and the symbolic space where we can verbalize, reflect on and begin to understand the recurring patterns and self-regulation strategies that so far have shaped the patient's life 'behind her back' in the external reality (Dantlgraber 1989:991).

It is an important element of the psychotherapeutic stance that the therapist occupies a position as a participant observer in and of the interpersonal field in the therapy, where everything that happens between patient and therapist as well as in the patient and the therapist, here and now, can and should in principle be used to understand the patient and her difficulties (see above). This is also one of the most demanding tasks in psychotherapeutic work, because the therapist has to be in sufficiently close emotional and psychological contact with the patient to be able to empathize emotionally with her emotions and her inner universe in general; at the same time, the therapist also has to be able to achieve sufficient distance from the patient (and own reactions, own resonance) to arrive at a clear understanding of her (and his own reactions), her situation and how the interaction with her, in the present moment, reflects aspects of her difficulties, personality functioning and general psychological functioning (cf. Greenson 1967:279). The position as participant observer combines an internal and an external perspective on the patient's unconscious and core difficulties, as they are manifested in the therapeutic space.

The therapist uses himself and his own emotions, reactions, subjective experiences and countertransferences in the interaction with the patient to understand and explore the patient's inner psychological life and unconscious, while simultaneously seeking to conceptualize, think about and thus objectify the patient's unconscious and pathology, as they are manifested in the therapeutic space by drawing on available treatment theory, pathology, developmental and personality psychology and so on. This balancing act cannot be put on a formula or reduced to an array of specific techniques. An attitude that is too detached and analytical would risk jeopardizing the empathic contact with the patient by eroding the necessary subject-subject relationship and thus the basis of the psychotherapy. On the other hand, if the therapist is too empathic and personally (over-)involved in the patient and her difficulties, he risks being emotionally flooded and losing the necessary analytical distance as well as the psychotherapeutic stance. This sort of over-involvement and lack of boundaries in the contact with the patients is not only unprofessional and risks the collapse of the psychotherapeutic space; it also carries a real risk of over-burdening the therapist and thus leading to burn-out.

The therapist's role as participant observer breaks with traditional—illusory—ideas about the therapist as a detached, objective and neutral observer who gathers and analyses information about the patient without being present as a subject or influencing what plays out in the therapeutic space, 'the observed'. As mentioned earlier, the therapist's interaction with and openness to being influenced by the patient provides an invaluable source of information about the patient and her difficulties (Mitchell 1997:74f). Moreover, as mentioned, it also gives the patient the experience of affecting and influencing the therapist's actions and reactions in the therapeutic space, which enhances the development of the patient's perception of herself as an actor in her life and in the world.

Varying Manifestations of the Psychotherapeutic Stance

As mentioned, the psychotherapeutic stance is not defined by a particular content; it is not a specific technique where the therapist has to say or do anything in particular, unlike what is often, to varying degrees, the case in manualized specific therapeutic methods. It is not a specific activity but instead a certain way of being in the relationship and relating to what happens in the therapeutic space, which cannot be standardized or developed solely via theoretical studies. The psychotherapeutic stance brings nuanced psychological thinking and multiple possible perspectives into the understanding of the patient, including the fact that psychological phenomena can have multiple meanings and functions and stem from an interaction between many different factors. In doing so, it seeks to avoid the pitfall of an overdetermination of human experiences and behaviour (Schafer 1983:8). The psychotherapeutic stance is not a permanent fixture in the sense that, once established, it will necessarily endure or find the same specific expression throughout. In principle, the psychotherapeutic stance has to be re-established at the beginning of each session as soon as the patient and therapist have settled in and are ready to begin the therapy. The 'margins' of the session—when the patient has just arrived to the therapist's office, before the session begins, just after it ends, and until the patient leaves the office again—constitute a kind of transitional zone where what happens cannot, or can only partially, be characterized as psychotherapeutic work; the relationship has a different character, and the therapist does not similarly deal with what happens in a psychotherapeutic manner. In these transitional situations, the therapist should endeavour not to appear artificial or inauthentic or rigidly hold on to his role as psychotherapist and instead temporarily step into something that is closer to an everyday relationship with the patient.

Just as the therapeutic process is in constant motion, the specific manifestations of the psychotherapeutic stance will also vary throughout. Both patient and therapist may, for various reasons, be tempted to turn the therapeutic relationship into an 'everyday' relationship, where the therapeutic task is pushed into the background in favour of a more enjoyable chat and exchange of pleasantries, where the therapist may for example resort to only living out the position as the good, non-frustrating and non-demanding object, which in the moment is more pleasant for the patient, but which does not help to bring about change. Many patients would like to get rid of their problems as quickly as possible, ideally through a quick-fix that is not too painful or too taxing in terms of requiring them to confront painful experiences, unacceptable aspects of the self or contact with powerful emotions. In relation to this issue, it is the therapist's responsibility to confront the patient with the fact that dealing with more severe psychological difficulties often takes a hard and prolonged therapeutic effort.

Especially in working with patients with severe relational difficulties, the therapist should appear as both a new and a familiar object to the patient. The therapist should (temporarily) enter into the role he is offered by the patient, while at the same time being different enough and able to break out of this role in a way that, on the one hand, does not lead to the patient being scared off by meeting a therapist whose behaviour is radically different from anything she knows and is able to handle and, on the other hand, provides new relational experiences that can help correct her existing perceptions of self, others and interpersonal relationships. If the therapist openly rejects the assigned role, refusing to accept and contain the patient's transferences, projected aspects of self and mental states, there is a risk that the patient will feel misunderstood, threatened and insecure and might break off the therapy. In order for the patient to have new experiences and integrate them into her existing perceptions of reality there has to be an appropriate balance between familiar and novel elements. Although it may seem paradoxical, it can be emotionally overwhelming and frightening to feel seen and understood and to experience intense emotional contact for someone who has never had that experience before, or who associates being seen with being abused; or having contact with subsequently being abandoned, exploited or having her boundaries violated. Juggling these different roles requires considerable flexibility from the therapist and, not least, a certain ability to determine what the individual patient needs in the moment and to attune his approach accordingly. That contains a number of paradoxes or seemingly contradictory demands to the therapist and the therapeutic stance, as described by, among others, the German psychoanalyst Zwiebel (2004:843f, 2007:47f).

Zwiebel (2004, 2007) has argued that the psychotherapeutic stance contains certain bipolarities, where the therapist continuously has to find the right balance in the way he relates to the individual patient. At the same time, he has to be able to contain these apparent contradictions and the complexity associated with working with psychotherapy, particularly long-term psychotherapy with more severe disorders. He has to be authentically present as a person and gratify some (especially emotional-relational) needs in the patient while maintaining his professional position, including the competent use of different interventions and attuned frustration of some of the patient's needs. The therapist should both invite dialogue and reciprocity (symmetry) in the therapeutic relationship and preserve a certain authority and the option of asymmetry when necessary.

On the one hand, the therapist should avoid having specific goals for the patient, holding back to see what the patient brings into the therapeutic space, and on the other hand, he should keep an eye on the overall goal of the therapeutic work, pursuing it and actively structuring the work, maintaining focus on certain themes when needed, and things are difficult. The therapist should remain open-minded and curious and meet the patient with a humble, not-knowing, inquisitive attitude, without, on the other hand, denying that he actually has considerable knowledge about and experience with psychological disorders, psychotherapy and what people with psychological disorders may need in various situations. The not-knowing attitude signals openness and invites dialogue. It is very different from ignorance. The patient knows more about what he or she thinks, feels and experiences than the therapist does, regardless of the therapist's lengthy training and experience. Assuming the role of the expert who fully comprehends the nature of the patient's problem raises the risk that both the therapist and the patient stop thinking.

Threats to the Psychotherapeutic Stance

Being in this complex area can be difficult and taxing for the therapist, and he should be prepared for the relatively frequent occurrence of what Zwiebel (2004:845) calls ‘problematic situations’, where he temporarily loses his capacity for listening to the patient in a balanced manner and becomes (too) focused on uncertainty, not-knowing, ambiguity and internal contradictions in what plays out in the therapeutic space. He gets tense and may have feelings of mild anxiety, guilt or shame over not (yet) knowing how to understand what is happening in the therapeutic process, and how best to handle it (failing to live up to his own professional ideals). Alternatively, the therapist may feel powerless, empty, inadequate, isolated (without contact with the patient) and lost in inner phantasies or forced and unproductive pseudo-reflection. This may be combined with observing the problematic situation, trying to take action to handle the problem by implementing insufficiently thought-out interventions, or with a mental state (countertransference) characterized by a vague sense of inner turmoil, bodily tension or emotional arousal without a readily discernible source (Zwiebel 2004:852).

Regardless how these problematic situations specifically manifest in the therapist, it is important to maintain the psychotherapeutic stance—also in relation to one’s own reactions—allowing the problematic situation to play out while preserving the necessary calm, patience and faith that it will be possible to reach an understanding of what it is happening. In the few cases where it proves impossible to achieve an understanding, and where the problematic situation endures and develops into an impasse in the therapy, it may be necessary to seek supervision. Generally, access to competent supervision is a key condition for safeguarding the therapeutic space, the psychotherapeutic stance and the therapist’s mental balance and ability to think nuanced thoughts (preserving ‘a mind of one’s own’) under pressure.

As mentioned, both patient and therapist may feel the urge to convert the therapeutic relationship into a personal, intimate one, especially in long-term and more intensive therapy, or to simply allow the psychotherapeutic process to transition into less demanding, supportive conversations, which are more pleasant for both parties. For the therapist, this may be related to an ambivalence towards the psychotherapeutic stance, which may make it tempting to adopt a more comfortable and less demanding attitude, and towards countertransferences and his own unmet needs that are pushing to be lived out or satisfied in the therapeutic space. When this happens, it is absolutely crucial that the therapist maintains the therapeutic stance and avoids acting on these recurring dynamics in the therapeutic relationship (this is particularly true for urges to convert the therapeutic relationship into a personal, intimate one) and instead uses them as a basis for verbalizing and understanding the patient and his or her relational needs and dynamics (‘Why won’t you give me what my parents never gave me?’, ‘Why won’t you be the close friend or partner that I never had?’, ‘Why can’t you give me the hugs I need but never had?’ and so on), supplemented with necessary reflections on his own potential contribution to and personal involvement in the dynamics that emerge (‘Why is it so difficult for me to preserve my professional boundaries with this patient?’, ‘Why is it hard for me to adopt a position as the demanding and frustrating object with this patient?'). The therapist thus has to remain aware that the psychotherapeutic stance is vulnerable, both because it may be challenged or even attacked (devalued) in various ways by the patient, and because of the therapist's own possible ambivalence towards the particular way of relating that is associated with the psychotherapeutic stance towards the patient and towards what plays out in the therapeutic space, including the possibility of one's own internal conflicts and unmet needs being actualized and triggering an urge to abandon the psychotherapeutic stance (Löchel 2013).

It may thus be tempting for the therapist to give into the patient's potential wish and his own urge to convert the relationship into one that is essentially non-therapeutic, in part because it may feel like a release of the inner tensions in the therapeutic relationship, as Zwiebel (2007:47f) has described. It may also be perceived as a way to create a more comfortable and uncomplicated relationship with a higher degree of pure symmetry and reciprocity—a relationship where the therapist can live out any unconscious desires or phantasies of being the pure and unwaveringly good object that does not frustrate the patient or make demands but simply accommodates the fragile other's immediate needs (perhaps connected to more or less unconscious phantasies of being able to cure the patient with limitless love). The main problem is that in the long run, this is completely incompatible with maintaining the psychotherapeutic stance, and in its more radical forms (involving personal, intimate contact) it is ethically unacceptable.

If the therapist abandons the psychotherapeutic stance for prolonged periods, the therapeutic space will collapse, and it will no longer be possible to carry out psychotherapeutic work; at best, the relationship may lend itself to supportive conversations or various types of counselling. Abandoning the psychotherapeutic stance for short durations—for example just before and after a treatment session, when the real relationship can move to the foreground (the therapist partially steps out of his role as a therapist and is authentically present with other self-aspects)—is not in itself a problem, just as it may, in certain situations, be relevant to advise the patient on how he or she might handle a specific problem (particularly patients with a weak social network). That may actually help the patient to see, in glimpses, other aspects of the therapist and encounter him or her as a normal person who contains other sides than the ones that are expressed in the psychotherapeutic space.

On the other hand, the psychotherapeutic stance is so important in the therapy, not only because it serves a crucial purpose in the process in itself, but also because it helps the therapist delimit himself and thus maintain his integrity and ability to hold on to himself and his professional role. It is important to be able to preserve the reality principle and the therapeutic framework, also when intense emotions and primitive (immature) object relations dominate the therapeutic space, or when the therapist and the psychotherapeutic stance are attacked by a patient who wants a different kind of relationship and demands immediate gratification of certain needs instead of engaging with difficult experiences and trying to understand herself better or taking on the demanding task of being in therapy (Köhler-Weisker 1986:144f). The psychotherapeutic stance can thus help the therapist set his own personal identity and life apart from what happens in the therapeutic space, although he remains—and must remain—emotionally and (in a sense) personally involved in the therapeutic work and in the interaction with the patient.

Personal Qualities

As a basis for adopting and maintaining a psychotherapeutic stance, the therapist has to have a number of interconnected personal qualities, social skills and professional and methodological competences (cf. Koch 2013:25f). The more personal qualities and social skills shaping the ability to practice psychotherapy include the following, among others (see also Chaps. 7 and 11):

- A well-developed ability to focus systematically on the patient's needs, relational patterns and mental states. Well-developed empathy or emotional resonance.
- A good and stable mentalizing capacity, a capacity for dynamic and psychological thinking—also in situations characterized by emotional arousal and interpersonal conflict.
- An ability to be personally (authentically) present in the contact with a wide range of patients and a sense for when it is possible to communicate which subjective experiences to which patients and how, with a view to using these experiences in the therapy—an ability that is closely linked to having a sensitive ethical compass and a keen sense of personal boundaries, one's own as well as the patient's.
- A sense of humour and ability to laugh at oneself and tragicomic elements combined with a well-developed sense for when it is fitting to invite or accept a humorous angle on what the patient says and what happens in the therapeutic space. The humour must never be sarcastic or in other ways mean in relation to the patient, just as the therapist must never laugh at the patient, only with him or her. This includes an awareness that humour, especially irony, requires a high level of mentalizing, and that not everyone is capable of playing with multiple meanings of verbally communicated messages, which is a condition for using humour (see Knox et al. 2017; Valentine and Gabbard 2014).
- Personal tolerance, which, among other things, is a condition for the ability to accept and respect a wide spectrum of patients, who may have lives, histories and values that are quite far removed from one's own personal life and experiences.
- Affect tolerance, an ability to contain and manage (regulate) a wide range of affects and mental states, including intense ones, that the therapist will encounter in working with different patients. More severely disturbed patients in particular often find it difficult to contain themselves and their own mental states, which makes the therapist's ability to tolerate, contain and reflect on affects without acting them out particularly crucial. One of the characteristics that set competent therapists apart from most patients is the ability to experience a wide range of affects and mental states, including the same affects and mental states as the patient, but less intensely and in way that lets them be used as a basis for reflecting on and understanding the patient instead of being acted out or flooding the therapist's psyche.
- An ability to contain and manage interpersonal conflicts and interpersonal and psychological complexity, also in situations where the therapist may feel personally offended, unfairly criticized or misunderstood by the patient. Especially in

working with severely disturbed patients, including patients with personality disorders, it is essential that the therapist is able to contain and avoid acting out the powerful negative reactions that may arise when painful interaction patterns from the patient's relationships are actualized in her interactions with others in the form of, for example, intense idealization or devaluing of the therapist (Castonguay and Beutler 2006:358). A low tendency to take offence (a thick skin) and the ability to avoid taking powerful transferences and projections personally are thus key qualities for the psychotherapist.

- A consistent awareness of own needs, desires, impulses, norms (prejudices), phantasies and urges that might disturb the therapy process unless they are registered and managed by the therapist. A well-developed capacity for (self-)reflection and self-insight.
- An emotionally and otherwise fairly satisfying life outside the therapeutic space that may help protect the therapist against acting out inclinations to satisfy emotional and other needs in the interaction with the patients. This in no way implies that the therapist should deny how profoundly interesting and personally rewarding it can be to work with psychotherapy.
- A fairly balanced professional and personal self-confidence and a capacity for self-criticism and for containing criticism from others, examining one's own (unavoidable) missteps and learning from them, including a realistic assessment of one's own personal and professional strengths and weaknesses.
- Endurance, persistence, inner calm and curiosity about human psychology and relational processes. Engagement in others and an ability to adapt (one's therapeutic style, one's language) to a wide and diverse range of patients, including sudden shifts in their current states and needs.
- Continuous attention to own reactions to the patient and the patient's communication in the therapeutic space, which may negatively influence the therapy process and outcome if they are left unreflected and acted out, but which may also hold valuable information about the patient's difficulties if they are decoded and used in a reflected manner. On a more general level, this is associated with balanced self-regulation and self-control.
- An ability to register and work with shifts and developments in the therapeutic relationship and alliance that may be related to the actualization of the patient's object relations and the repetition of patterns from the patient's interpersonal relationships. An ability to strive to understand the underlying meaning and background of the patient's actualized and communicated mental states, relational patterns and desires, which, in part, requires the therapist to remain continuously updated on the newest and best (what is presented as the newest knowledge is far from always the best or the best-founded knowledge) scientific knowledge about what might play out in and complicate interpersonal interactions, including how people tend to repeat patterns and difficulties from earlier relationships in their current relationships and in the relationship with the therapist (cf. Strupp 1986:519).
- An ability to form trusting relationships and a secure base for the patient, which is the condition for any form of therapeutic work with difficult issues.

The therapist's personal development and the development of his or her more personal qualities with key relevance for the therapeutic work, including selecting the right candidates to practice psychotherapy in the first place, constitute perhaps the most important and most overlooked factor in the field of psychotherapy today (cf. Coughlin 2017:10), dominated as it is by a focus on specific technical competences and the narrow acquisition of standardized treatment methods. More specifically, it implies that psychotherapists must undergo therapy themselves, and that they must have the opportunity to learn from the practice of skilled therapists in their field. Moreover, supervision should always include attention to the therapist's own emotions, own mental states, internal conflicts, defences, perceived needs and urges and personal limitations. Psychotherapeutic practice also requires certain more professional and specific methodological (more technical) competences, such as:

- Theoretical knowledge of psychopathology, general psychology, psychotherapy and the latest empirical research findings of relevance to the practice of psychotherapy and, not least, an ability to translate this theoretical knowledge into an understanding of specific patients, issues and the contribution of contextual factors in the individual case.
- Knowledge of, experience with and an ability to implement a wide range of psychotherapeutic interventions.
- Ability to establish a psychotherapeutic space and defend it against threats or attacks from the patient, the therapist or (therapeutically problematic) organizational-bureaucratic requirements.
- Ability to read, contain and verbalize the patient's mental states in the present moment and to link them to the patient's behaviour.
- Good timing and an ability to solve specific (interpersonal and other) problems that arise in the therapeutic space.
- Attention to and an ability to decode nonverbal communication, including facial expressions, body language, variations in tone of voice and so on (see this chapter).
- Ability to decode the patient's defence mechanisms, as they are manifested here and now in the therapeutic space, and to assess when it is appropriate to direct shared attention at them versus refraining from doing that out of concern for the patient's emotional balance (arousal level and preserving the patient's ability to thing).
- Ability to communicate with both clarity and nuance.

As human beings, we tend to react to others' appearance and behaviour based on a collection of basic ideas about what is right and wrong, what is socially acceptable or unacceptable behaviour in a given situation and how people ought to live and be. These ideas are informed by a certain worldview and certain ideas about human ways of living. Here, it makes a big difference what intentions we attribute to others as the basis of their behaviour, as it is typically much easier to tolerate and accept acts that may seem unacceptable, strange or morally offensive if we believe them to be motivated by what we perceive as understandable reasons (cf. Nida-Rümelin 2016:253f). The psychotherapeutic attitude towards the patient differs, in that ordinary social norms and ideas about what is socially acceptable behaviour are to some extent suspended in the psychotherapeutic space, which gives the patient a high degree of latitude to say just about anything to the therapist without the therapist taking it personally, reacting with moral outrage or otherwise punishing or judging the patient.

Psychotherapeutic practice gradually builds experience with containing many different kinds of people, mental states and behaviours, just as it trains the therapist to think nuanced thoughts about the virtually endless number of motivations people may have for acting in a certain way or for perceiving themselves and the world the way they do. The therapist is trained in linking the patient's actions with his or her subjective experiences, mental states and internal psychological dynamics, which makes it easier to contain the patient's communicated experiences and behaviour. Even if the psychotherapist regards his patients as (to varying degrees) freely acting and morally responsible subjects, he does not hold them morally responsible for what they say and do, the way they would be outside the therapeutic space. The main task in the therapeutic space is not to hold the patient morally to account or to act on what the patient says or does in the therapeutic space, but rather to make sense of and understand the background for the patient's behaviour and experiences. This is a unique characteristic of the psychotherapeutic space and of the psychotherapeutic stance.

10.2 Aristotle—Qualified *Phronesis*

Is psychotherapy a craft or a scientifically informed discipline? And if we were to define it as either one or the other, what would that mean, what does that mean for the education and evaluation of psychotherapists? It is far from simple to answer questions such as these, which have roots in ancient Greek philosophy, where Plato emphasized scientific and intellectual understanding as the basis of practice, while Aristoteles was more interested in experiential wisdom and a more craft-based approach to the world and to practice (Nida-Rümelin 2014:88f). The key in this context is that the two cannot be separated: the good psychotherapist needs both theoretical scientific training and good judgment based on personal development and experience. Unfortunately, our late modern society and educational institutions are predominantly focused on scientific theoretical and verbalized knowledge and on the development of standardized and, broadly speaking, technological methods for solving well-defined problems that can be standardized, while knowledge forms that cannot be similarly verbalized, standardized and evidence-based—such as the knowledge underlying the experienced psychotherapist's good judgment and ability to establish and repair a therapeutic relationship with patients with severe attachment disorders—do not enjoy anywhere near the same status in our educational institutions.

As explained in previous sections, psychotherapy can be said to unfold on two fundamentally different levels at once: a largely action-oriented and technical level and a level that is more based on personal processes or subjectivity. At the technical level, the therapist uses a number of methods that are, to varying degrees, standardized and specific in order to make a diagnosis, assess the patient's functioning level and establish a therapeutic framework, a formalized cooperation with the patient and so on, just as the therapist relies on a number of technical interventions directed at the individual patient's main difficulties. To a large extent, the therapist may acquire these competences of a more technical nature via formalized training, although their optimal specific implementation in the therapy naturally requires good judgment and sensitivity, which go beyond what can be formalized.

The more personal level of psychotherapeutic practice involves the authentic meeting between patient and therapist as two equal human beings that cannot be planned or controlled via formalized rules or techniques. It is a meeting that goes beyond their formalized roles as patient and therapist. It depends to a high degree on the therapist's good judgment, emotional responsiveness, context sensitivity and other, more personal, qualities that do not similarly lend themselves to being developed or learned via formalized education or training but are primarily developed via interpersonal contact, personal and professional experience and contact with persons (experienced, competent therapists) with well-developed judgment, sensitive responsiveness and so on (cf. Stehr 2017:257ff). Even if the therapist's more personal involvement in, sympathy for and dedication to the patient is not part of his formal job description, by all indications, the more personal level of the therapy is absolutely crucial for the course and outcome of therapy.

In a culture dominated by globalization, the competition state and technology fetishism, education tends to be dominated by the idea that students should primarily acquire specific competences and tools that can immediately be translated into specific problem-solving in the labour market. Meanwhile, more open concepts of knowledge—the idea that it may be worthwhile to acquire knowledge that cannot be immediately linked to specific competences and problem-solving tools—may be perceived as an inessential, unproductive luxury, 'a road to nowhere', that we cannot afford (Zakaria 2015:15f). Large sections of our late modern society are increasingly dominated by a largely instrumental approach to knowledge and education, where we overlook that education should do much more than simply fill up the student with specific knowledge and problem-solving methods; perhaps it should primarily teach students to think, make nuanced assessments of diverse situations and choose among different options. This includes the development of good judgment and a nuanced sense of what happens in and between people and, to some extent, learning elements of craft-based knowledge.

Becoming a competent psychotherapist thus takes more than completing a formalized professional therapy training programme with a focus on acquiring general theories and specific technical skills. Prospective therapists should also study social science, the humanities, including classical and modern art, different cultures and, perhaps not least, fiction and drama, which contain some of the most nuanced descriptions of human psychology and what can happen in interpersonal relationships (Greenson 1967:403; Freud 1926/1959:280f; Mar et al. 2006). Some aspects of the professional therapist's knowledge thus have a different character than scientific and empirical knowledge; it has a large element of 'lived' knowledge that cannot be readily verbalized but is actualized in the specific situation (Zwiebel 2007:90). For example, empathic understanding depends on a nuanced sense of the other that emerges spontaneously in the situation as a form of actualized emotional responsiveness or involvement in the other's inner life and state. Moreover, knowledge of scientific psychological theory can of course, to a considerable degree, expand and add nuance to the therapist's empathic understanding of his patients.

One of the challenges related to craft-based or tacit knowledge is precisely that it is, to some extent, tacit, unverbalized, which makes it harder both to convey and to test (Polanyi 1966). However, it is not impossible, for example, to get a little closer to articulating what the psychotherapeutic stance involves. The present book, hopefully, serves as an illustration of this point. We also need to take a critical look at technical rationality (Schön 1983:21ff) and the related notion that science will be able to come up with technical answers to all human problems; a mindset that increasingly dominates late modern society. There is reason to challenge the widespread notion that the practice of clinical psychology should be centred on the implementation of science-based technical solutions, where positivist epistemology is infused into professional practice (Schön 1983:31).

Clinical practice is inevitably characterized by unpredictability and an absence of clear-cut answers to what is the one correct solution to complex problems (informed by the very notion that there is one, and only one, correct solution). The psychotherapist has to be able to contain and handle this anxiety-provoking uncertainty (Kemmis 2012:152), in part by approaching it as a cause to reflect, rather than perceiving uncertainty as a threat and its admission a sign of weakness (cf. Schön 1983:69). On the one hand, we can never offer a detailed prediction of the course of the psychotherapeutic process, just as it will never unfold in accordance with a prior plan; for that, interpersonal interactions are far too complex. On the other hand, it is the therapist's responsibility to establish a psychotherapeutic space and a therapeutic process that promote the patient's development (Stehr 2017:260). In this effort, the therapist's practice must be framed by the psychotherapeutic stance and adhere to general ethical and technical therapeutic guidelines for psychotherapeutic practice.

In his principal ethical treatise, *The Nicomachean Ethics*, Aristotle (2009:102f) writes, 'And let it be assumed that there are two parts which grasp a rational principle—one by which we contemplate the kind of things whose originative causes are invariable, and one by which we contemplate variable things.' He similarly distinguishes between theoretical and practical wisdom, which, broadly speaking, correspond to our scientific knowledge and human judgment, common sense or *phronesis*. Although Aristotle's reflections primarily concern ethical and political issues, they also have relevance for our understanding of what is required for practicing psychotherapy, that is, how practitioners need to be able to reconcile or integrate theoretical-scientific knowledge and personal judgment.

As a species, human beings are capable of attaining objective insight into the world, including into aspects of human psychology and psychological disorders, via the sciences. And as individuals we have the capacity to develop into rational beings with good judgment, capable of using intuition and reflection to achieve a goal without having to rely on a manual. According to Aristotle, wisdom is the most perfect form of knowledge, and the wise person has both acquired scientific knowledge and developed good judgment, which is used, in part, to translate this theoretical knowledge into practical action in specific situations (see also Chap. 7). Wisdom 'must be intuitive reason combined with scientific knowledge' (Aristotle 2009:108). Having theoretical knowledge of what is 'the right act' is not same as being able to perform it in practice in the given situation; that takes the right character and a number of more personal qualities. It takes practical wisdom and judgment to be able to translate theoretical insight into the right actions—a character and a sense of judgment that some people, but far from all, will be able to cultivate, to varying degrees, with training and experience.

Thus, there is a difference between being able to state universal principles and empirical research findings and knowing them or internalizing them in a way that lets them be converted into rational and thoughtful action in the given situation. Thus, 'while young men become geometricians and mathematicians and wise in matters like these, it is thought that a young man of practical wisdom cannot be found. The cause is that such wisdom is concerned not only with universals but with particulars, which become familiar from experience, but a young man has no experience, for it is length of time that gives experience' (ibid.:110). With Aristotle, then, we can say that young psychologists, psychiatrists and prospective psychotherapists rarely have the wisdom—the experience, inner calm and firmly founded judgment—required to practice psychotherapy at the highest level. However, they may be able to develop these qualities via training and experience.

With regard to interpersonal relationships and what plays out in the psychotherapeutic space, what is the right action cannot be determined once and for all, across different individuals and situations; it cannot be standardized. It is therefore up to the individual in the specific situation to use his or her reason and make the right decision about what needs to be done. It is thus far from sufficient for someone who wants to work with psychotherapy to have theoretical scientific schooling, although that is a necessary condition for practicing therapy in a qualitied manner. According to Aristotle (2009:109), someone who is without theoretical scientific schooling and knowledge of the rules guiding the proper action, who instead has experience, practical wisdom and nuanced knowledge of particulars may in some cases be more effective in practice than someone who merely possesses theoretical knowledge of the rules for the right action. 'Therefore we ought to attend to the undemonstrated [not scientifically validated] sayings and opinions of experienced and older people or of people of practical wisdom not less than to demonstrations; for because experience has given them an eye they see aright,' as Aristoteles (2009:113f) puts it. This recommends that qualitative researchers examine and seek to specify what it is that experienced and exceptional psychotherapists have to offer, and what they do in their therapeutic practice (see Chap. 7). Further, there is reason to respect experienced therapist's psychotherapeutic skills, developed over many years of psychotherapeutic work, even if they may not be able to verbalize their skills, let alone have credentials from years of scientific schooling. Finally, there is reason to be critical of the radical empiricist idea that all scientific understanding rests on empirical data alone (Nida-Rümelin 2006:27), for example in regard to a book such as the present that seeks to define and explore the psychotherapeutic stance.

Sensitivity to Context and Individual Cases

Thus, to be converted into highly qualified actions in practice, it is necessary to combine theoretical scientific knowledge with judgment and experiential insight into the given practice, that is, into the many subtleties and special concerns that are inevitably at play in the individual case, and which cannot be put on a formula. The specifics of what is the best way to help another human being deal with psychological difficulties cannot be deduced from universal principles or technologized guidelines for what is, theoretically, the correct act/intervention, even if these guidelines may be helpful on a general level in the sense by shaping and qualifying one's reflections on what to do. Human behaviour in specific situations will always be influenced by a large number of internal and external conditions in the given situation, which renders them inherently unpredictable. The same is of course also true of the patient's behaviour in the therapeutic space, which makes it similarly impossible to predict or formulate detailed general guidelines for the therapist's response. Even the most detailed guidelines would not even get close to predicting what is going to happen in the therapist's interaction with the patient; hence, they cannot be used as detailed instructions for the therapist about how to handle a specific situation with a specific patient. The psychotherapeutic stance offers a general framework or structure for how the therapist should relate to and understand what happens in the therapeutic space, in specific situations and in interaction with the individual patient. In that sense, the psychotherapeutic stance may serve as a kind of basic structure or framework for the therapist's judgment.

A person with good judgment knows a great deal about how to do the right thing in the right way and at the right time, based on a nuanced and correct assessment of the facts (Flanagan 1996:63). Therapeutic judgment and practical wisdom in the therapeutic work constitute an ability to determine exactly when to do what, and how. Knowing what to do in a given situation also involves being able to determine when not to implement a strategy that is normally effective. It is the ability to distinguish, to avoid simplistic and unreflected generalizations and to activate and apply one's general knowledge in the given case based on a nuanced understanding of the unique nature of the present moment and context. Judgment is rooted in an ability to reflect, think nuanced thoughts and consider before taking action, in contrast to acting impulsively or in accordance with standardized procedures that only involve a limited capacity for independent thought.

Good judgment is an ethically framed intellectual virtue, which is variable and context-sensitive, not a form of knowledge that can readily be made explicit and directly passed on to others. The risk is that we begin to perceive good judgment as a form of knowledge that can be formalized and conveyed via conventional teaching formats rather than an ability to think and carry out nuanced evaluations that is primarily developed in the meeting with practice. Knowing that therapeutic practice requires the use of Socratic questions or the stimulation of the patient's mentalizing capacity is one thing; knowing or being able to determine exactly when and how this should be done in the work with this particular patient, with his or her unique characteristics, is something else entirely and much more complicated. Among other things, that involves a conscious or non-conscious (more intuitive) assessment of what the patient needs right now, how to avoid acting in ways that the patient may perceive as a repetition of maladaptive interaction patterns from his or her past life, and how specific interventions are attuned to the patient's current functioning level.

For example, the therapist must have a sense of the individual patient's tolerance for anxiety and continuously pay attention to the patient's current anxiety level as a gauge for the degree to which the patient feels exposed and threatened in the present moment (Dantlgraber 1989:979). The patient's anxiety level is part of the therapist's basis for determining how to intervene in the moment—where a more supportive, holding and validating intervention is needed to lower the patient's anxiety level, or whether there is a basis for a more explorative intervention, perhaps with a focus on what is happening in the therapeutic relationship here and now, which the therapist knows from experience can raise the patient's emotional arousal and anxiety level. All these decisions defy standardization and can only be based on the therapist's judgment and practical wisdom.

This process also includes an evaluation of what is the core of the individual patient's difficulties, which requires both extensive theoretical knowledge and disciplined judgment and the ability to differentiate between what is important and what is not important in the specific situation (including in what the patient is displaying and saying in the here and now), where the therapist has to weigh a variety of factors and concerns in the specific situation and make a balanced decision. This stands in contrast to the disorientation and the tendency to a mindless adherence to formalized rules or guidelines that may be the result when the therapist is not able to see 'what is at stake.' Even if some patients have a single, well-defined problem (diagnosis), where there may be some justification for pointing to certain tried-and-tested treatment methods, that is far from the norm. The typical patient, especially at the more severe end of the psychiatric spectrum, has multiple comorbid disorders and difficulties that are not readily delimited, just as behavioural symptoms and disorders that manifest in a similar manner may have fundamental differences in aetiology and underlying psychological dynamics that call for different interventions and therapeutic strategies. For that reason too, the therapist's good judgment and ability to define the unique core(s) of the issue in the individual patient and intervene on this are crucial for the course and outcome of the therapy.

The therapist's judgment is associated with a capacity for nuanced assessment of novel situations, which in principle occur constantly in the therapeutic space, where the therapist has to draw a considered connection between the general and the specific. In practice, that means a well-considered application of general knowledge in the given situation that considers the unique aspects of the individual patient and of the situation. These assessments provide the basis for the therapist's balanced decision concerning how best to help the individual patient. Good judgment thus also involves an awareness of the vulnerability of universal principles, theoretical knowledge and empirical research findings in the encounter with clinical practice, which is often more complex than the general categories that are used, for example, in quantitative psychotherapy research (Hibbert 2012:65). It takes strong judgment to be able to translate universal principles to the individual patient and therapy.

Equanimity

It could be argued that *phronesis*—equanimity and judgment—also includes the ability to register and allow emotions and other mental states to be present in oneself, reflect on what they reveal about oneself, others, the current situation or the world and, not least—by exercising judgment—determine what to do with these emotions and mental states. Should the therapist act on them, and if so, how? Should the decision serve good, long-term goals rather than immediate needs gratification or impulsive acting out (cf. Schmitt 2012:49)? This aspect of human judgment is essential for the therapist's work in the therapeutic space.

Judgment requires an ability to contain and acknowledge the complexity of reality, to consider the greater context and to contextualize the diagnosed problems, including refraining from acting out immediate urges and instead weighing various concerns before taking action (Nida-Rümelin 2015). It is necessary to pause and examine the situation before deciding what to do. This points to the importance of equanimity—the willingness to consult with others when necessary, which is based on an awareness of one's own strengths, weaknesses, personal boundaries and limitations, and taking the necessary time to make optimal decisions rather than focusing on quick decisions and quick results. Of course, it may sometimes be essential to act quickly, for example if a suicidal patient walks out in the middle of a session, or if escalating conflicts in a group threaten to turn into physical violence or otherwise become destructive to the therapy. It also requires a recognition of the limits of one's own competencies and a willingness to identify and work towards rectifying professional deficits (Sellman 2012:116). Moreover, the practitioner's judgment may be enhanced through a realistic understanding of the way in which organizational conditions and formalized requirements outside his or her influence frame and potentially constrain the practice.

Some have perceived Aristotle's concept of *phronesis* and the exercise of human judgment as a way to escape the abstract, rationalistic, potentially inhumane and technical rationale and approach to the world that characterized aspects of modernity in favour of a more holistic, experiential and practice-oriented thinking (Radke-Uhlmann 2012:3). That would be a simplification, however, as the qualified exercise of judgment requires factual knowledge and a capacity for rational thinking. It is thus an illusion to imagine that it might be possible to realize our practical reason by jettisoning theoretical scientific knowledge and approach to the world. The art lies in combining the two: theoretical and practical wisdom. Transferred to the craft of psychotherapy, this means that qualified therapists need both theoretical scientific training and the development of good judgment, which enables them to translate the theoretical scientific and practical knowledge in qualified specific acts in practice, with an eye for nuance and the unique characteristics of the specific situation and in the individual patient. This may also be described as an ability to contextualize one's knowledge, that is, to interpret and translate knowledge into practice in light of a nuanced decoding of the specific situation. Practical reason is built on sand if one does not know what to look for, or what it means, due to incomplete factual knowledge about the practice context (Radke-Uhlmann 2012:8). In that sense, practical and theoretical wisdom, factual knowledge and judgment, are inextricably linked. In the therapeutic space, neither aspect can find a qualified expression without the other.

The art lies in striking the right balance between, on the one hand, the necessary disciplining of the therapist's practical wisdom and judgment, based on factual knowledge and familiarity with formalized guidelines (in contrast to the unbounded and thus unqualified creativity, where 'anything goes') and a capacity for critical reflection on these and, on the other hand, maintaining a large space for the individual therapist's creativity, judgment and professional decision-making (in contrast to the uninhibited urge to control the individual therapist's work by means of standardization and formalized guidelines for 'the right treatment', which undermines the therapist's creativity). The therapist has to find a balanced position that avoids, on the one hand, a mindless insistence on the veracity of a particular theory and the use of certain categorizations and standardized methods in the meeting with all patients and, on the other hand, an insistence on the unique character of the individual patient and the therapeutic meeting and the unassailability of the hermeneutic method to a degree where common scientific knowledge and therapeutic recommendations are disregarded as irrelevant and useless, because they are seen to fail to capture the uniqueness of each patient. The psychotherapist's absolutely necessary 'intelligent disobedience' (Pollmann 2005:9) in relation to standardized guidelines for psychotherapeutic work rests on strength of character, a firm grasp of factual knowledge and well-developed judgment and should not be dictated by a purely emotionally motivated disinclination to follow rules and guidelines or unqualified impulsivity in the therapist's actions in the therapeutic space.

On the other hand, it is important to bear in mind that practicing psychotherapy requires strong personal and ethical qualities—the development of an ability to see, understand and take qualified action in interaction with people in need. This requires, among other things, the ability to imagine others' experience and perceptions—an empathic ability to see reality from someone else's perspective—and a capacity for dynamic and psychological thinking. The therapist has to acknowledge, recognize and be open to his or her own vulnerability, which is also a reflection of a fundamental human vulnerability and may help to inoculate the therapist against contempt for weakness, fear of the unfamiliar, unknown and irrational and the tendency towards cynicism and dehumanization of others that may emerge as a form of self-defence when people are under prolonged pressure (Nussbaum 2010:10f), for example when they work in severely understaffed healthcare institutions. The therapist who is open to his or her own vulnerability and more primitive sides is better equipped to imagine and register what is happening in the patient.

In light of this, it is obviously problematic that our current educational institutions are increasingly focused on ensuring that students accumulate knowledge and specific technical skills as quickly as possible, while the development of personal qualities and good judgment receives less and less attention. The emphasis is on the ability to reproduce theory and empirical findings and to solve simple specific problems using various techniques that are fairly simple to operationalize and test, while more personally embedded skills, including good judgment and social skills, which are crucial for psychotherapeutic practice, are pushed to the periphery in an education system that is increasingly driven by the goal of bringing the students through to graduation and into the job market with a certificate in hand documenting that they have passed certain formalized tests of their ability to reproduce theory and empirical findings. We need therapists with theoretical, scientific and technical skills as well as personal judgment. Currently, however, our education systems and the prevailing understanding of psychotherapy are characterized by a serious imbalance between, on the one hand, the development of judgment and personal qualities (*bildung*) and, on the other hand, the acquisition of theoretical knowledge, scientific methods and technical competences. This imbalance stems from an overly one-sided focus on the latter, on the development of technical competences, the acquisition of scientific methods (predominantly from the health and natural sciences) and (sadly, to a lesser degree) theoretical knowledge, at the cost of the individual therapist's personal development (*bildung*) and professional judgment.

The development of therapists' ability to think—of their judgment—requires an institutional culture in our educational and healthcare institutions that prioritizes nuanced thinking (Hibbert 2012:69)—institutions with the space and time for the individual therapist's judgment to develop and be exercised without being seriously constrained by rigid demands for short-term efficiency and for adherence to formalized guidelines or the use of specific methods in the treatment of patients with specific diagnoses.

10.3 Responsiveness

The American psychotherapy researcher William Stiles (Stiles et al. 1998; Stiles 2009) has described what he calls the therapist's responsiveness, which is a key condition for any kind of psychotherapeutic work, regardless of the specific choice of therapeutic model. Responsiveness also represents a common therapeutic factor and is an element or a manifestation of the therapist's judgment. Responsiveness may also be viewed as a psychotherapeutic meta-competence in the sense that it deals with the therapist's ability to apply therapeutic methods with the proper timing and sense for what the individual patient needs here and now. Responsiveness is thus not a specific therapeutic technique that can be manualized but a specific manifestation of the therapist's empathic capacity and judgment. This means that the therapist varies his or her approach to the patient and his or her choice of specific interventions depending on the specific patient, situation and context. In addition to sensitivity and empathy—the ability to read the patient's current state and needs—responsiveness requires a high degree of self-regulation, in the sense that the therapist has to be able to regulate what he does in the interaction with the patient to attune to the patient's current state and needs and thus help her, also in situations with high conflict and arousal levels.

Responsiveness is related to the therapist's sensitivity to the patient's strengths (psychological resources) and weaknesses (deficits), which may vary considerably over time and with the specific context. Responsiveness may, for example, involve the therapist attuning aspects of his or her interpersonal style to the individual patient's attachment pattern (cf. Hardy et al. 1998) and matching the choice of treatment strategy and specific interventions and the regulation of psychological and emotional closeness in the therapeutic relationship in the moment to the level of maturity in the patient's defences (cf. Despland et al. 2001), ego strength and current mentalizing capacity (Bateman and Fonagy 2006:154ff). More specifically, for example, this may mean that the therapist meets a patient who is very emotional and easily emotionally overwhelmed in a different way than a patient who tends to be more intellectualizing and protects herself from getting into contact with difficult emotions by means of rationalizations and a one-sided focus on cognitive aspects in her perception of reality; the former patient needs the therapist to be more structuring and to encourage rational thinking, while the latter needs the therapist to try to activate her attachment system and stimulate more emotional reactions in the therapeutic process. The goal is to enhance the integration of the patient's cognitive and emotional 'knowledge' about reality and thus help the patient to achieve a more nuanced, deeper and more complex understanding of the world.

In relation to this point, Bateman and Fonagy (2016:197f) speak of 'contrary moves', where the therapist, through his actions in the interaction with the patient, seeks to improve the balance and integration in the patient's approach to the world by doing and inviting different responses than the patient is used to in his or her interactions with the world. It may also involve stimulating a patient who mainly sees others' needs and perspectives on reality (focused on understanding others) to become more aware of and pay attention to his or her own needs and perceptions of reality (understanding him/herself) by systematically focusing their shared attention at this in the therapeutic space. Similarly, when working with more self-centred patients, who are primarily aware of their own needs and perceptions of reality, the therapist may at times insist on also focusing the shared attention on how others might perceive reality, and what needs others might have. Further, there may be a need for the therapist to wonder aloud and introduce a doubt if the patient appears very convinced of the 'truth' of his or her own (rigid) perceptions of reality, while there may, conversely, be a need to promote and validate some of the patient's perceptions of reality, self and others when working with patients who are plagued by profound insecurity and a lack of confidence in their own sensations and experiences. Here, too, the therapist devises a strategy and picks an approach in the meeting with the patient that is attuned to the individual patient and based on a nuanced understanding of how this particular patient functions and what he or she needs.

Responsiveness also implies that empathy is not always manifested only by being friendly and accommodating towards the patient, it may also be necessary to be more confrontational and insist on maintaining a focus on themes that are difficult and painful for the patient. Any notions that the therapist always has to be the good and explicitly nurturing person who never subjects the patient to anything that might be difficult or, at times, painful may thus be countertherapeutic and be nourished by the therapist's own difficulties with giving up the position as the 'unwaveringly good object', who never does anything that might hurt or be difficult for others, even if it may be necessary for the sake of realizing more long-term goals. This issue is related to the challenge that any therapeutic stance, approach and technique, including the position of the (unwaveringly) friendly and empathic object, risks being used defensively to satisfy the therapist's own needs and protect the therapist from anxiety-provoking situations. That is also why the therapist's responsiveness and ability to decode the individual patients current state and needs and, not least, attune the interventions accordingly are so crucial for the therapeutic process.

The timeframe for the therapist's display of responsiveness may range from a few seconds to a complete therapy process, from minor adjustments in the therapist's way of meeting the patient in the present moment to the choice of general treatment strategy and patient-therapist matching (Stiles et al. 1998:440f). The therapist's responsiveness is thus expressed in the ongoing assessment of the patient and what plays out in the therapeutic space, the adherence to a treatment strategy that is attuned to the patient and his or her difficulties and resources (including mentalizing capacity, anxiety and frustration tolerance) and intervening in ways that are aligned with the patient's current state and need. The therapist's responsiveness is thus related to his or her ability to determine when (timing) to do what and exactly how and to the continuous attunement of what he or she does in the interaction with the patient based on the development of the therapy—the therapeutic process—and the patient's state, including what the patient needs in the here and now.

Three aspects of the therapist's empathy are closely related to responsiveness in the meeting with the patient (Hatcher 2015:748f): (1) The therapist's affective response in the interaction with the patient, based in part on his general emotional responsiveness and his ability to read and sense the patient's current emotional state, (2) the therapist's ability to take on the patient's perspective on the world and use it as a basis for understanding the patient's experience, situation and inner universe and (3) the therapist's capacity for self-regulation, which may be necessary to avoid maladaptive acting out in handling the emotional arousal and stress that may result from entering into what is sometimes a severely traumatized universe with profound mental anguish and dysfunctional relationships. These aspects of empathy are necessary for the therapist to be able to read what the patient is experiencing, how the patient feels (his or her emotional balance in the moment) and what the patient needs. Hence, they are a condition for the therapist to act responsively in the interaction with the patient.

Responsiveness is related to the fact that human behaviour is normally influenced by the context where it is played out, including the characteristics and behaviour of the persons we interact with in the moment. In that sense, not only the therapist but also the patient is responsive, which implies a possibility of mutually reinforcing feedback loops in the patient-therapist interaction. Patient and therapist will inevitably influence each other. The opposite to responsive behaviour is the ballistic action (Stiles et al.1998:440), which is pre-determined (standardized) and is carried out independent of feedback and the current context (with no use of context-sensitive judgment). For example, the inexperienced or incompetent therapist may inadvertently intervene in a way that is inherently ballistic and unresponsive when he says something to his patient that is the more or less verbatim repetition of a suggestion in a manual or from his supervisor without the necessary consideration for the specific patient's current state and needs, including that the specific intervention that might have been helpful in the previous session (which was the basis for the therapist's discussion of the process with his supervisor) is not necessarily appropriate the next session, when the patient is likely to be 'somewhere else', as the therapeutic process moves on.

It is difficult to imagine a successful psychotherapy conducted by a therapist who merely initiates these ballistic actions. Good psychotherapy requires responsiveness, where the therapist's clinical decisions are informed but not specifically determined by knowledge in a manner that is independent of the current context and which trumps the therapist's qualified assessments in the present moment—a context-sensitive, rather than a ballistic (pre-determined) use of knowledge. Most of the relational factors that appear to be associated with a good treatment outcome (see Chaps. 4 and 6) can be seen as reflective of various elements of therapist responsiveness (Stiles 2013:35).

The 'good-enough' therapist's responsiveness, that is, the ability continuously to attune the interventions to the individual patient, fairly independent of the choice of any specific (and, to varying degrees, standardized) therapeutic method, is presumably an important part of the explanation why it has not been possible to identify a link between the therapist's degree of adherence and the treatment outcome (see Chap. 5), just as it would also inevitably blur any differences in the effect of different standardized therapeutic methods. That undermines some of the underlying assumptions of the RCT-based efficacy study, including that the performed treatment can be viewed as an independent variable that can be controlled by the use of treatment manual and various forms of adherence and competence evaluations of the participating therapists' work, without sufficient awareness that competent therapists will—and must—vary the way they work, depending on the given patient and context (Stiles 2009). Similarly, the responsiveness of good therapists can make it difficult to identify consistent (linear) connections between, on the one hand, different patient, therapist and process characteristics and, on the other hand, treatment outcome (Stiles et al. 1998:444). Two patients will never receive exactly the same therapy. However, in principle, many outcome studies are based on an implicit ballistic assumption that this is the case—that patients who are randomly assigned to a given treatment method will receive the same treatment, or that all the other aspects that have a significant influence on the treatment outcome are more or less evenly distributed in the treatment groups that are being compared (Stiles et al. 1998:440; Stiles 2013:33).

References

Allison, E., & Fonagy, P. (2016). When is truth relevant? *Psychoanalytic Quarterly, 85,* 275–303.

Aristotle (2009). *The nichomachean ethics*. Oxford, UK: Oxford university press

Bateman, A., & Fonagy, P. (2006[2007]). *Mentaliseringsbaseret behandling af borderline personlighedsforstyrrelse*. Copenhagen, Denmark: Akademisk Forlag.

Bateman, A., & Fonagy, P. (2016). *Mentalization-based treatment for personality disorders: A practical guide*. Oxford, England: Oxford University Press.

Beebe, B., & Lachmann, F. M. (2014). *The origins of attachment: Infant research and adult treatment*. London, England: Routledge.
Bollas, C. (1987). *The shadow of the object*. New York, NY: Columbia University Press.
Bonaminio, V. (2008). The person of the analyst, interpreting, not interpreting, and countertransference. *Psychoanalytic Quarterly, 77,* 1105–1146.
Buechler, S. (2004[2009]). *Psychotherapeutische Tugenden. Elementare Gefühle und gelebte Werte in der relationalen Psychoanalyse* [Psychotherapeutic virtues. Elementary feelings and lived values in relational psychoanalysis]. Gießen, Germany: Psychosozial-Verlag.
Castonguay, L. G., & Beutler, L. E. (2006). Common and unique principles of therapeutic change: What do we know and what do we need to know? In L. Castonguay & L. E. Beutler (Eds.), *Principles of therapeutic change that work* (pp. 353–370). New York, NY: Oxford University Press.
Coughlin, P. (2017). *Maximizing effectiveness in dynamic psychotherapy*. London, England: Routledge.
Dantlgraber, J. (1989). Die psychoanalytische Haltung als Stufe in der Übertragungs-/Gegenübertragungsbeziehung [The psychoanalytic attitude as a step in the transference-countertransference relationship]. *Psyche, 43,* 973–1006.
Despland, J.-N., de Roten, Y., Despars, J., Stigler, M., & Perry, J. C. (2001). Contribution of patient defense mechanisms and therapist interventions to the development of early alliance in a brief psychodynamic investigation. *Journal of Psychotherapy Practice and Research, 10*(3), 155–164.
Flanagan, O. (1996). *Self expressions. Mind, morals and the meaning of life*. New York, NY: Oxford University Press.
Freud, S. (1959). The question of lay analysis. Conversations with an impartial person. In J. Strachey (Ed. and Trans.), *The standard edition of the complete psychological works of Sigmund Freud* (Vol. 20, pp. 177–258). London, England: Hogarth (Original work published 1926).
Gorkin, M. (1987). *The uses of countertransference*. Northvale: Aronson.
Greenberg, J., & Mitchell, S. A. (1983). *Object relations in psychoanalytic theory*. Cambridge, MA: Harvard University Press.
Greenson, R. R. (1967). *The technique and practice of psychoanalysis*. London, England: Hogarth Press.
Hardy, G. E., Stiles, W. B., Barkham, M., & Startup, M. (1998). Therapist responsiveness to client interpersonal styles during time-limited treatments for depression. *Journal of Consulting and Clinical Psychology, 66,* 304–312.
Hatcher, R. L. (2015). Interpersonal competencies: Responsiveness, technique, and training in psychotherapy. *American Psychologist, 70,* 747–757.
Hibbert, K. (2012). Cultivating capacity. Phronesis, learning, and diversity in professional education. In E. A. Kinsella & A. Pitman (Eds.), *Phronesis as professional knowledge: Practical wisdom in the professions* (pp. 61–71). Rotterdam, The Netherlands: Sense Publishers.
Jørgensen, C. R. (2008). *Identitet. Psykologiske og kulturanalytiske perspektiver* [Identity. Psychological and culture analysis perspectives]. Copenhagen, Denmark: Hans Reitzels Forlag.
Jørgensen, C. R. (2009). *Personlighedsforstyrrelser. Moderne relationel forståelse og behandling af borderlinelidelse* [Personality disorders. Modern relational understanding and treatment of borderline disorder] (2nd ed.). Copenhagen, Denmark: Hans Reitzels Forlag.
Jørgensen, C. R. (2012). *Danmark på briksen. Et psykologisk perspektiv på Danmark og danskerne i det senmoderne* [Denmark on the therapist's couch. A psychological perspective on Denmark and Danes in later modernity]. Copenhagen, Denmark: Hans Reitzels Forlag.
Kemmis, S. (2012). Phronesis, experience, and the primacy of praxis. In E. A. Kinsella & A. Pitman (Eds.), *Phronesis as professional knowledge: Practical wisdom in the professions* (pp. 147–161). Rotterdam: Sense Publishers.
Kernberg, O. F. (2016). *Psychoanalytic education at the crossroads: Reformation, change and the future of psychoanalytic training*. London, England: Routledge.

Knox, S., Butler, M. C., Kaiser, D. J., Knowlton, G., & Hill, C. E. (2017). Something to laugh about: Humor as a characteristic of effective therapists. In L. G. Castonguay & C. E. Hill (Eds.), *How and why are some therapists better than others?* (pp. 285–306). Washington, DC: American Psychological Association.
Koch, E. (2013). Verstehen [Understanding]. In R. Sannwald, M. Schulte-Markwort, & F. Resch (Eds.), *Psychotherapeutische Fertigkeiten* (pp. 23–37). Göttingen, Germany: Vandenhoeck & Ruprecht.
Köhler-Weisker, A. (1986). Zum Begriff der Haltung des Psychoanalytikers am Beispiel einer Fokaltherapie [On the concept of the psychotherapist's stance as an example of focal therapy]. *Jahrbuch der Psychoanalyse, 18,* 143–173.
Küchenhoff, J. (2013). *Der Sinn im Nein und die Gabe des Gesprächs. Psychoanalytisches Verstehen zwischen Philosophie und Klinik* [The meaning of no and the gift of conversation. Psychoanalytic understanding between philosophy and clinic]. Weilerswist. Germany: Velbrück Wissenschaft.
Leuzinger-Bohleber, M. (2007). Forschende Grundhaltung als abgewehrter „common ground" von psychoanalytischen Praktikern und Forschern? [The explorative attitude as repelled 'common ground' of psychoanalytic practitioners and researchers?] *Psyche*, *61*, 966–994.
Löchel, E. (2013). Ringen um psychoanalytische Haltung [Achieving the analytic attitude]. *Psyche, 67,* 1167–1190.
Mar, R. A., Oatley, K., Hirsh, J., dela Paz, J., & Peterson, J. B. (2006). Bookworms versus nerds: Exposure to fiction versus non-fiction, divergent associations with social ability, and the simulation of fictional social worlds. *Journal of Research in Personality, 40,* 694–712.
Mitchell, S. A. (1997). *Influence and autonomy in psychoanalysis*. Hillsdale, MI: Analytic Press.
Nida-Rümelin, J. (2006). *Demokratie und Wahrheit* [Democracy and truth]. Munich, Germany: C. H. Beck.
Nida-Rümelin, J. (2014). Der Akademisierungswahn. *Zur Krise beruflicher und akademischer Bildung*. Hamburg: Edition Körber-Stiftung
Nida-Rümelin, J. (2015). *Die Optimierungsfalle. Philosophie einer humanen Ökonomie* [The optimization trap. The philosophy of a human economy]. Munich, Germany: BtB-Verlag.
Nida-Rümelin, J. (2016). *Humanistische reflexionen* [Humanistic reflections]. Berlin, Germany: Suhrkamp Verlag.
Nussbaum, M. C. (2010). *Not for profit. Why democracy needs the humanities*. Princeton, NJ: Princeton University Press.
Ogden, T. H. (2016). Destruction reconceived: On Winnicott's 'The use of an object and relating through identifications'. *International Journal of Psychoanalysis, 97,* 1243–1262.
Polanyi, M. (1966). *Den tause dimensjonen. En introduksjon til taus kunnskap* [The tacit dimension. An introduction to tacit knowledge]. Oslo, Norway: Spartacus Forlag.
Pollmann, A. (2005). *Integrität. Aufnahme einer sozialphilosophischen Personalie* [Integrity. Establishing a social-philosophical personal identity]. Bielefeld, Germany: Transcript Verlag.
Radke-Uhlmann, G. (2012). Phronesis als philologische Tugend [Phronesis as philosophical virtue]. In G. Radke-Uhlmann (Ed.), *Phronesis—die Tugend der Geisteswissenschaften* (pp. 3–29). Heidelberg, Germany: Universitätsverlag Winte.
Schafer, R. (1983). *The analytic attitude*. New York, NY: Basic Books.
Schmitt, A. (2012). Phronesis—eine andere Art des Erkennens [Phronesis—a different form of insight]. In G. Radke-Uhlmann (Ed.), *Phronesis—die Tugend der Geisteswissenschaften* ((pp. 31–81)). Heidelberg, Germany: Universitätsverlag Winter.
Schön, D. A. (1983). *The reflective practitioner: How professionals think in action*. Aldershot, England: Arena.
Sellman, D. (2012). Reclaiming competence for professional phronesis. In E. A. Kinsella & A. Pitman (Eds.), *Phronesis as professional knowledge: Practical wisdom in the professions* (pp. 115–130). Rotterdam, The Netherlands: Sense Publishers.
Stehr, H. (2017). Psychodynamische Psychotherapie als interpersonaler Entwicklungsraum—das 'etwas mehr' als Behandlungstechnik [Psychodynamic psychotherapy as interpersonal development space—The 'something more' as therapeutic technique]. In Neumann, E., & Naumann-

Lenzen, M. (Eds.) *Psychodynamisches Denken und Handeln in der Psychotherapie. Eine intersubjektive und verfahrensübergreifende Sicht* (pp. 251–266). Gießen: Psychosozial-Verlag.
Stern, D. N. (2004). *The present moment in psychotherapy and everyday life*. New York, NY: Norton.
Stiles, W. B. (2009). Responsiveness as an obstacle for psychotherapy outcome research: It's worse than you think. *Clinical Psychology: Science and Practice, 16,* 86–91.
Stiles, W. B. (2013). The variables problem and progress in psychotherapy research. *Psychotherapy, 50,* 33–41.
Stiles, W. B., Honos-Webb, L., & Surko, M. (1998). Responsiveness in psychotherapy. *Clinical Psychology: Science and Practice, 5,* 439–458.
Strupp, H. H. (1986). The nonspecific hypothesis of therapeutic effectiveness: A current assessment. *American Journal of Orthopsychiatry, 56,* 513–520.
Symington, J., & Symington, N. (1996). *The clinical thinking of Wilfred Bion*. London, England: Routledge.
Treurniet, N. (1997). On an ethic of psychoanalytic technique. *Psychoanalytic Quarterly, 66,* 596–627.
Valentine, L., & Gabbard, G. O. (2014). Can the use of humor in psychotherapy be taught? *Academic Psychiatry, 38,* 75–81.
Winnicott, D. W. (1971). *Playing and reality*. New York NY: Tavistock.
Zakaria, F. (2015). *In defense of a liberal education*. New York, NY: Norton.
Zwiebel, R. (2004). Der Analytiker als Anderer: Überlegungen zum Einfluß der Person des Analytikers in der analytischen Praxis [The analyst as 'other': Thoughts on the influence of the analyst's personality in the analytical practice]. *Psyche, Zeitschrift für Psychoanalyse, 58,* 836–868.
Zwiebel, R. (2007). *Von der Angst Psychoanalytiker zu sein* [On the fear of being a psychoanalyst]. Stuttgart, Germany: Klett-Cotta Verlag.

Chapter 11
Channels of Communication and Levels in the Therapeutic Relationship

Psychotherapy is normally perceived as a form of talk therapy, which might give the impression that psychotherapy is solely or mainly about the content of the verbal communication between patient and therapist. However, that is far from the case. The process is much more complex, and the pathways to psychotherapeutic change include much more than the explicit content of the patient and the therapist's conversation. It is thus important to attend to and include these other aspects in one's understanding of the psychotherapeutic stance.

11.1 Verbal and Nonverbal Communication

> The psychiatric interview is primarily a matter of vocal communication, and it would be quite a serious error to presume that the communication is primarily verbal. The sound-accompaniments suggest what is to made of the verbal propositions stated (Sullivan 1954:7).

> Psychotherapy is not making clever and apt interpretations; by and large it is a long-term giving the patient back what the patient brings. It is a complex derivative of the face that reflects what there is to see (Winnicott 1971:137).

One of the key characteristics of the psychotherapeutic stance is, as mentioned, that the therapist listens to the patient on several different levels and under consideration of different contexts (here-and-now and there-and-then, the conscious and unconscious intentions behind the patient's communication on different levels in here-and-now, actualization of the patient's implicit relational knowledge and so on). It is possible to identify at least three channels of communication between patient and therapist: verbal communication, nonverbal communication and the therapist's countertransferences, including the communication that is implied in the psychoanalytic concept of projective identification (see below). Similarly, we can distinguish between five levels in the relationship between patient and therapist—levels that, to some extent, accompany or may be considered in relation to the three channels of communication: the real relationship, the therapeutic alliance, the professional role

C. R. Jørgensen, *The Psychotherapeutic Stance*,
https://doi.org/10.1007/978-3-030-20437-2_11

relationship, transference and countertransference (see below). The five relational levels are relevant to any form of psychotherapy, although their relative weights may vary considerably, depending on the specific patient's issues (degree of disorder, level of personality organization), the duration of the therapy and, not least, the choice of specific therapeutic method, where some methods claim—somewhat naively, especially in work with more severe psychological pathology—that transference and countertransference can largely be ignored and do not constitute key aspects of the psychotherapeutic work.

All these channels of communication and levels in the therapeutic relationship contain potential mechanisms of change (see the section on corrective emotional experiences in Chap. 3) and opportunities for achieving a better and more nuanced understanding of the patient, provided the therapist understands how to use them in his or her work. The three channels of communication, broadly speaking, include the following:

- *Verbal* communication refers to the explicit content of the patient's and the therapist's verbal communication: what they talk about. Naturally, this includes the therapist listening to the explicit content of the patient's stories but also that he or she assesses their structure and quality: are they well structured, clear and understandable—or are they incoherent, vague, confused, unclear and a little difficult to follow, and if so, why?
- *Nonverbal* communication includes the way things are said (tone of voice, pauses, silence, tempo, volume), body language (posture, movements), facial expressions (incl. eye contact), clothing (including unusual or very heavy makeup, tattoos, piercing, personal hygiene and so on) and other forms of nonverbal communication (including any physical touching) between patient and therapist, including nonverbally communicated requests or invitations to certain forms of reactions from the other and nonverbal reactions to the other's verbal and nonverbal communication in the present moment. This may also be referred to as the subtext and latent messages (intentions) or meanings in the patient's and the therapist's statements, behaviour and general appearance (cf. Gullestad and Killingmo 2013:167; Kiesler 1996:205). As for the therapist's nonverbal communication to the patient, it is important to pay attention to how it is possible to hold, contain and show nurture and empathy for the patient via the use of voice, tone, facial expressions and other emotional signals in the therapist's way of interacting with the patient, just as the patient will read the therapist's nonverbal signals with a view to discerning how he reacts to what she says and shows in the therapeutic space, that is, whether he can contain it, is overwhelmed or distances himself from it. Besides, the therapist will always communicate elements of 'who I am' and aspects of his unconscious to the patient via his nonverbal communication.
- The therapist's countertransferences are defined in slightly different ways by different writers, but broadly speaking, the concepts refer to the therapist's emotional and other reactions to the patient and the emotions, perceptions, impulses, urges, desires and other types of mental states that arise in the therapist in the therapeutic space in the interaction with the patient (see below and Chap. 7); this includes how

the therapist immediately feels about and reacts to what the patient says (feeling overwhelmed, sad, impressed, detached, empty, confused, concerned, caring, upset and so on). These reactions and mental states are assumed to relate, to varying degrees, to the patient's behaviour, verbal and nonverbal communication and mental states; thus, they are regarded as a form of communication of the patient's inner psychological life (mental states, internal object relations, implicit relational knowledge and so on) that is conveyed to the therapist without conscious intent. This channel of communication also influences the therapist's perception of the mood or atmosphere in the therapeutic space and in the interaction with the patient, which typically varies with, among other aspects, the patient's mental states and the (internal and external) object relations that dominate the therapeutic relationship at any given time. The therapist's ability to contain and process the countertransferences that are activated in the interaction with the patient may in itself contain important mechanisms of change, just as the therapist's ability to receive, experience and mirror a wide range of mental states, including intense ones, can have a key impact on the course and outcome of the treatment. The therapist's countertransferences are closely linked to the therapist's empathy and related to what is known as mirror neurons in neuropsychology.

When people engage in face-to-face contact, they inevitably continuously send messages to each other via the various channels of communication. Both sending and receiving messages are active processes that are inevitably affected by one's subjectivity. When people communicate, they not only convey explicitly verbally represented messages, but also messages about how the verbally communicated message should be understood, what the (actual or desired) relationship is between the interlocutors as well as more emotional (nonverbalized) aspects, just as each party in the communication sends messages related to his or her self-perception, self-perceived status in relation to the other and attempts to define their mutual relationship. Nonverbal communication is often the primary channel for more emotional and relational messages, including messages about the perception of self and other (Kiesler 1996:204ff).

Generally, we are somewhat less aware of our nonverbal communication, which is also not under nearly the same degree of conscious (intentional) control. Nonverbal communication and what plays out in the transference and the countertransference may be viewed as a form of communication between the patient's and the therapist's unconscious (Nacht 1962:210), which may hold importance for the therapeutic process and the treatment outcome. Moreover, nonverbal communication is often more ambiguous and hence far more open to interpretation than verbally communicated messages. All patients convey important messages via their nonverbal communication, but as a rule of thumb, the nonverbal communication and the therapist's countertransferences (including projective identification, see later) will carry more weight and constitute more important channels of communication concerning the patient's difficulties the more severe the patient's pathology is. Thus, the more severely disturbed the patients are that a therapist works with, the more attention he or she generally needs to pay to their nonverbal communication and his or her own countertransferences.

The relationship between the different channels of communication and their impact on the therapist's experience and perception of the patient can be illustrated with a parallel to the way we normally experience films. When we watch a film with strong auditory content, the film music and sound effects will often have a big impact on our emotional experience of and reactions to the images on the screen, our understanding of the film's narrative and what seems most important in the film (its main focus), even if we are not necessarily consciously aware of it. What happens in one channel of communication (sound) has a major influence on how we perceive and process what happens in another channel of communication (images). However, if we deliberately focus our attention on the sound and begin to register consciously how it affects us and reflect on how the director uses certain kinds of music and other sound effects to strike a certain mood and convey certain experiences and emotional reactions, the sound loses much of its impact on our film experience. In a sense, we lose the holistic film experience, as we gain other experiences we would not have had without this analytical detachment in relation to the sound elements. Similarly, the very act of deliberately directing one's attention at the patient's nonverbal communication and one's own countertransferences—and reflecting on how the communication and the reactions that occur in these channels of communication may be understood—can in itself reduce their impact on our emotional reactions and behaviour in the interaction with the patient quite considerably, just as we gain insight into some of the 'effects' the patient often (unconsciously) uses in interactions with others and the reactions that often arise in others when they interact with the patient.

Choice of Primary Focus

The therapist's reactions to the patient may of course be related to the patient's verbal and, especially, nonverbal communication, and hence, in practice, it may be difficult to achieve a precise delimitation of the three channels of communication. Often, what the patient communicates by nonverbal means, and which is activated in the therapist's countertransference, is more emotionally intense and more important than what the patient explicitly communicates in his or her verbal communication, in part because the patient may find it hard to verbalize key aspects of his or her difficulties (which are mentally unrepresented, unconscious and stored in the procedural memory, see below), or because the patient, for various reasons, does not want to tell the therapist about the most painful or embarrassing (shameful, experiences associated with guilt and so on) elements of her difficulties, actions and experiences. It is therefore crucial for the therapist not only to focus on what is, in a sense, the easiest, namely the verbal communication, but also to remain continuously focused on what sort of relationship the patient seeks or invites, what role or position the patient seeks to place the therapist in, what desires and needs the patient implicitly communicates and seeks to satisfy in her interaction with the therapist, what emotions and mental states dominate the interaction with the patient, and what perceptions of self and others (in this case, the therapist) appear to underlie the patient's interactions with the therapist.

Does the patient primarily seek to establish a narcissist relationship, where the therapist is expected to support her self-esteem and help regulate and stabilize her self, while the therapist develops a sense that his subjectivity and existence as a separate individual with his own emotions and thoughts are of no significance or are not noticed by the patient? Does the patient perhaps rather invite a semi-symbiotic relationship, where she is very dependent on the therapist's mirroring, support and positive attention? Or is a generally more mature relationship formed, with a higher degree of reciprocity between two clearly delimited, separate individuals, where the patient recognizes and relates to the therapist as a subject with a unique individuality, not merely as a function or as someone who is there to satisfy certain needs in the patient (Zwiebel 2013:200f)?

Further, incongruences may exist between what is communicated via the three respective channels. Both patient and therapist may try to communicate one message via the verbal communication, while the nonverbal communication and the person's appearance in the moment seem to carry other, perhaps contradictory messages. Similarly, it is important to notice any rapid shifts between very different or perhaps even incompatible messages communicated in one or more of the three channels of communication, which may reflect a lack of internal integration (identity diffusion) in the patient and a painful confusion or inadequate control over contradictory impulses or self-components in the patient. For example, a patient may describe how many people she has begun to see (after initially feeling very lonely) and explain that she no longer feels that she has any difficulty making contact with others. At the same time, the therapist develops a sense of lack of contact and emptiness (in the countertransference), which might reveal something about the quality of the relationships the patient is talking about; they may be more superficial relationships without the deeper personal and emotional contact that the patient has been missing and (is still) seeking, even if that may not be what she talks about or what she herself is consciously aware of (perhaps because it is too painful for her to realize that the relationships she describes are superficial and lack any deeper emotional contact). Perhaps the patient, at the beginning of a session, talks about all the new things she has initiated which make her happy, but later in the same session she describes feeling empty and melancholic and lacking initiative—a shift that may initially seem confusing, and which may reflect a similar confusion in the patient and illustrate the big fluctuations in her functioning level, self-perception and emotional state. In these situations it may be important for the therapist to help the patient verbalize and explore fluctuations and the confusion they cause. The therapist must remain aware of the need of adopting a psychotherapeutic stance towards all aspects of what is communicated in the three channels of communication in the therapeutic space.

Structured and Actualized Affects

In relation to the three levels of communication the patient's (and the therapist's) affects and other mental states may be brought into the therapeutic space in two different ways, what Gullestad and Killingmo (2013:116) call *structured* versus *actualized affects*. The former of the two concepts refers to verbalized narratives about more 'digested' affects that the patient, to varying degrees, has already placed into a meaningful context, has some distance to, is able to think thoughts about and communicates via verbal communication, while the latter refers to affects and other mental states that are actualized here and now in the therapeutic space as a result of the processes playing out in the transference, in the verbal therapeutic work and in the interaction between patient and therapist here and now in general.

Actualized affects and mental states have not yet been similarly verbalized or organized, understood, digested and placed into a meaningful context and are thus primarily expressed (communicated) via nonverbal channels of communication. They constitute more raw affects and mental states (what Bion calls beta-elements, see the section on projective identification below), which are lived out, dominate or take over the patient's psyche when they are activated, and which it will often be part of the therapist's task to help the patient become aware of, verbalize (represent mentally), validate, organize and place into a meaningful context, where the patient is better able to decode what the affects signify. For example, the patient may start out the session with an expression of anger, avoid eye contact with the therapist and react with intense irritation to everything he says and does, as if it is profoundly moronic and only serves to illustrate that the therapist has understood nothing at all, although this does not seem to have any obvious connection to what happened in the previous session. The patient does not say that she is angry, let alone who she is angry with or why—but she is clearly angry, and it is not immediately evident who she is angry with, or why, only that she is obviously venting the anger in the relationship with the therapist.

The therapist's first task therefore is to bring up (verbalize) this anger explicitly and invite the patient to explain what made her angry, frustrated, upset or whatever may be driving the actualized anger that is now being lived out. This may in itself improve the patient's ability to become aware of and verbalize her affects and other mental states and will also further her understanding of what led to these affects here and now, perhaps in connection with the actualization of past experiences and reaction patterns in the therapeutic space—all processes that may help the patient move from 'being' her affects to 'having' affects, which she will be better able to regulate and use as a basis for a greater self-understanding and understanding of the world.

Generally, actualized affects and mental states in the therapeutic space take precedent over structured affects. Focusing on what is happening in the patient, the therapeutic relationship and the therapeutic space here and now—actualized mental states—should have a higher priority than working with the patient's narratives about past experiences with related structured affects, just as affects and other mental states should generally take priority over (narratives about past) behaviour. At the same time, the focus on the patient's actualized affects must always be attuned to a continuous assessment of the patient's current state and needs, as the focus on the patient's actualized affects in the present moment may sometimes be anxiety-provoking and increase the patient's arousal level beyond what is optimal, especially if the therapist is not sufficiently validating in his interaction with the patient and her actualized mental states. Further, the therapist should bear in mind that for many patients it can be difficult and associated with shame to confide in the therapist, focus on her mental anguish and intense mental states here and now and thus reveal her vulnerable emotional state to another person. Finally, the balance between structured and actualized affects in the patient contain information about the patient's general psychological functioning level. With patients who are more poorly psychologically structured (deficit pathology) the therapeutic space and work will be more dominated by actualized affects, and the patient may at times struggle with structuring, digesting and verbalizing his or her affects and mental states.

A patient describes a conflict she had with her mother the previous day; the explicit content of her story is dominated by the anger she feels towards the mother. While she is describing the conflict she becomes increasingly emotionally affected and begins to cry, even though the content of her story continues to be dominated by how angry she is with her mother. While the therapist initially listened primarily to the what the patient was saying, in part in order to form an impression of what matters most to the patient right now, he now focuses their shared attention explicitly at the patient's actualized affect: 'I can tell that you are very moved and upset when you speak about the conflict with your mother.' At first, the patient reacts by saying in a tone dripping with self-contempt: 'Yes, damn it, I always begin to bawl,' which for various reasons can be assumed to reflect how she has previously been met by, especially, her mother when she was upset, that is, with contempt and demands to 'pull yourself together.' Then the focus shifts to how the patient has during much of her life missed having a mother who understood her and whom she could lean on and receive support from when she was sad. This makes her sad, but at the same time she is also furious with her mother for not, as the patient sees it, being there for her, 'the way a mother should be there for her children.' Meanwhile, she is also moved by being seen by the therapist—that he sees that she is upset and does not meet her with contempt or demands to 'pull yourself together.' Instead the therapist invites her to talk about it, which represents a deviation from a recurring pattern in her relationships with significant others and thus enables the patient to have a corrective emotional experience in the therapeutic relationship; 'I don't have to be alone with my pain; there are other people who can see, contain and help me when I am sad.' Afterwards, it may be relevant to return to the patient's anger with her mother to examine the cause of it.

11.2 Explicit Declarative Memory and Implicit Procedural Memory

As mentioned earlier, it is a key point in Freud's classical psychoanalysis that experiences and perceptions that are repressed become part of the so-called dynamic unconscious. The content of the dynamic unconscious may be a contributing factor to the development of psychopathology in the form of symptoms and maladaptive behaviour. In natural extension of this, the pathway to recovery is seen to go through removing the repression and uncovering unconscious perceptions and conflicts, mainly through the attainment of insight via the therapist's interpretations of the patient's material—that is, primarily via the content of the explicit verbal communication. In light of what we now know about the human memory, this model of pathology and of the curative therapeutic processes is at best incomplete (see Chaps. 4 and 8). Especially in case of more severe psychopathology, uncovering, remembering and attaining insight into (possibly repressed) past experiences in themselves thus probably do not have a significant impact on treatment outcome; in particular, patients with a more fragile ego can be difficult to reach and help via more abstract and content-focused analytic interpretations of the patient's material (cf. Cremerius 1979:586). What happens in the interaction between patient and therapist in connection with the therapeutic work, which goes well beyond the content of the verbal communication and influences other parts of human memory end recollections of specific events, is far more important.

It should also be remembered that contemporary psychoanalytic psychotherapy, compared to classical psychoanalysis, is focused much more on the treatment of personality pathology (often referred to as 'early disorders' or 'deficit pathology'), where the effort to remove repression and uncover the unconscious moves into the background in favour of efforts to diminish splitting, establish nuanced mental representations of significant experiences and enhance integration within the patient's self or personality (Küchenhoff 2010:94). Finally, one might ask whether the dominant forms of pathology may have changed over time, so that psychological disorders related to repression and suppressed needs play less of a role today and have, in part, been supplanted by pathologies associated with internal fragmentation and perceived meaninglessness and disorientation in relation to identity diffusion. That is a complex question that lies outside the scope of the present book (see Jørgensen 2002, 2008, 2009, 2012, 2014).

Broadly speaking, we can distinguish between two key memory systems that are relevant to our understanding of the mechanisms of change in psychotherapy (Lemma 2003:76ff). One is the explicit declarative memory, which includes the autobiographical memory, specific facts about our life and person and episodic memories—all memories that are or can be readily verbalized and accessed consciously. This memory system enables us consciously and intentionally to recall facts and specific events from our life ('knowing that'). The other is the implicit, procedural and, in a sense, more emotion-driven memory system, which primarily contains unverbalized experiences, non-conscious habits, ways of reacting in different situations, non-conscious behavioural norms and matrixes for handling interpersonal relationships associated with what could be called implicit relational knowledge ('knowing how', implicit thinking and action strategies). The content of the procedural memory is unconscious, not because it has been repressed but because it was typically never mentally represented. In that sense, the content of this memory system is the result of a kind of non-conscious learning of ways to orient ourselves in the world and relationships, which is manifested in specific behaviour, not in conscious memories. The specific background of the procedural memory cannot readily be recalled.

Large parts of our relational experiences, which may be a contributing cause of the development of maladaptive patterns in interactions with others and thus of the development of psychopathology, are stored in our implicit procedural memory (Lyons-Ruth 1999:578). Our internal working models for interactions with others and knowledge about how to act in various contexts are thus not primarily stored in the form of easily recalled or evoked declarative knowledge or memories about the specific events that led to these relational working models. To a certain extent, the declarative and the procedural memory act as two separate systems, which means that changes in the declarative memory are not necessarily accompanied by corresponding changes in the procedural memory, which is much more important for both the development of and the recovery from (especially more severe) psychopathology (Lyons-Ruth 1999:589). Recalling specific events that are stored in the declarative memory and attempts to verbalize individual elements within the procedural memory will therefore not necessarily have any therapeutic effect in terms of leading to any major changes in the procedural memory. On the other hand, the effort to uncover and verbalize specific events in the patient's life and to verbalize parts of the procedural memory should be seen as a relational event in the therapeutic space, which has the potential to change the patient's procedural memory; importantly, this potential stems from the specific way in which this happens, rather than the specific content that is uncovered and verbalized.

Hence, the patient's way of relating to the therapist and the patient's behaviour in the interaction with the therapist is the therapist's primary windows into the patient's procedural memory and thus to curing the patient's pathology. The content of the patient's procedural memory—the patient's working models or implicit relational knowledge for interactions with others—is manifested in the form of actualization or performance of specific acts in the interaction with the therapist (Klöpper 2014:68). Similarly, the specific interaction between patient and therapist, including, not least, the therapist's therapeutic stance and way of relating to the patient, are key mechanisms of change and have a major impact on the patient's benefit of the treatment—an impact that by all indications is somewhat bigger than that of the specific insight (in a narrow content sense) that the patient attains in the therapeutic work. The procedural memory can thus be viewed as a system for implicit relational regulation that is not readily accessible to the conscious mind (explicit declarative memory), and which is primarily changed via the nonverbal interaction between patient and therapist, including the therapist's reception and psychological processing of the patient's self-parts and mental states, as they play out in the therapeutic space, as well as the therapist's regulation of the affective atmosphere in the therapeutic space, including the successful management of the problems that arise in the therapeutic relationship.

On the other hand, failed attempts at managing the problems that arise in the therapeutic relationship (ruptures in the alliance) and failures in the therapist's attunement to the patient and in his ability to contain the patient, will often confirm the elements of the patient's procedural memory that are part of the background for the patient's difficulties and thus exacerbate the patient's state. Recurring patterns in the patient's interactions with others are manifested via the patient's way of being, psychological functioning and interactions with the therapist, which gives rise to a sort of 'dialogue-in-action' that is only partially conscious and verbalized but which may be crucial for changes in the patient's procedural memory. The therapist's ability to contain and process the patient's difficulties, as they are manifested in the therapeutic space and the therapeutic relationship—the continuous emotional exchange and attunement between patient and therapist—is crucial for changing the patient's procedural memory. This has very little to do with the use of any specific treatment techniques, while the therapist's more personal qualities, including his ability to remain emotionally balanced and in contact and to maintain the psychotherapeutic stance in handling what happens in the therapeutic space, may be crucial.

Moments of Meeting in the Therapeutic Space

Thus, over time, the specific interaction between patient and therapist in the therapeutic space, which enables the patient to have new corrective emotional experiences in the interaction with the therapist, can lead to changes in the patient's procedural memory and hence in the patient's working models (internal object relations) for interactions with others, including in the patient's dominant perceptions of self and others. Moments of emotionally intense intersubjective contact between patient and therapist hold the potential for changing the patient's procedural memory and implicit relational knowledge outside (or at least partially outside) the verbal communication and the declarative memory (Stern 2004; Stern et al. 1998). One of the key characteristics of these moments of meeting, which are characterized by close and intense intersubjective contact is that the therapist is personally and emotionally present as a subjective fellow human being in a manner that clearly goes beyond the implementation of a standardized therapeutic technique. The technocrat therapist, who is not authentically present in a meeting with the patient but merely carries out a series of technical procedures, will not have the same ability to establish these meetings, which are so crucial for the treatment outcome. On the other hand, these moments in the therapeutic space also contain a risk that the therapist fails to seize and use them appropriately or that he spontaneously reacts in ways that confirm the patient's maladaptive perceptions of self and others or otherwise hampers the patient's progress. It is therefore essential for the therapist to realize that these moments may occur and to be as well prepared as possible to handle them, even though such preparation is only partially possible and depends to a high degree on the therapist's more personal qualities, which only have limited responsiveness to formalized training.

The intense intersubjective meeting is thus often associated with situations where something unexpected happens. The patient does or says something that calls for the therapist to do something novel, which is not described in the formalized method and, to some extent, to step outside the method (Stern et al. 1998:913). These are situations where the right response from the therapist is not formally given. The standardized method does not describe how the therapist should handle the situation; the therapist finds himself outside the comfort zone of his normal role as therapist and has to show spontaneity and creativity. The therapist thus reveals aspects of his self and offers an authentic emotional or personal response to the patient (ibid.:917) in something that approaches a real relationship (see below) and which may thus break the patient's perceived loneliness (Safran 2017). Hence, moments of meeting cannot be manualized, let alone emerge during routine work, where the therapist adheres to a strict implementation of a standardized method. At the same time, establishing moments of meeting will often involve that the therapist partially (and temporarily) steps outside his professional role, while still maintaining the psychotherapeutic stance and preventing the therapeutic relationship from turning into a different kind of relationship, including beginning to offer certain services to 'the special patient' or beginning to (expect to) receive something in return from the patient for the proffered help. This is a demanding balancing act, but not an impossible one. It is possible to do this 'well enough', being authentically present emotionally and as a person in the contact with the patient, without becoming unnecessarily personal or overstepping the boundaries of acceptable behaviour in professional therapeutic work. Authenticity by no means implies telling the patient whatever one thinks and feels, without a filter, or violating boundaries in one's spontaneous reactions to the patient. The process has to remain disciplined, reflected and guided by considerations of what the patient needs right now and with respect for the patient's personal boundaries (cf. Mitchell 2000:127).

The patient's yearning for emotional and psychological (intersubjective) contact—the yearning to be seen, heard and share significant subjective experiences—is often an important driver of the therapeutic work and may also help break the patient's experience of psychological-mental loneliness (Stern 2004). This contact may of course be established in connection with the normal therapy work, but as Stern (2004) and The Boston Change Process Study Group (Bruschweiler-Stern et al. 2010), among others, have described, moments in the therapeutic space characterized by particular emotional intensity and moments where the normal contact and rhythm of the process are breaking up (also referred to as 'present moments' or 'now moments'), contain heightened opportunities for establishing a therapeutically significant meeting or a contact between patient and therapist that holds the potential for change, provided the therapist (and the patient) can seize the opportunity. The patient's implicit relational knowledge, including her perceptions of self, others and what being in contact with others involves, is actualized and open to revision. What actually happens in the exchange between patient and therapist will determine whether the possibility for positive change in the patient's implicit relational knowledge is realized. Below, two examples of sudden ruptures in the therapeutic contact are outlined; in one, the therapist reacts in a way that probably prevents the realization of a moment of meeting, while in the other he manages to react in a way that leads to an intense moment of meeting between patient and therapist that enables positive change in the patient.

A patient recently became a mother. She is alone with the child and does not have a strong social network where she can find someone to look after her child, and because she is keen to continue in therapy as soon as possible after the delivery, she takes her weeks-old infant, with her to the therapy. This was not arranged ahead of time, but the therapist spontaneously says that it is okay. At the beginning of the session, she happily shows the therapist her baby and then puts the child down to sleep, without major problems, and the session begins in more or less the same way as a normal session would. Later, during the session, the child wakes up and becomes increasingly active, which naturally affects the session, in the sense that the conversation begins to turn to the infant in a way that is pleasant and very close to how such a situation would normally be handled in a private context outside the therapeutic space. After a short while, the patient picks up the baby and prepares to breastfeed him. The therapist reacts slightly surprised and spontaneously (a little too quickly), without thinking much about it, asks the patient whether they should take a break so she can go into an adjacent room and feed the child without the therapist being present. The patient reacts clearly negatively to this proposal, as if the therapist had told her she could not breastfeed in the therapist's office, or as if the therapist could not contain the idea of her breastfeeding in the therapeutic space and thus, in a sense, breaking the therapeutic boundaries, which was correct—in the situation, the therapist did have difficulty determining how to react to the fact that the patient began to breastfeed her child. Even though, in formal terms, it could be argued that the therapist's response was appropriate, he clearly did not react spontaneously to this sudden situation in the therapeutic space in a manner that allowed for a moment of meeting and might contribute to changing the patient's perception of herself, of others' perception of her and of interpersonal contact. Instead the therapist was a little too preoccupied with preserving the therapeutic frame, boundaries and formal guidelines for what can happen in the therapeutic space.

Another patient who has periodically had serious difficulties regulating her affects and handling interpersonal boundaries—she alternates, confusingly, between avoiding contact and allowing others to get too close—enters the therapy room and immediately begins to take off her shoes. She also moves her chair a little and says to the therapist that today she would like to sit cross-legged on the floor if he does not mind (and that it is okay, if the therapist wants to join her on the floor). She explains that she has discovered that it gives her an inner sense of calm, and also, that is her typical seating position when she has important conversations with her friends. The therapist reacts with slight surprise, but spontaneously says that it is okay if she is more comfortable sitting that way today (without implying that she will necessarily be able to change the arrangement in the therapeutic space in this way in the future), but that he is going to sit in his normal chair. After a brief initial phase where they both laugh a little at the fact that the patient is sitting on the floor, while the therapist is sitting in his chair and is thus raised above her, the session proceeds fairly 'normally' (with no discernible impact of the somewhat unusual arrangement), and after about half an hour the patient spontaneously gets up and sits in her chair again. Throughout the session the mood is intimate and emotionally unencumbered, while the patient begins to work with a very painful experience. The therapist refrains from thematizing or offer any overly psychologizing interpretations of the patient's urge to sit on the floor (he quickly decides to wait until a subsequent session to address how they might understand the patient's urge to sit in a different manner than normal). Naturally, this incident in the therapeutic space could be understood in many different ways. Growing up, she felt as if she were in prison, stifled by the rigid rules in her family, and in light of this history it seems obvious to perceive the patient's behaviour as a more or less unconscious test of the therapist and his ability to grant her freedom (avoid confining her to a prison of rigid rules). Of course, it could also be perceived as the patient's attempts to alter the nature of the therapeutic relationship (or to be more grounded and thus improve her self-regulation). The therapist apparently passes the test, and the incident strengthens his contact with the patient and also allows for a liberating element of humour (moments of meeting). Had the therapist stuck rigidly to the formal treatment setting, insisting that the patient had to sit in her chair, the patient might have perceived this as an indication that the therapist, like her parents, was intent on keeping her locked up in a prison of rigid rules. He would probably have failed the test, which in all likelihood would have impaired his contact with the patient.

The use of humour also contains the potential for establishing an emotionally intense meeting with the patient that goes beyond the normal therapeutic contact without becoming unnecessarily private or violating the patient's boundaries, provided that the therapist is able to use humour with the necessary sense of the patient's individual personality, sense of humour and boundaries. Humour can bring in spontaneity and an emotional lightness, while strengthening the alliance by giving the patient and therapist a shared third element to laugh at together (Valentine and Gabbard 2014). Besides, the use of humour—provided the timing and content are attuned to the patient—can help resolve conflicts and pent-up affects, just as it may enable patient and therapist together to take a step back from the patient's perceived difficulties and observe them from a new perspective (Sultanoff 2013:389f; Knox et al. 2017).

That these elements, which are potentially crucial for treatment outcome, lie beyond the use of a formalized treatment technique in no way means that the content of the verbal communication does not matter, since the verbal communication typically acts as the central medium for establishing an emotional intersubjective contact between patient and therapist. Talking about experiences that are painful and emotionally significant for the patient in ways that increase the patient's trust in and perception of the contact with the therapist will strengthen her experience of being seen, heard, validated and understood by the therapist. An emotional contact may be established between patient and therapist that temporarily goes far beyond what is communicated via the verbal communication alone, and which may for example enable a positive change in the patient's self-image and identity as she internalizes her perception of how the therapist sees and perceives her.

Speaking with another human being who listens attentively and with interest, lets the patient speak out and invites shared reflection can in itself be effective, fairly independently of the specific topic of the conversation. And it may be absolutely crucial for the establishment of the intense intersubjective contact. However, the intersubjective meeting in itself is more important for the patient's long-term change process than the specific topic, provided it is perceived as emotionally significant to the patient, is focused on the patient and his or her difficulties and contributes to the intersubjective contact. There is reason to assume that establishing intense intersubjective contact is relatively more important in therapy with more severely disturbed patients and patients with attachment and personality disorders, who typically have severe relational difficulties. On the other hand, it is relatively less important in therapy concerning milder symptom disorders with less comorbidity. Here too, however, establishing intersubjective contact is important for the effectiveness of the more disorder-specific and symptom-focused interventions, although there should not be the same intensity of focus on or work with elements of the therapeutic relationship with patients who do not have major relational difficulties, and where there are no major problems in the therapeutic relationship (Caspar and Holtforth 2009:64).

11.3 Real Relationship, Professional Role Relationship and Therapeutic Alliance

In a sense, the therapist is present in the therapeutic space in two versions in relation to the patient: as a subject and a fellow human being in a real relationship and in the role of therapist, defined by the therapeutic frame. Similarly, the patient is present both as an equal fellow human being in a real relationship and in the role of patient, who is similarly defined by the therapeutic frame (Zwiebel 2013:198f). We may also speak of the more personal versus the more technical dimension of therapy. The real, personal relationship refers to the more immediate, 'genuine' and realistic aspects of the therapeutic relationship, which are not determined by transferences, the patient's history or other factors outside the relationship that cause the patient's perception of the therapist to be distorted or influenced by the 'presence' of other (past) persons in the therapeutic space (Gelso 2011:12). The real relationship is a relationship between adult, mature individuals, none of whom are seeking the gratification of immature needs or trying to drive the relationship towards asymmetry. It could be argued that the moments of authentic intersubjective contact between patient and therapist that, by all indications, appear to be crucial for the course and outcome of therapy occur primarily in the real relationship. The real relationship may also be connected to a form of meta-alliance (a key condition for the ability to work with severe ruptures in the alliance) or shared implicit knowledge about the relationship that exists parallel to transferences, countertransferences and the formal roles of patient and therapist (Stern et al. 1998:916).

The real relationship is in no way unique to the psychotherapeutic relationship, but it is important in all forms of psychotherapy, although there is considerable variation in how much importance it is attributed, just as, in quantitative terms, it typically plays a relatively smaller role (but still exists and is important) in therapy with more severely disturbed patients, where the patient's transference and difficulties with establishing a symmetrical and trusting relationship play a more prominent role. That does not mean, however, that the therapist's ability to be authentically present, spontaneous and 'alive' is less significant in the work with these patients. The real relationship is not attributed any major importance in classical psychoanalysis, while more humanistic and experientially oriented therapies traditionally consider the real relationship as central to the therapy (Gelso 2011:13). Contemporary versions of psychoanalysis with a relational and intersubjective orientation also place significantly greater emphasis on the real relationship (the meeting between patient and therapist) than more classical psychoanalysis (Gelso 2011:70).

The psychotherapeutic stance involves meeting the patient as an equal subject, using the real relationship as one of several carrier waves in the therapeutic work. The therapist speaks *with* the patient as an equal subject, not *about* the patient in a way that implicitly objectivizes him or her (Ogden 2016:9f), with the primary goal of understanding the patient, not explaining the patient's difficulties with reference to any objective mechanisms outside the patient's subjectivity. The patient must *never* feel that the therapist merely sees him or her as a case or a diagnosis. Objectivizing the individual can lead to an instrumental approach to the patient, characterized by a lack of empathy and of any deeper understanding and recognition of the patient's subjectivity. The second important carrier wave for the treatment is the therapeutic alliance, which is more unique to the psychotherapeutic relationship (see below). Most patients can make very precise and apt observations about their therapist, which cannot, in any way, be reduced to distorted perceptions determined by transferences or projective perceptions. The notion that most patients are 'in the grip of their emotions' and only have access to pathologically distorted perceptions of the therapist must be viewed as a relic from a time when the relationship between patient and therapist was viewed far more as being based on asymmetrical authority, than is the case today. Hence, the real relationship should also be included in our understanding of the therapeutic relationship, even though the patient's way of relating to the therapist, to varying degrees, will also be coloured by the patient's characteristic relational difficulties.

The psychotherapeutic space defines a certain context for the psychotherapeutic relationship, setting it apart from all other types of relationships. Within this context, patient and therapist are assigned their characteristic roles as respectively, the patient seeking help, who is expected to speak to the therapist about very personal and private experiences, and the therapist as the professional helper who makes him/herself and his or her time available to the patient within a given setting and then, to the best of his or her abilities, listens to, tries to understand and seeks to help the patient resolve his or her psychological difficulties. In some regards, this is a highly personal relationship within an impersonal professional framework, where the therapist typically gets quite close to the patient's inner and emotional life but, then, only has contact with the patient within the pre-determined therapeutic context. Conversely, the patient gains very little direct or explicit insight into the therapist's personal life and any emotional challenges.

As human beings, patient and therapist are equal, but in practice the psychotherapeutic relationship can become quite asymmetrical, and the patient may feel dependent on, exposed to and subordinate to the therapist. On the other hand, the therapeutic relationship offers the patient an opportunity to play out and thus gain a better understanding of his or her difficulties in relation to perceived authority figures and problems concerning control and submissiveness, closeness and distance, establishing trust and entering into and remaining in a prolonged, emotionally significant relationship. Any unresolved conflicts or difficulties that the therapist has with regard to these and related issues may, of course, become actualized in the therapeutic relationship and influence the therapist's actions in the therapeutic space, which may indirectly offer the patient a sense of the therapist's personality, inner life and any emotional difficulties. Especially patients in long-term psychotherapy may thus develop a fairly in-depth and accurate understanding of the therapist's psychology, strengths and weaknesses.

The therapist is inevitably placed into a position as a form of authority figure in an asymmetrical relationship. Rhetorically, one might say that the only thing the therapist does not have the authority to do is to suspend his or her structurally determined position of authority, although this position may of course be managed in many different ways (McWilliams 2004:152). One should not deny the existence of this structural reality. If the therapist feels a strong urge to do so, he should consider what it may say about him, that is, how it might be related to his own challenges in regard to exercising authority. The inherent rules of the therapeutic space concerning both the patient's and, especially, the therapist's actions, prescribe certain conditions for the therapist's role. With increasing experience comes a gradual internalization of this role, and with time (often relatively quickly, in the span of a few years) one finds one's own voice and way of living out the role that is compatible with who one is as a person, and which thus feels authentic and also appears more authentic in the eyes of the patients. This involves, to varying degrees, liberating oneself from aspects of the theories, therapeutic models and specific methods that one identified within during therapeutic training and developing a personal way of meeting and communicating with the patients while also improving one's ability to listen to the patients relying on one's unique inner resonance (Löchel 2013:33). The therapist who merely plays the part of a therapist without the necessary personal authenticity, and who asks questions and (mechanically) intervenes in certain ways because that is what is prescribed in a given manual or set of clinical guidelines has little chance of success as a psychotherapist (cf. McWilliams 2004:52). On the other hand, perhaps especially more experienced therapists, who believe they know all the ground rules of psychotherapy and, with some justification, believe that by embracing an unassailable ethical attitude they are free to take a more creative approach to the therapeutic process need to watch out for the risk of ruptures in the psychotherapeutic frame and stance as well as any maladaptive deviations from the normal procedures for competent psychotherapeutic work (Jacobsen and Mortensen 2017:126).

According to the prevailing view today (Bordin 1979), the therapeutic alliance is defined by a basic consensus between patient and therapist about the goals of the therapy and about how these goals should be pursued (therapeutic method). It could be argued that this reflects a remarkably rationalistic and goal-focused understanding of psychotherapy (Rønnestad and Skovholt 2013:42). In addition to this more cognitive-rational aspect, the therapeutic alliance also includes a mainly emotional bond between patient and therapist (Bordin 1979), which in the patient is associated with a fundamental trust in the therapist, a conscious or unconscious identification with the therapist and the treatment and elements of what could be called, borrowing Freud's terms, a positive 'inoffensive', contemporary transference rooted in reality (see Chap. 9)—a transference of positive experiences from earlier relationships on to the therapist and the therapy. The therapeutic alliance links the patient to the therapist as a person, to the therapy process and to the common therapeutic endeavour and thus helps to stabilize the therapeutic relationship, lay the foundation for a positive attitude towards the therapist and increase the chances that the therapeutic work can continue, even when conflicts arise in the therapeutic relationship, and when the patient is frustrated, dissatisfied or angry with the therapist and feels like terminating the treatment.

The therapeutic alliance enables the patient to maintain a fundamentally positive attitude towards the therapist and the therapeutic work, also when conflicts arise in the therapeutic relationship, when the patient is frustrated with certain aspects of the treatment, perceives a lack of progress and so on (cf. Sandler et al. 1992:37). One should expect to be able to establish an alliance fairly quickly and without major difficulties with most patients who have mild problems and patients without severe attachment problems. Here it is not normally necessary to focus especially on establishing a sustainable therapeutic relationship, as it largely happens on its own, unless the therapist makes major missteps.

Working with more severely disturbed patients and patients with severe relational and attachment disorders is much more complicated, as the core of these patients' difficulties will typically be manifest in the therapeutic relationship and hamper the establishment of a therapeutic alliance. Here, the therapeutic alliance will be more fragile and subject to lasting ruptures or threats of dissolution (the patient terminating the therapy). This presents a complex situation, since these patients' difficulties will play out in the therapeutic space in a way that hampers the establishment of a stable relationship or alliance, which is a necessary condition of the therapeutic process. That makes it absolutely crucial to meet this challenge with a psychotherapeutic stance and to see the establishment of a therapeutic alliance or the development of the therapeutic relationship—and not least the obstacles to these goals—as a key task in the therapy.

The patient's difficulties with trusting and establishing a stable attachment to the therapist and live out the core of his or her difficulties in the interaction with the therapist here and now in the therapeutic relationship thus contain important therapeutic material and possibilities for initiating important development processes in the patient, which makes the development of the therapeutic alliance the therapist's primary priority. Generally, ruptures in the alliance will be related to negative transferences and the actualization of problematic elements from the patient's internal object relations in an interplay with suboptimal responses from the therapist, and the response should be framed by the psychotherapeutic stance. In that sense, ruptures in the alliance are interactional events that involve both the patient and the therapist, both of whom contribute to their occurrence. Ruptures in the alliance may also be related to resistance to the therapy and with the patient's activation of defence mechanism in response to anxiety or a perceived threat to the self in the therapeutic space.

In connection with ruptures in the alliance the main therapeutic task is thus to focus on the problems that have arisen in the therapeutic relationship. The therapist has to register and direct the shared attention at these ruptures in the therapeutic alliance, and healing the ruptures becomes a key efficacy factor in the therapy and an opportunity for the patient to have corrective emotional experiences, change his or her perception of self, others and relational conflicts/difficulties and change his or her way of being in relationships, including his or her understanding of relational processes and normal strategies for managing relational difficulties (based in the procedural memory). In addition to becoming the key focus of the treatment, as recurring relational patterns in the patient play out in the therapeutic space and become the focus of the therapeutic process, which in itself contains significant mechanisms of change, healing ruptures in the alliance also serves to diminish the risk of treatment drop-out and prolonged impasses in the therapeutic process.

Healing Ruptures in the Alliance

In descriptive terms, ruptures in the alliance can be defined and, to some extent, observed as implicit or explicit disagreement between patient and therapist about the goals and/or method of the therapy and as problems that arise in the emotional bond (the mutual trust and mutual positive perceptions) between patient and therapist. Patient and therapist will often agree on whether a rupture has occurred in the alliance, but this cannot be assumed always to be the case. Sometimes the patient perceives a rupture in the alliance, while the therapist does not share the experience, and vice versa. Patient-perceived ruptures in the alliance and problems in the therapeutic relationship in particular can have a negative impact on the treatment process and outcome, unless they are resolved. Safran and Muran (2000) have dealt in depth with how to register and handle ruptures in the alliance with a psychotherapeutic approach, where working with the ruptures in itself becomes the top priority and the main efficacy factor in the therapeutic work.

How the therapist should deal with ruptures in the alliance cannot be standardized. The most important feature is for the therapist to adopt and maintain a psychotherapeutic stance in relation to problems that arise in the therapeutic relationship/alliance and to view them as the result of something that happened in his interaction with the patient and as a shared problem that the two have to solve together. With that approach, the problems can be used to facilitate the understanding of some of the difficulties the patient often experiences in interactions with others.

Generally, we may distinguish between two types or manifestations of ruptures in the alliance, associated with the balance between, on the one hand, the need for integrity, agency and control (autonomy, freedom), and, on the other hand, the need for contact and emotional relatedness (security) in the individual patient (Safran and Muran 2000:141f; Muran et al. 2010:322). It is not without its problems to focus solely or predominantly on the manifestations of ruptures in the alliance in the patient, since in fact, the therapist may be the first to withdraw from contact with the patient or to struggle with handling powerful negative emotions in relation to the patient and so on, but that discussion will not be addressed further in the present context. The two types of ruptures in the alliance, according to Safran and Muran (2000), are:

(1) A form where the patient withdraws from the therapeutic work. The patient becomes unengaged, merely appears to go along (passively and superficially) with the therapist's agenda without actually contributing to the therapeutic work. This may be seen as a form of pseudo-alliance, where the patient gives up his or her need for clear integrity and agency in an attempt at least to maintain contact with the therapist and the sense of security it brings.

(2) A form, where the patient explicitly expresses the dissatisfaction, anger or contempt she feels towards the therapist and the therapeutic work. Perhaps the patient complains about a lack of progress in the therapy and thus airs considerations about breaking off the treatment. Here the patient maintains his or her need for agency and integrity at the cost of his or her need for contact and positive attachment with the therapist.

In both manifestations of ruptures in the alliance, the therapist's capacity for nuanced both/and thinking and for maintaining a balanced psychotherapeutic stance may come under pressure, which leads to a risk of primitive either/or thinking, an urge to defend oneself against perceived attacks from the patient or to counterattack—perhaps by withdrawing emotionally from the patient. The therapist's ability to maintain multiple equally valid perspectives on reality may be threatened when he feels personally attacked, devalued or cut off from contact with the patient or when he finds that the therapeutic space is flooded by powerful (evacuated, acted-out) affects from the patient.

Ruptures in the alliance always occur between the patient and the therapist (they cannot be isolated to the patient), and thus, the therapist's ability to manage his or her own countertransferences, including continuously observing and regulating his or her own reactions—particularly hostile and negative feelings towards the patient—in the therapeutic space, impact the development of ruptures in the alliance. Especially in connection with ruptures in the alliance where the patient discreetly withdraws from contact and the therapeutic work, the therapist has to bear in mind that the patient's (passive-aggressive) embrace of the therapist's agenda does not indicate a good alliance. However, the patient's behaviour may illustrate how he or she manages perceived power relations, which is an issue that must be handled by psychotherapeutic means. These considerations underscore the importance of ensuring an atmosphere in the therapeutic space that makes it possible for the patient to criticize the therapist and to play out and work with any issues associated with being in what the patient perceives as an asymmetrical relationship. If that is not possible, the therapy may be reduced to an unchallenged power relationship, where the patient unconsciously repeats a tendency to submit to perceived authority figures (possibly only until it becomes too much for her, and she breaks off the relationship without warning), which may be part of the background for the patient's difficulties but which is not addressed in the therapeutic work (Cushman and Gilford 2000:991).

A contributing factor to ruptures in the alliance may stem from the therapist's inadequate ability to attune his or her stance and way of handling the therapeutic relationship to the balance between the need for agency/integrity and relatedness/security in the individual patient, in a way that respects both needs to a degree that is acceptable to the patient. The balance between the two needs in the individual patient may be influenced by individual temperament and factors in the patient's history. An example could be a patient who has a strong need for the therapist explicitly to acknowledge that she can get by on her own, and who may be provoked when she finds that the therapist questions this, perhaps because he asks about how realistic some aspects of her plans are. That may be perceived as a provocation that makes the patient attack the therapist and accuse him of not having faith in her ability to get by on her own, which echoes how, for much of her life, she has found that her father and other significant persons underestimated her ability to cope and defend herself. It could be a patient who becomes passive and taciturn—maybe with some passive-aggressive irritation—or, alternatively, loses herself in stories that go on and on and do not seem relevant, whenever the therapist tries to hold her to the need to work with certain painful experiences the patient had with a man since the previous session. Here, the patient does not directly signal that she does not wish to talk about it, but she does so indirectly by failing to engage with the therapist's interventions and by changing the focus of the conversation. The patient's way of withdrawing from contact or attacking the therapist when ruptures occur in the alliance will typically be characteristic of the way the patient generally tries to manage perceived frustration (lack of gratification of central needs), abandonment and perceived conflicts (Safran and Muran 2000:143). The patient's actions in connection with ruptures in the alliance can thus give the therapist a valuable sense of the organization of the patient's inner psychological life, internal object relations, implicit relational knowledge and defences.

Regardless how ruptures in the alliance become manifest, the therapist should first verbalize how he or she perceives the common problem in the therapeutic relationship with reference to specific aspects of his or her own and the patient's behaviour in the therapeutic space. This should be phrased in terms that clearly reflect that they describe the therapist's subjective experience, which invite a symmetrical dialogue about a shared solution—'My experience is that at…', 'As I see it…', 'I'm thinking that…'—and the patient's subjective perception of the situation should be explicitly validated. The focus should be on specific elements in the interaction here and now, not on abstract and general formulations or past events. The therapist may stop and go back to the point in the therapy process when the rupture in the alliance appeared to occur or became manifest in order to explore, with the patient, what they both experienced. The immediate goal of this verbalization and shared investigation of ruptures in the alliance is not to make the patient change or to signal to the patient that she did something wrong. The primary goal is to make the patient curious, interested and more conscious about what happens in relationships and, in the long term, to strengthen the patient's understanding of how his or her stressful experiences and difficulties may be linked with dynamic-relational and psychological processes (Safran and Muran 2000:116). At the same time, the negative emotions that typically emerge in connection with ruptures in the alliance are verbalized and processed (detoxed) to prevent them from becoming an obstacle to a positive re-attunement between patient and therapist.

In some cases, it may be necessary for the therapist to invite a dialogue about partial changes to therapy goals and methods, just as the therapist may invite a shared effort to resolve any misunderstandings, including, not least, that they examine together what specifically led up to the current problems in the alliance. Here, the therapist explicitly takes responsibility for his share in the difficulties that have occurred, later accompanied by open questions about whether the patient finds that the process surrounding current ruptures in the alliance contain elements of recurring patterns that she has experienced in other relations. The successful resolution to misunderstandings and the conflicts they lead to can in itself offer a corrective experience for the patient: 'Okay, so it is possible to resolve conflicts by talking about them.' Another key element in Safran and Muran's work about a psychotherapeutic way to handle ruptures in the alliance is that the therapist meta-communicates about their communication and relation, meaning that the therapist takes a step back from what is happening in the therapeutic relationship in the present moment and (from a triangulating position) invites a conversation about their mutual communication, more processual aspects of their mutual communication and the character of their relationship.

Attuning with the Patient's Primary Needs

Both when the patient withdraws from the therapy process and when she engages in a more explicit conflict with the therapist, it can sometimes be relevant for the therapist to verbalize the challenges that may exist, both with regard to needing to mark one's own boundaries and needs, including the need for control and delimiting one's self-identity, and with regard to one's need for the contact and security that can only come from close relationships with significant others. Being in relationships inevitably involves compromises and the balancing of different concerns, needs and so on. In those cases when a rupture in the alliance is dominated by the patient's withdrawal from engagement in the therapy work, it will be helpful for the therapist to acknowledge that it appears to be important for the patient not to damage their relationship, but that the patient may be afraid of her own anger or 'greed' or, alternatively, that asserting herself and her own boundaries might cause dissatisfaction or counterattacks from the therapist or in other ways be fatal to the relationship. The main purpose is to articulate and recognize what may be the reasons behind the patient's inclination to withdraw instead of communicating her frustration or dissatisfaction more directly.

If ruptures in the alliance are primarily manifested through the patient's explicitly stated dissatisfaction, criticism and visible detachment from the therapist, it may be relevant for the therapist explicitly to recognize the patient's need to assert herself, mark her boundaries and keep the therapist at arm's length. The therapist may explain that it is understandable if the patient feels the need to protect herself instead of simply letting the therapist in, because she needs to test whether she can trust the therapist, whether he is competent and knows what he is doing; whether she can trust the therapist not to take advantage if she opens up, lets down her guard and allows the therapist to get closer (Safran and Muran 2000:26). It may also be helpful for the therapist to propose what he might have said and done—or perhaps failed to say and do—that might have made the patient feel the need to mark her boundaries. Here, the therapist verbalizes and reflects on his own possible missteps without becoming unnecessarily defensive or apologetic (cf. Tuckett 2005:40). The main purpose in this context is to formulate what may be behind the patient's contribution to the rupture that has occurred in the alliance, while the therapist also explicitly acknowledges his own contribution to the current problems in the therapeutic relationship.

With a phrase borrowed from psychoanalysis, the therapist might generally 'go with' the patient's resistance (or defence) by verbalizing that the resistance is understandable—especially in light of the patient's history. The therapist registers and reflects on the patient's resistance rather than (directly) trying to counter or overcome it, which may of course be an indirect attempt to enable the patient to reduce her resistance. At the same time, the responsibility for the ruptures in the alliance is not placed exclusively on the patient; there is no attempt to reduce it to the patient transferring or repeating old reaction patterns (which de facto also attributes responsibility to the patient); instead it is seen as something that emerged in their mutual interaction and which can subsequently be used as a basis for understanding the patient's relational difficulties, that is, how the patient often reacts to and attempts to handle perceived problems in relation to significant others.

In connection with the thematization of ruptures in the alliance and processes in the therapeutic relationship here and now, one should always—as in any other context—attune one's interventions, including the degree of closeness and emotional intensity, to the patient's current state and functioning level. For example, it should be expected that patients with a poorly integrated identity (severe identity diffusion) may become emotionally flooded and experience anxiety in connection with prolonged intensive thematization of the therapeutic relationship in the present moment. Similarly, patients with severe attachment disorders, especially disorganized and, not least, anxious-avoidant attachment, may be overwhelmed by to much emotional and psychological closeness in the relationship with the therapist. In either case the patient typically reacts by withdrawing from the contact, in the worst case breaking off the treatment unless the therapist manages to attune his approach to the patient's functioning level (Mertens 2015:181). Further, the alliance may be so fragile that the therapist has to open the conversation about the topic by verbalizing his perceived difficulties with handling the rupture that has occurred in the alliance and his struggle to preserve the possibilities to help the patient: 'Right now I have the experience that whatever I say or do, it's going to be wrong and might add to the distance between us—that your experience is that I don't understand you, which may well be true. How does that match your experience of what is happening between us right now?'

Especially when working with more severely disturbed patients and patients with various forms of attachment disorders, ruptures in the alliance will be an unavoidable as well as a necessary part of the therapeutic work. When the therapist focuses on ruptures in the alliance the patient learns that it is in fact possible to handle even intense interpersonal conflicts without the self or the relationship breaking apart. That produces an experience that it is possible to handle ruptures in the alliance and offers ideas for what the patient can do to heal ruptures in relationships outside the therapeutic space.

11.4 Handling Transference

The therapist must continuously bear in mind how what happens in the therapeutic relationship and in the interaction with the patient will contain actualizations of recurring patterns from the patient's relationships outside the therapeutic space, which are central to the patient's psychological difficulties. As mentioned earlier, the transference concept was originally introduced by Freud. This has been outlined above (see Chap. 9). The primary focus here is therefore on how the therapist meets the patient's transferences with a psychotherapeutic stance.

Key aspects of the patient's difficulties will be '(re-)enacted' and played out in the patient's way to relate to and interact with the therapist. This takes the form of the patient's transference of parts of her inner life and of her perceptions of herself, significant others and interpersonal relationships from past and current relationships outside the therapy on the therapist and on the interaction with the therapist here and now. The therapist should therefore continuously pay attention to what is happening in the interaction with the patient in the here-and-now and meet it with a psychotherapeutic stance, attempting to verbalize and incorporate it in the therapy.

Historically, the dominant understanding of the transference concept has moved from viewing the transference as something that springs solely or predominantly from within the patient—meaning that the patient re-enacts relational patterns and dramas from his or her history in the interaction with the therapist, regardless of the therapist and regardless what specific therapist the patient might interact with—to viewing it more as part of an interactional process that the therapist, to varying degrees, influences by his behaviour and personal presence. Thus, the understanding of transferences has gone from a one-person understanding, where the therapist as an external and objective observer interprets the patient's transference (often with reference to the patient's early relationships), to a two-person understanding, where the transference is regarded as a common current construction that the patient and therapist should work strive to understand together, here and now (Körner 2013:41f). Representatives of contemporary relational psychoanalysis (Sassenfeld 2015:286ff) have criticized Freud's classical transference concept (see Chaps. 8 and 9) for being rooted in an objectivizing one-person psychology that does not to a sufficient degree see the patient-therapist interaction as a meeting between two subjects, both of whom influence what plays out in the therapeutic space.

From the vantage point of a contemporary relational (intersubjective) understanding, the transference is always also a reaction to or is actualized by something actual in the therapist. It reflects the patient's attempts at meaning-making and the patient's immediate emotional reaction to the therapist and can therefore not be reduced to simple distortions in the patient's perception of the therapist or regarded merely as pathological and unrelated to actual (external) reality (Wachtel 2008:21). Rather, the patient's experience in the therapeutic space is selective and, to varying degrees, locked into a particular perspective on reality, and the patient's reactions to the therapist in certain situations are quite powerful and slightly unexpected or unpredictable for reasons that are potentially understandable in light of the patient's previous relational experiences and implicit relational knowledge. In patients with more severe pathology, the transference may give rise to more idiosyncratic experiences of the therapist, where the therapist's contribution to the actualization of the transference plays a relatively smaller role, although it does not go away. Also, the behaviour of patients with more severe disorders may be dominated by the patient's transference of reaction tendencies and patterns from relationships outside the therapeutic space to the therapy.

Generally, the main focus of the work with the patient's transferences should always be on what is playing out in the therapeutic relationship here and now (common reflections on and dialogue about how we can understand what is happening between patient and therapist in the here-and-now), with a secondary focus on how that might contain elements of recurring patterns from the patient's other current relationships. In some cases, but far from always, it may be appropriate, as a final element to examine possible connections to the patient's early relationships. The main point is that the therapist should continuously meet what happens in the therapeutic relationship with a psychotherapeutic stance and invite the patient into shared attention and reflections on it. Similarly, the specific content of the patient's transference is less important than the shared effort of patient and therapist to achieve a nuanced understanding of what is happening in the therapeutic relationship and in the patient's relationships in general.

Mapping Possible Transference Dynamics

Knowing that recurring patterns in the patient's relationships and thus the core of the patient's pathology will be actualized in the therapeutic space, before the start of therapy (during the assessment) we should seek to map the main elements of these patterns, including how any previous therapy courses were concluded. The purpose of this is to anticipate any likely dynamics in the therapeutic relationship, prepare the patient to expect that patterns from her other relationships and previous therapy course might repeat themselves in the current therapeutic relationship, as this can help diminish the risk of drop-out when the patient again experiences relational conflicts or frustrations in the therapeutic relationship, which might otherwise lead to the premature termination of therapy. Before the therapy begins, the therapist discusses with the patient that when she begins to experience frustration or signs of a repetition of the identified maladaptive interpersonal patterns in relation to the therapist, she should see that as a manifestation of her difficulties and thus as a unique opportunity for working with these difficulties. Whenever possible, she should tell the therapist about these experiences, so that they can address them together and try to understand what is happening in their relationship. Any problem that arises in the therapeutic relationship should thus be met with a psychotherapeutic stance, which means regarding it as a specific manifestation of the patient's general difficulties, without, however, placing the responsibility for the problem solely with the patient, casting it as the patient's fault or simply viewing it an expression of the patient's disturbance, while the therapist has no share in the problem that has arisen in the therapeutic relationship.

Based on the patient's specific stories about important experiences with significant others and on the patient's interactions with the therapist here and now, the following points, among others, are investigated (cf. Luborsky 1984; OPD Task Force 2008:54ff; Levenson 1995:48ff):

- How the patient perceives herself in the interaction with significant others; the patient's specific behaviour and self-perceptions in interactions with others.
- What needs the patient—consciously or unconsciously—seeks to gratify in her relationships with others.
- What conflicts and frustrations the patient experiences in interactions with others; the patient's ability to balance needs for integrity (individuation, autonomy) and attachment (dependence and relatedness), between needs for control and the urge to submission, between needs for attention and nurture versus self-reliance and the urge to get by on her own, being independent of others and so on—and how the patient specifically attempts to handle these frustrations and conflicts.

- How the patient experiences others in her interactions with them; what reactions the patient expects (imagines) from others, and what reactions she has actually experienced in specific situations (the two are not necessarily the same), including how others react to the patient's relational needs; whether the needs are gratified or frustrated, and how.
- What emotions and other mental states and subjective experiences the patient often has in connection with interactions with significant others, including what self-regulation strategies (including defences) the patient typically uses in connection with these mental states.
- How others perceive the patient in interpersonal interactions, including the therapist's perception of the patient in the therapeutic space.
- How the patient treats herself or 'behaves towards herself' in connection with interpersonal interactions (contempt, hate, love, nurture, protection and so on).
- How others perceive themselves and react emotionally, when they interact with the patient, including the therapist's own experiences in the countertransference (see below).

Based on this and other gathered information about recurring patterns and themes in the patient's interpersonal relationships a dynamic relational focus in the patient's interactions with others is formulated—a focus (patterns and themes) that one would generally expect to see actualized in the transference and thus repeated in the interaction with the therapist; the patient will tend to perceive and react to the therapist in certain ways and have certain expectations and desires in the interaction with the therapist, without necessarily knowing why. This may also be seen as a precursor to uncovering the patient's more or less unconscious implicit relational knowledge (knowledge about 'how to be together with others') stored in the procedural memory.

A young woman begins in psychotherapy. During the initial stage of the therapy, it is difficult for the therapist to make eye contact with her, and he gets a vague sense of a lack of contact; it is difficult to determine 'where the patient is at', 'who she is', and what is emotionally important to her. The therapist also finds that he has to put a great deal of energy into determining what is actually, more specifically, the core of the patient's problems. Gradually, a picture emerges of a woman who her whole life has seen herself as odd, awkward, broken and wrong (a perception related to the way she perceives others' perception of her, linked with a profound sense of shame and a feeling of inadequacy because she cannot live up to others' expectations), combined with a perceived necessity to keep up a facade that signals that she is fine, and that she does not need other people (cf. the patient's self-perception in interactions with others). For much of her life, she has had a powerful but unmet need for contact and both physical and emotional closeness with others, at the same time as she is afraid that she might be overwhelmed by the intense emotions she comes into contact with when she is close to others. She associates contact and closeness with fear of being abandoned, humiliated or hurt or of hurting others. Contact is associated with a high degree of vulnerability and vague, almost paper-thin boundaries between herself and the outside world, and with the risk of harm to both self and others.

The patient has a need to 'be seen' and receive attention from others, but she is also afraid that this might reveal how empty she really is—that behind her well-functioning facade she a void, nothing, and has nothing to give to others (cf. the patient's needs and the challenges she experiences in interactions with others). When she occasionally tries to get into contact with others, she finds that they become uncertain and are unable to contain her, so they withdraw; according to her, they think she is 'too much' and that she does not respect their boundaries (which may be difficult to imagine, based on her cautious behaviour so far in the therapeutic space). At the same time she is overwhelmed by contempt for the other's insecurity; she seems to find it impossible to contain that others are insecure in their contact with her (which might be associated with a sense that when she lacks control over the situation, the other must be in charge, linked with a vague fear that 'something fatal' might otherwise happen); she withdraws and can no longer deal with the person (cf. the patient's perception of others' reactions and behaviour in interactions with the patient). When her attempts at establishing contact fail, and she or the other becomes frightened and retreats, she feels self-loathing and self-contempt because she perceives herself as being 'completely useless' (cf. how she treats herself in connection with interpersonal interactions).

Finally, the therapist, as mentioned, senses a remarkable lack of contact, an absence of emotional contact, but gradually also more and more moments of initially very cautious, then gradually more intense emotional contact. The therapist also notes that he puts great effort into establishing contact (cf. the therapist's countertransferences and analytical eye for them) and tends to perceive himself as a failure and as inadequate but also as being a little 'too much' in his attempts to make contact with the patient (cf. others' emotional reactions in interactions with the patient). Overall, a picture thus emerges of a patient and an interpersonal field characterized by a strong desire for contact that also contains a high degree of fragility, insecurity and a tendency to feel wrong and 'too much' and to protect herself from abandonment and from being flooded by powerful emotions (which the patient struggles to regulate) by withdrawing from contact, being alone and hiding behind an almost impenetrable wall of self-reliance ('I don't need anyone or anything'). This image plays out and gradually becomes more nuanced in the therapeutic relationship, and over time it also becomes possible to break this pattern of failed attempts at contact which exacerbate the patient's experience of 'too much'.

What is Playing Out in the Therapeutic Relationship Here and Now?

In the specific work with the transference, the therapist continuously pays attention to what is happening in the therapeutic relationship here and now, and how it might be connected to recurring patterns and relational issues in the patient—to internal object relations and an implicit relational knowledge that is currently actualized in the patient right now, colouring her self-perception and her perception of the therapist and influencing the way she acts in the interaction with the therapist. In this process, the therapist may consider the following questions, among others:

- What role am I placed in/assigned by the patient right now?
- How does the patient perceive me right now?
- How does the patient perceive herself right now?
- What does the patient want and expect me to do right now?
- What needs is the patient seeking to have gratified?
- What internal drama in the patient am I on the verge of becoming a part of right now?
- What type of relationship is the patient inviting me into, and from which position (in an actualized object relation) is the patient speaking to me right now?
- How am I affected by what is happening right now, and how am I reacting to it on a subjective personal level?
- What reactions is the patient inviting from me right now?
- How do I normally react in situations similar to the one that is playing out in the therapeutic space right now?
- What affects and other mental states are present and dominant in the patient, in me and in the therapeutic space?
- Are there emotions or other mental states that the patient and I avoid in the therapeutic space?
- What defensive strategies is the patient and am I using right now, and why?

The key task in the work with the patient's transferences is not, as in classical psychoanalysis, to (re)construct the possible roots of the transferences by going far back into the patient's history; instead it involves using the transference (and the countertransference) as a basis for working together with the patient to investigate, verbalize and think nuanced thoughts about which elements from the patient's other relationships with significant others are playing out and being re-enacted in the therapeutic space right now. What is happening between the therapist and patient right here, right now, is clearly much more important than what it might reveal about the patient's early relationships (cf. Thomä and Kächele 1985:70f). Probably the single most important mechanism of change in the transference work, however, is that the therapist manages to avoid playing along in a fully unfolded and unreflective repetition of maladaptive patterns from the patient's life, and that the patient thus achieves new corrective and emotionally intense experiences that may over time, change her dominant perceptions about (mental representations of) self, others and relationship and, not least, her implicit relational knowledge.

Based on interpersonal theory we can conceptualize and understand some of the internal psychological and interpersonal processes that play out in relation to the patient's transferences in the therapeutic space from a slightly different perspective (Kiesler 1996). Here, the basic point is that most people have a fairly stable self-image, developed in early relationships, which frames the way they act in interactions with others. Typically we act in ways that are compatible with this self-image (with its accompanying perceptions of others), and which tend to evoke responses from others that confirm and reinforce our established self-image. More or less unconsciously, we thus act in ways in interactions with others, that invite responses that confirm and validate our existing self-image (identity) and our way of being in the world—a process that, when it is successful, (at least in the short term) reduces anxiety, supports our self-esteem and satisfies our needs to experience the world as reasonably predictable (Kiesler 1996:84f), but which in other regards (especially in the long term) can be quite maladaptive and lead to low self-esteem.

The typical patient has a self-image that is negative, rigid and fixed in many regards (in part because it is very difficult to make new experiences that might correct this image due to epistemic mistrust). Because this negative self-image frames the patient's behaviour in interactions with others, it tends to evoke reactions from others that confirm and strengthens it. Hence, it is a key therapeutic task to notice these self-perpetuating negative processes, that is, how the patient acts and thus unconsciously invites certain reactions from the therapist, and how this might be connected to the patient's self-perception. When the therapist deviates from the pattern and fails to react in a way that matches the patient's unconscious invitation and instead appears as a new object which also helps the patient to verbalize and understand recurring patterns in relationships, this challenges the patient's negative self-image and her simplistic perceptions of others and of how she might benefit from relationships. That process may be quite anxiety-provoking in the moment, but in the long term it can be a catalyst for positive changes.

Transference in Time and Space

When working with the patient's transferences, the therapist may find it helpful to bear in mind that transferences may operate in two different dimensions (Mitchell 1997:104f):

- *Transference as temporal displacement*—from past to present; object relations (perceptions of self, others and relationships) and defences against them from the patient's history are actualized and re-enacted, to varying degrees, in the interaction with the therapist here and now. This dimension is usually the dominant one in less severe disorders and is primarily described in classical psychoanalysis (see Chap. 8) and in parts of the theory on object relations (Caligor et al. 2007:69ff).
- *Transference as spatial displacement*—from internal to external, from self to other; the patient projects or evacuates parts of her inner world into the therapist. Arguably, transference and projection begin to merge here, and drawing a precise distinction between the two becomes conceptually challenging. This dimension is typically at play in connection with more severe disorders and is best described in Kleinian psychoanalysis (Weiss 2009). It is often associated with projective identification (see the next section).

Normally, the patient's transferences will play a bigger role and dominate the therapeutic space more in work with more severely disturbed patients, just as one should expect it to be harder to establish and maintain a good therapeutic alliance, in part because the therapeutic relationship is continuously flooded with powerful transferences and projections, just as self-perpetuating bad cycles may occasionally develop in the interaction between patient and therapist. The bad cycles cannot be reduced to a mere actualization of the patient's pathological internal object relations and repetitions of the patient's relational patterns or to patient transferences alone but are also related to the therapist's (not always optimal) reactions and behaviour in the countertransference. Historically, the patient's internal object relations and implicit relational knowledge have developed via the internalization of core elements of the patient's relationships with significant others in the form of the establishment of mental representations of self (in relation to others), others (in relation to self), interpersonal relationships (between self and others) and the related affects, which are subsequently activated and influence the patient's subjective perceptions of others and his or her way of being in interactions with others, including the therapist.

Specific Manifestation and Functioning Level Determine Handling Approach

In patients with a fairly high functioning level, transferences may be manifested in the form of more'digested' or processed perceptions and thoughts about the therapist, which the patient, to varying degrees, is able to verbalize. By contrast, transferences in therapy with more severely disturbed patients is more likely to be expressed via the patient's unreflected behaviour (acting out) in the therapeutic space and in the interaction with the therapist, which the patient is not consciously aware of or able to verbalize (cf. also structured versus actualized affects). In the latter context, the therapist should therefore be particularly attentive to what is playing out in the therapeutic relationship, the atmosphere in the therapeutic space and so on. The transference offers a window for the therapist to gain insight into and change the patient's implicit relational knowledge, internal object relations and procedural memory (which are not readily verbalized), when these parts of the patient's psychology are brought to life in the interaction with the therapist.

Some studies suggest that especially with personality disorders of medium and high severity it may have a big impact on the treatment outcome that the therapeutic process focuses explicitly on the transference, while attention to the transference serves more as an underlying carrier wave for the process in the work with less severe disorders, where the focus can be directed more towards the patient's relationships outside the therapeutic space (Høglend 2014:1062). Thus, patients with more severely disturbed object relations have been found to benefit more from dynamic-relational therapy, which explicitly includes work with the transference (the relationship to the therapist here and now), compared to a dynamic-relational approach that does not involve a focus on the therapeutic relationship, both when measured post-treatment and at the three-year follow-up (Høglend et al. 2006, 2008). Interestingly, women have generally been found to benefit more than men from working with what plays out in the therapeutic relationship (Ulberg et al. 2012).

Working with the possible connections between key elements of the current interaction with the therapist and the patient's past relationships presupposes the existence of a stable inner space in the patient for symbolization and psychological thinking. Establishing meaningful links between past, present and future presupposes that these three temporal dimensions or categories exist as fairly distinct entities, unlike a perception of timelessness or of the past as ubiquitous (for example as a result of a defect repression barrier) and a porous distinction between self and other, which is often found in patients with more severe psychological disorders (Weiss 2009:123). In patients with more severe (deficit) psychopathology, the key issues, as mentioned earlier, are not necessarily mentally represented. The patient does not speak about his or her difficulties (through verbal communication) but shows or 'is' them in her interactions with the therapist (through transferences, nonverbal communication and actualizations in the therapist's countertransferences); also, at times, her perception of the therapist may be influenced by extensive transferences and projections related to an inadequate distinction between internal and external, self and other and an inadequate inner space for symbolization and nuanced psychological thinking.

In that case, it will therefore not be similarly meaningful to work with the (re)construction of links between the patient's past relationships and current interaction with the therapist, just as it may be difficult for the patient to have new corrective experiences in the interaction with the therapist, since the patient's perception of the therapist is at times very influenced by her own projected perceptions. Instead, the attention should be focused on verbalization and on shared reflection on what is happening in the patient and in the therapeutic relationship here and now. That is pursued by verbalizing mental states and interpersonal processes and by explicitly distinguishing between internal and external, patient and therapist, and, not least, by the therapist containing and processing the patient's projected self aspects before he attempts to verbalize them and 'return them' to the patient once she is ready (se section on projective identification).

11.5 Working in and with Countertransference

Historically, there have been many and fairly different perceptions, delimitations and definitions of the countertransference, which has contributed to some degree of confusion and lack of clarity about the concept and how to understand the phenomena it seeks to capture (see also Chap. 7). As is the case with many other psychological concepts, different authors have used the same term to refer to fairly different phenomena without necessarily offering even a fairly precise and satisfactory definition. As mentioned earlier, the concept of countertransference generally refers to the reactions and emotional states the therapist experiences in therapy and in the interaction with the patient. There is disagreement about, one, the extent to which these reactions arise in the interaction between patient and therapist versus how much they can be attributed to the patient and thus mainly reveal something about him or her and, two, whether the countertransference includes all or just certain aspects of the therapist's reactions and emotional states in the therapeutic space and, three, how the countertransference should be handled.

Meeting one's countertransferences with a psychotherapeutic stance involves acknowledging that one is inevitably personally and emotionally affected by working with the patients, and that the patients are affected by seeing their therapists be affected by the interaction with them. The therapist should continuously register how he or she is affected by the work with the individual patient and reflect on how it might be understood, including how his or her own reactions may be related to factors within him/herself as well as in the patient and thus may contain information about the patient's current state, difficulties and needs. In most cases the therapist only becomes consciously aware of and able to reflect on his or her countertransferences once they have already been acted out to some extent in the interaction with the patient. The countertransference is an important element of the therapist's capacity for empathy, affective resonance and sensitivity (receiving emotional aspects of the patient's communication) and role-responsiveness (readiness and ability to take on the role or relational position he or she is unconsciously assigned by the patient in connection with the patient's actualization of internal object relations) in the interaction with the patient. Core elements of the patient's implicit relational knowledge (procedural memory), that is, elements of the patient's recurring relational patterns that have never been mentally represented and verbalized will often be actualized in the transference and the countertransference, and thus it can be a key element in understanding the patient's relational difficulties to 'listen to' one's own countertransferences.

Resonance

The German sociologist Rosa's (2016:282ff, 2018) work contains some very interesting reflections on how resonance, a concept from the science of physics, can be translated to interpersonal relations. His reflections are also interesting in connection with the understanding of resonance in the therapeutic relationship, as resonance can be viewed as an important aspect of the countertransference and the patient's possibility of experiencing emotional contact with others (in this case, the therapist), which is essential for human beings' psychological life and development. In physics, resonance refers to the phenomenon that when an object is made to vibrate at a particular rate or frequency, other nearby objects that can also be driven to vibrate will begin to do so, not at quite the same frequency, but at their own particular frequency. Each object thus vibrates with its own unique 'voice'. Moreover, they may potentially enhance each others vibrations. It is thus not a simple echo or a linear mechanical influence but a phenomenon that occurs in the interaction between interacting objects. Translated to social processes, it describes a special mode of being in the world, a certain way of relating to the world, where subjects enter into relations with each other in a very specific manner. This requires that the interacting subjects are capable of resonating with others and to act as a resonance box for others, let themselves be touched and 'reply to' others' vibrations. And they inevitably do so in their own voice. Thus, resonance is not about one-to-one objective mirroring of the other but about a way of being brought to 'vibrate' that both mirrors the other and contains elements of one's own subjectivity.

When the therapist opens up, invests him/herself and lets him/herself be psychologically and emotionally affected by the patient, he makes himself available as a resonance box for the patient and the patient's vibrations in the therapeutic space (cf. Zwiebel 2007:174). This is a process that is related to what happens when the therapist contains the patient's unintegrated, split-off and evacuated self aspects, as they are communicated via the different channels of communication. Similarly, processes unfold when the therapist temporarily assumes the role he or she has been assigned in the patient's currently dominant (actualized) internal object relations and identifies with core aspects of the patient's inner universe and mental states in the here-and-now. That requires an ability and a readiness to temporary and controlled regression in the interaction with the patient (Zwiebel 2007:83), where the therapist's personality, emotional resources and current mental states (inner balance) inevitably influence both the ability to act as a resonance box and to maintain the necessary psychotherapeutic stance towards the resonance, including continuing to function as a therapist (cf. the therapist's ability to alternate between an experiencing/perceiving and an analysing position).

The therapist's emotional, bodily and mental resonance in the meeting with the patient opens opportunities for hearing, feeling and sensing the patient's moods and mental states and other aspects of the patient's inner life, which thus become accessible to verbalization, shared reflection and psychological processing. On the other hand, the resonance box does not have unlimited capacity, as the therapist also has to maintain a clear delimitation from and the measure of distance to the patient that are conditions for the psychotherapeutic stance, the therapist's analytical position and the continued existence of a (third) position outside den current interaction between patient and therapist that may catalyse reflections on what is happening in the therapeutic relationship here and now (Zwiebel 2007:173f). The therapist needs to preserve and defend a space where he can think freely (a freedom that may be jeopardized in symbiotic relationship and in a relationship that is governed exclusively by current emotions and sensations), and where he is able, together with the patient, to 'play with' different perspectives on what is playing out in the therapeutic space. This is also the condition for the therapist to make meaning in the resonance—the mental states—he or she experiences in the contact with the patient and to include it in his or her understanding of the patient. With reference to modern mentalizing theory, we may say that the therapist has to be able to preserve the ability to mentalize the affects and other mental states that are activated in him/herself in the interaction with the patient. A related concept here is mentalized affectivity, where affective and cognitive knowledge are integrated (Bateman and Fonagy 2016:108).

As Rosa (2016:293) argues, the experience of resonance can connect body and mind, the spiritual and the corporeal, self and other/world and, potentially, emotions and intellect. Both individual subjectivity and intersubjectivity are constituted in resonance relations, and neither identity (integrity) or attachment (a sense of community) is possible without perceived resonance. The psychotherapeutic space thus represents an extremely powerful resonance box in our late modern culture on a par with art, religion, intimate relationships and nature (although these are far from always equally powerful)—a space that may, however, be hampered or, in worst cases, destroyed by calls for increased efficiency and standardization. Resonance is only possible when the interpersonal relationship and contact is regarded as a goal in itself, without being polluted by objectivizing the other (for example when categorizing/diagnosing the patient takes priority over the meeting with the patient as a human subject) or a calculating, manipulative and controlling approach to the other. Similarly, resonance requires openness, time and that the therapist is able to engage in and experience a broad spectrum of both bodily and emotional states.

Experiencing resonance is probably a fundamental human need (in contrast to alienating relationships, without contact, where the world is perceived as unresponsive, silent or even hostile, Rosa 2016:306) and an important driver of psychological development. Hence, experiencing the therapist's emotional attunement to herself in the therapeutic relationship is in itself efficacious for the patient. The experience of resonance is related to an experience of mutual influence and recognition as a subject, being mutually emotionally affected and having importance for and influencing each other. It is a mutual tuning into and attuning to one another, related to the way we continuously attune to each other physically, for example in dance or in sexual contact. In the therapeutic space the therapist's psychotherapeutic stance (by virtue of the unique, disciplined way of opening him/herself to the patient) helps enable resonance experiences in the patient. For patients with severe psychological disorders, the contact with the therapist may be the first time in their life they experience resonance, which may be an exceptionally positive experience (in part because it promotes an experience of existing and mattering to another human being); however, in some cases it can also be potentially overwhelming—as one patient, who had a borderline personality disorder, said to his therapist towards the end of a long-term (four years) course of psychotherapy: 'You are just so super-present—I feel that you see and recognize me on all cylinders, which is super-neat, but also overwhelming, almost too much, sometimes.'

Proposals for Definitions and Handling

From Freud first wrote about countertransference more than a century ago until today, we have generally moved from a very narrow definition, where the countertransference was regarded as an unambiguous obstacle to the therapeutic process that had to be minimized, to a somewhat broader understanding where the countertransference, to varying degrees, is viewed as unavoidable and as an element of the therapist's empathy that enables understanding of the patient's inner life and history (Akhtar 2013:82f). We may distinguish between at least four different definitions of countertransference (Hayes et al. 2011:240):

1. The *classical* understanding, which we find in Freud's work, where the countertransference includes the therapist's unconscious reactions to the patient's transference with roots in the therapist's own unresolved conflicts, and where it is the therapist's responsibility to overcome the countertransference to prevent it from being acted out in the interaction with the patient or influencing the therapeutic work. Freud writes about 'the "counter-transference", which arises in him as a result of the patient's influence on his unconscious feelings, and [...] [the analyst] shall recognize this counter-transference in himself and overcome it' (Freud 1910/1957:144f). He further views the countertransference as a manifestation of the therapist's resistance to the therapeutic work (Sandler et al. 1992:102). From a contemporary perspective, Freud's understanding of the countertransference must be regarded as somewhat simplistic, outdated and lacking an understanding for how the therapist may use his or her own emotional sensitivity in the therapy process. It could also be argued, however, that the countertransference in practice reflects how the therapist's unconscious, via evenly

suspended attention, 'listens to' and understands the patient's unconscious, which Freud viewed as a key aspect of therapeutic work (cf. Freud 1912/1958:111).

2. At the opposite end of the scale to Freud's very narrow understanding is a very broad '*totalistic*' understanding, where the countertransference in principle includes all the therapist's reactions to the patient that may potentially contain valuable openings to furthering the understanding of the patient, provided the therapist captures and analyses these reactions in him/herself. This definition is so broad as to be nearly meaningless in its undifferentiating attribution of everything that happens inside the therapist in the therapeutic space to the patient. It also disregards how the therapist's personality, subjectivity and emotional balances inevitably influence his or her reactions to the patient in the here-and-now.
3. Further, there is an understanding of the countertransference as being *complementary* to the patient's transference. Here, the focus is on how some of the therapist's reactions in the therapeutic space may occur because the patient, in the actualization of his or her internal object relations, in his or her behaviour and in assuming certain roles or interpersonal positions, invites certain (complementary) reactions from the therapist, corresponding to the roles that generally have shaped and continue to shape the patient's interpersonal relationships. The reactions that this evokes in the therapist thus offer a nuanced in vivo insight into the patient's inner universe, relational style and relational patterns, including what reactions the patient typically evokes or meets in others. This includes situations where the patient's behaviour is influenced by projective identification, and the therapist receives evacuated aspects of the patient's self (Ogden 1979), just as the therapist can gain insight into the patient's key perceptions of self (self-representations) and of significant others (object representations) in the patient's interactions with others (Racker 1968). This view of the countertransference clearly invites the therapist to use his or her own reactions and what he or she experiences in the interaction with the patient in the therapy process, although the therapist's own share in these reactions—how the therapist's own relational history and internal object relations influence his or her reactions in the therapeutic space—are not adequately discussed and considered.
4. Finally, we may point to a *dynamic-relational* understanding of the countertransference, which in many regards (descriptively) is not far from the complementary view, but which goes further in recognizing the countertransference as a shared construction, a phenomenon that emerges and unfolds in the interaction between patient and therapist and which thus cannot be unambiguously attributed to the patient. The therapist's own needs, unresolved conflicts and tendency to act or react in certain ways (the therapist's character) has to be included in the understanding of his or her mental states and actions in the therapeutic space—yet still with the primary goal of using his or her countertransferences to further the understanding of the patient and what happens between patient and therapist in the therapeutic space, where it is also acknowledged that the therapist's listening, experience and way of understanding the patient is always, to varying degrees, coloured by the therapist's history and internal (partially unconscious) reality. The therapist perceives and reacts to the patient in ways that, in part, are

triggered by the patient's unconsciously communicated expectation of/wish for certain reactions from the therapist and, in part, can be related to the therapist's more subjective reactions to the patient's communicated messages, behaviour and person (Kiesler 1996:228f).

The former three views of the countertransference are fully or largely associated with a one-person psychology, while the dynamic-relational view springs from a two-person psychology (see Table 8.2). Regardless exactly how the countertransference is defined, the very fact that the therapist verbalizes and, together with the patient, seeks to understand aspects of his or her countertransferences and what is happening in the therapeutic relationship and the shared interaction here and now, can help develop the patient's capacity for mentalizing, nuanced verbalization and thinking thoughts about mental states, subjective experiences and interpersonal interaction.

Objective and Subjective Countertransference

In order to determine which parts of the countertransference might contain valuable information about the patient and the patient's difficulties, we basically need to distinguish between countertransferences that spring mainly from the patient's and the therapist's psychology. With inspiration from Winnicott (1949), we may distinguish between objective and subjective countertransferences, where the former are objective in the sense that they are largely reactions to the patient's actual personality and actions in the therapeutic space and to the patient's way of relating to the therapist, while the latter may be labelled subjective because they are mainly related to the therapist's own unresolved conflicts, unconscious processes, urge to have certain needs satisfied and tendency to act in certain ways in interaction with others. The subjective countertransference may be said to be related to the therapist's subjective involvement in the interaction with the patient and a manifestation of the therapist's own 'pathology' or non-neutrality in the therapeutic space. The objective countertransference is primarily induced by the patient's behaviour in the therapeutic space and can, to some extent, be generalized to the way other people typically react and behave in interactions with the patient (Kiesler 1996:230).

Although this countertransference dichotomy is both theoretically and heuristically valuable, it is difficult or de facto impossible to apply with any precision in practice. That is not the main point, however. The main point is that the therapist should be consciously aware of the following:

(1) The therapist may have desires, needs and perceptions in relation to the individual patient and to the therapeutic process; this is okay, provided it does not dominate the therapeutic space or determine the therapeutic work.
(2) The therapist is emotionally and in other ways affected by therapeutic work, and in the interaction with the patient he or she is inevitably drawn into (re-)enacting aspects of the patient's inner life and recurring relational patterns. Temporarily this may involve acting in ways in interaction with the patient that catch the therapist by surprise and do not live up to what he or she would consider 'competent therapeutic behaviour', which may be shameful and associated with an urge to deny or otherwise disregard it. It is important to remember that this happens

to all therapists—including the most experienced and competent—and that the best way of dealing with it is to embrace that it happens and to reflect on how it may be understood (preserving the psychotherapeutic stance and the ability to play with multiple perspectives on one's own experiences and reactions) and how it may best be handled, possibly in dialogue with a colleague or supervisor.

(3) The emotions, reactions, inclinations to act in certain ways and mental states that the therapist experiences in the therapeutic space emerge in the interaction with the patient, and, to varying degrees, they spring from both the patient's and the therapist's own psychology (transference tendencies) and objective life circumstances (cf. Yeomans et al. 2002:111f).

(4) The therapist should continuously register these reactions and mental states in him/herself and reflect on (possibly in a dialogue with a supervisor) which parts of the countertransference are primarily about him/herself (are subjective) or show something about how the patient feels, the patient's inner universe (mental states currently dominant object relations) and which reactions the patient typically meets or evokes in interactions with others. It is also important to note that in some cases it can be a challenge—but an important one—to remain in emotional contact with the patient in situations with intense countertransferences that may cause distress and inner tension in the therapist.

In itself it is thus not essential to be able to distinguish unambiguously between subjective and objective countertransferences. The key is to be conscious of the indisputable reality and complexity of countertransferences, continuously to register one's own desires, reactions and mental states in the interaction with the patient and, not least, repeatedly to pause and reflect on how these actualized desires, reactions and mental states can be understood and reveal something about either the patient or oneself. Are there signs that what is happening in the therapist right now contains substantial elements of recurring patterns that the patient described in other relationships, or, on the other hand, that the therapist's subjective experience and action urges in the moment contain elements of recurring patterns from the therapist's other relationships, other courses of therapy, current life or history? Does there appear to be a clear and meaningful connection between the therapist's experiences in the countertransference and the patient's experiences here and now, or does the therapist's subjective experience appear to be of a more personal nature and thus a manifestation of subjective countertransferences? (Gorkin 1987:115).

Consistently asking this kind of question about one's own experiences enhances one's ability to consider and, to some extent, disregard one's own subjectivity in the effort to understand the patient and what plays out in the therapeutic space. To the extent that one is capable of making this sort of distinction, the countertransference and what plays out in the therapeutic relationship otherwise—including the patient's transferences and ruptures in the alliance and how these might be linked to the patient's difficulties with establishing and maintaining trust—can serve as an in vivo laboratory for exploring recurring patterns in the patient's relationships and the interpersonal source of the patient's difficulties. Besides, the attention on these processes can help maintain a continuous internal dialogue and therapeutic process in the therapist that enhances his or her ability to contain and digest (psychologically process) the occasionally powerful (primitive, regressive) processes that are played out in the therapeutic relationship.

In a session a patient talks for quite a long time about various, somewhat unspecific study plans. The patient's tone of voice is atypically monotonous, and even though the therapist asks a number of specific questions about her plans and how her thinking about education might be linked to what happened earlier, when she began several different programmes without getting even close to completing any, the therapist registers that he gets bored, loses interest and has difficulty maintaining attention on what the patient is talking about. Gradually, he gets increasingly annoyed that the patient keeps talking about the same topic, seemingly ignoring his invitations to focus on other and, in the therapist's assessment, more important underlying themes. In this situation, the therapist has to ask himself how he might understand his immediate reaction to the patient, and to what extent this reaction is about him respectively contains elements of (re-)enactments or actualization of patterns and relationships (including internal object relations) from the patient's life and thus reveal something about the patient and her difficulties.

Is the therapist getting bored because he needs stimulation after a poor night's sleep, or because he is generally impatient and feels the need to be effective? Is he getting annoyed with the patient because he feels ignored (and needs to be seen), because he feels that the patient has taken control over what is happening in the therapeutic space (and needs to be in charge), or because he finds that the conversation is not going anywhere, that it deals with something that is not important, and that they are wasting their time (combined with how he hates to waste his time)? What is the source of his irritation? Does it contain an element of critical attention to what the patient is saying about her ideas and plans—and if so, why? Or is it because a familiar pattern from the patient's life and relationships is about to repeat itself in the therapeutic space—where the patient over and over again has found that her mother was not interested in her, did not listen, lost interest and changed the subject whenever she told her about something that was important to her? And might the patient's own share in this matter be about how she talks about what is important to her, including that it is hard for her to listen and register how the other (previously the mother, currently the therapist) reacts to what she says, because she is worried that she might not be met with the interest from the other that she so desperately needs? Does the patient perceive the therapist's questions as criticism of her plans and ideas, just as she felt that her mother would always criticize her and doubt her ability to realize her (sometimes rather unrealistic) plans? Is she trying to protect herself from possible criticism by not really paying attention to the therapist's questions?

Another female patient talks about her relationships with varying men and begins to tell increasingly specific details about her sexual relations with the men, about her sexual desires, phantasies and needs. The male therapist registers how he is gradually captivated by the patient's sexual stories and wants to hear additional, and more specific, details. At the same he senses an increasing tension, inner turmoil and a fixation of his body, while on a more cognitive conscious level, he is aware that it is essential for him to remain conscious of and to protect the boundary between himself and the patient. In this situation, one might ask how the therapist's curiosity and urge to hear more should be understood. Does it spring from his general curiosity or sexual interest in the patient? Does it say something about the therapist's difficulties with sensing and drawing appropriate boundaries for closeness in relation to this particular patient or to his patients and other people in general? Or should the therapist's curiosity be understood in relation to the fact that for much of her adult life, the patient has worried about losing men who have become important to her, and that she has learned that the only way to capture their interest and keep them (avoid being abandoned) is to use her provocative sexuality and by providing sex? Should the bodily tension that the therapist registers be understood as a form of sexual tension that calls for release? Or does it rather mirror the patient's bodily sensation when she has to dissociate and block out sensations in her body in order to handle being sexually intimate with the many varying men in her life—interactions that do not gratify her sexually, but which she perceives as the price for contact and as a (rarely successful) strategy to avoid being abandoned? And what might the therapist's preoccupation with boundaries reveal, except that it is obviously important for him in a situation such as this one to be conscious of and maintain the ethical therapeutic boundaries for how to work with the patient's sexuality in the therapeutic space? Might the therapist's preoccupation with boundaries reflect a similar focus on—as well as intense confusion about—her own boundaries in the patient?

Naturally, these questions have no clear-cut answers. The key point is the importance of the therapist continuously asking him/herself this type of question about what is happening in the therapeutic relationship, how to understand his or her own reactions, and whether these reactions might offer insight into how maladaptive patterns (object relations) and experiences from the patient's life are being re-enacted in the therapeutic space. It may be important to stop these patterns and experiences (withholding reaction) or focus shared attention on them if they already occurred; also, it may be important to verbalize them and use them as a basis for understanding what it is the patient keeps experiencing, over and over, in his or her relationships with others.

Conditions for the Psychotherapeutic Use of Countertransference

In order to be able to use the countertransference as an instrument of understanding and to maintain the psychotherapeutic stance during periods, where the therapist's ability to think and keep a cool head (avoid unhelpful acting out) is under pressure from heavy countertransferences, the therapist should continuously alternate between a perceiving, participating and an analytical position in the therapeutic space (Gullestad and Killingmo 2013:155). Here it may be helpful if the therapist has undergone therapy him/herself to strengthen his or her self-awareness and ability to contain and regulate a wide range of affects and other mental states and translate them into something that is helpful in the therapy (cf. Heimann 1950:74). One of the goals of the therapist undergoing therapy him/herself is thus to enhance the therapist's disciplining of his or her subjectivity and ability to listen in a balanced way to the emotions and other mental states that are inevitably activated in intensive psychotherapeutic work without acting them out (Akhtar 2013:101). This also includes the ability to contain and handle one's own anxiety, shame and anger, which are activated in the meeting with the patient, in a constructive way, and it serves as the foundation for the ability to think rather than acting.

It is important for the therapist to permit all sorts of emotions and other mental states in him/herself and in the patient, including, for example, hate and fear (cf. Winnicott 1949:78) to prevent them from being suppressed or otherwise denied and thus acting in unseen ways to the therapist's actions in the interaction with the patient. This includes recognizing and accepting the emotional stress that may be associated with working with, especially, more severely disturbed patients and seeking supervision or continuing training when necessary in order to be in the therapeutic space and maintain the emotional contact with the patient. The psychotherapist's most important tool is his or her own personality and emotional sensitivity, which he or she may get to know better via his or her own therapy, which also offers a way to encounter mental states, sides of him/herself and aspects of being human that he or she may never have encountered before. For that reason, too, undergoing therapy may be a key element in developing the therapist's therapeutic competence (McWilliams 2004:66). With reference to Gelso (2011:49f), it is possible to identify a number of interlinked elements that are important in handling countertransferences:

- *Some degree of self-insight*. The therapist's ability to understand his or her patients and to distinguish between objective and subjective countertransferences may be hampered by a lack of understanding of him/herself and of what is at stake for him or her in the interaction with the patient. The therapist relies in part on his or her own inner world for understanding the patient, and his or her capacity for psychological thinking (mentalizing) and understanding complex psychological processes is fundamental to his ability to understand the patient; hence, an inadequate understanding of his or her own universe and psychology can limit or even distort the therapist's understanding of the patient.
- A well-developed capacity for verbalizing and conceptualizing—thinking nuanced thoughts about—internal psychological processes and interpersonal interactions. An ability to take a step back from experiences, perceptions, feelings and sensations in the moment, corresponding to the position of participating observer, where the therapist alternates between being or allowing him/herself to be involved in what plays out in the internal as well as the external arena in the here-and-now and taking a step back to reflect on it with assistance from clinical experience, psychological theory and empirical findings. Theoretical knowledge and understanding in itself is far from sufficient but has to be combined with a certain insight into own mental states, motives and reaction patterns to become truly useful in the therapeutic work. This also involves the ability to control and limit the acting out of countertransferences and avoid immediately translating intense emotional reactions into rash actions in relation to the patient. There is a big difference between, on the one hand, acting out a vague, unprocessed irritation or anger towards the patient in a verbal attack and, on the other hand, converting that irritation to an understanding of the patient and of what the irritation may be about, before it might be verbalized for the patient in a digested and detoxed form, where the

central message is not an attack on the patient but an effort to understand what the perceived irritation may reveal, and how it may further the understanding of the patient's difficulties (cf. actualized and structured affects, see above).

- Good capacity for empathy, for vicarious identification with the patient and his her inner universe and perception of reality. An ability to register the patient's needs, emotional states and reactions and any links between the patient's mental states and his or her behaviour in the moment. The optimal use and communication of empathy to the patient also requires that the therapist is able to remain separate from the patient without exaggerating his or her (mere vicarious) identification with the patient and his or her difficulties. If the therapist's ability to remain separate from the patient is compromises, and if the therapist's emotional state in the therapeutic space begins to fuse with the patient's, it becomes difficult to maintain the position as a participating observer that is so vital for the therapeutic work; the ability to take a step back and reflect on what plays out in the therapeutic space between patient and therapist (triangulation) collapses. Countertransferences that get out of control can thus undermine the therapist's empathy and capacity for congruent and marked mirroring of the patient—a mirroring that captures the patient's self and mental state in the moment, while it remains clear to the patient that it is her emotion and not the therapist's that is mirrored. Balanced self-regulation and affect regulation are thus important conditions for the therapist to preserve his or her capacity for marked and congruent mirroring, also in situations characterized by high emotional arousal in the therapeutic space.
- A well-developed ability to experience (open oneself to), contain and regulate a wide range of mental states, including anxiety and intense affects; a well-developed emotional sensitivity and ability to perceive resonance in relation to diverse mental states without the intensity becoming so high that the ability to take a step back and reflect is compromised (cf. Heimann 1950:75). The therapist has to dare to be affected by the patient and his or her occasionally both intense and painful emotional states and must be ready to be used emotionally by the patient without violating boundaries (Gorkin 1987:77f). To be able to preserve his or her empathy and ability to think, the therapist has to be able to experience anxiety and intense affects without activating defensive mechanisms, shut down emotionally or resort to action in order to escape overwhelming or painful affects. The therapist has to let the patient's transference unfold and allow it to affect the therapist's self, including being open to own countertransferences, unlike the therapist who, driven by anxiety and insecurity, shuts down his or her inner potential space and demands quick understanding or specific action. Moreover, the therapist has to be able to regulate the emotional arousal level in the therapy, for example by moving from a more explorative or confrontational approach to a more supportive and validating (possibly factual) one when the arousal levels gets too high, and the patient's (or the therapist's) ability to think is in jeopardy. This is particularly important when working with more severely disturbed patients and patients with a reduced capacity for self-regulation (under-regulation), who need the therapist's help to regulate powerful affects when they are activated in connection with the therapeutic work.

Any therapist can lose the ability to think and thus the ability to function as a therapist if his or her inner space is flooded by intense countertransferences (in the form of diffuse anxiety or inner turmoil, fear that the patient may commit or attempt suicide or physically attack him or her, or if the therapist fails to maintain appropriate boundaries in relation to the patient and so on). If this happens repeatedly, the therapist should seek supervision. Especially when working with patients with personality disorders, the countertransference may at times be characterized by diffuse (occasionally bodily) tension states and confusing subjective experiences that may at first seem confounding and difficult to verbalize (Rudolf 2005:143). Similarly, the patient may need to use the therapist as a waste bin or a storage space for evacuated experiences and aspects of the self, which he or she may manifest as loquaciousness, perhaps talking about seemingly very diverse experiences since the previous session, or by communicating intensely on several channels of communication at once, which may make the therapist feel 'filled up' and experience very strong countertransferences without necessarily being able to specify exactly what he or she is 'filled up' with (Weiss 2015:930).

Disclosing Countertransferences

It is neither possible nor meaningful to formulate standardized and specific guidelines for how the therapist should use and, possibly, communicate his or her countertransferences to the patient. On the more general strategic level, however, there are a number of different recommendations for whether and if so, to what extent and how the therapist should communicate countertransferences to the patient (Maroda 1994:84):

- A *conservative* position argues that countertransferences can only, at best, be a tool for the therapist's understanding of the patient but would only be a burden for the patient (shift the focus unnecessarily from the patient to the therapist) if it is explicitly disclosed.
- A more *moderate* position recommends occasionally disclosing one's countertransferences to more severely disturbed patients (not to more well-functioning patients).
- An approach that some have called *radical* recommends the continuous disclosure of countertransferences as a key part of therapeutic strategy.

A number of arguments can be made for the therapist to verbalize (parts of) one's countertransferences to the patient (Maroda 1994:87; Gorkin 1987), in part that it may contribute to the patient's understanding of what happens in interpersonal interactions, and how others perceive and react to her way of being in a relationship. It offers the patient an in vivo opportunity for understanding how she influences the therapist and others in general (Gorkin 1987:84f).

The disclosure of countertransferences can also demonstrate the therapist's honesty, authenticity and subjectivity (humanity) and show that the patient is being seen, matters and influences the therapist (and thus others in general). This may confirm the patient's sense of reality, rather than the therapist pretending, denying his actual experiences and reactions in the interaction with the patient and thus contributing to making the patient (even more) insecure about the validity of her own sensations and experiences. The therapist demonstrates his ability to be present as a fellow human being (a subject) and to enter into genuine contact when he speaks *with* the patient, not just *to* the patient (cf. Ogden 2016:175). If the therapist denies the reality of the countertransferences and insists on being the neutral therapist who is able to keep his person, his subjectivity and his own emotions completely separate from his work, he is at best reduced to a technocrat who will hardly be successful in treating more complex psychological disorders. At worst, this approach increases the risk that countertransferences—unbeknownst to the therapist—influence the therapeutic work negatively in the form of distorted perceptions of the patient, problems with being present for the patient (as a result of intense countertransferences) or contributing to constant repetitions of maladaptive interpersonal patterns in the therapeutic relationship.

Finally, verbalizing countertransferences can be said to illustrate the therapist's humanity (fallibility), which may make it easier for the patient to accept her own, including accepting her own perceived flaws and shortcomings. Similarly, the therapist can show the patient in vivo how to adopt a curious, explorative and playful attitude towards oneself and one's own reactions, thoughts, emotions and mental states. That is an attitude towards the self that the patient can gradually adopt and thus develop a more tolerant, accepting but also more curious attitude towards herself, her inner life and her reaction patterns. If the therapist chooses to verbalize parts of his or her countertransferences to the patient, it must always be done in a way that clearly maintains the focus of the therapeutic work on the patient, and which does not feel intrusive to the patient (where the patient experiences that now she has to contain and digest the therapist's subjective experiences, rather than vice versa, and so on).

Handling Silence

As mentioned, especially in working with more severely disturbed patients, it is important for the therapist to be present and visible as a person, including taking responsibility for keeping the therapeutic process moving, as much as possible, in a direction that is fruitful for the patient. Here, the therapist has to consider how episodes involving prolonged silence in the therapeutic space should be understood and attune his or her handling of it accordingly. Especially in some parts of the classical psychoanalysis, the patient's silence has been perceived as resistance to the treatment or as an aggressive attack from the patient on the therapist and the therapy. Although in some (fairly rare) cases, the patient may actually use silence as a way of controlling or disarming the therapist—an unconscious attempts to destroy 'the good object' and its ability to help the patient and a manifestation of the patient's negative transference (the therapist is put into the position of the bad object, which is to be held at bay and not let into the patient's inner universe and so on)—the patient's silence may also be driven by many other and very different dynamics. The therapist has to draw on his countertransference and knowledge of the patient to understand why the patient is silent or shows very limited response to his interventions and invitations to verbal contact. If the therapist becomes silent or struggles to know what to say, he has to examine what that may be about. Why is it suddenly hard to find the right words, and why has his communication with the patient hit an impasse?

The patient may, for example, perceive the therapist's (and her own) silence in the moment as a calm, pleasant space with room to sense herself and think—a caring way of providing space. On the other hand, the therapist's silence may also be perceived as a sign of a lack of understanding, an aggressive intent way of frustrating the patient, withholding help and care or a sign that the contact with the therapist is broken. In these cases, the patient may perceive the therapist's silence as a repetition of experiences of being abandoned, left to handle her painful difficulties alone (which more severely disturbed patients may perceive as an existential threat). Similarly, the patient's silence may be a sign that she is being reflective and is processing something that was just actualized, or that she needs time and space to take a breath before moving on with the current work or changing the focus. On the other hand, the patient's silence may also be an indication that she is lacking words, has nothing to offer the therapist (and others in general), is overwhelmed by a feeling of emptiness and meaninglessness and a sense of standing at the edge of a dark abyss, where the patient needs the therapist's active assistance to get back in contact and to verbalize, process and understand this (Akhtar 2013:25ff).

Finally, the patient's silence may occur because her inner universe right now is flooded by impulses and perceptions that she finds it impossible to talk about with the therapist, because in her mind they are forbidden, unbearable (and would only get worse or get out of control if they were verbalized), terrible, shameful or a sign of what a bad and evil person she is. Here too, the patient will need the therapist's help to break, reflect on and process the silence—a silence that the patient typically knows all too well from her life outside the therapeutic space. As with many questions in the therapeutic space the therapist needs to assess the specific situation and find a balanced way to handle it, which involves being aware that in appropriate amounts, silence can help provide contact to deeper layers of the self, just as eye contact can lead to deeper emotional contact between patient and therapist—provided the patient (and the therapist) has the necessary resources to sustain this contact with parts of herself and with the other.

To assess the character of a silence that has emerged the therapist has to listen to his or her own sense of the silence. What is the mood in the therapeutic space, what signals does the patient send about how she is feeling right now? And, not least—may it be fruitful to verbalize the silence, which in itself (for good and bad) can help break it, and try to talk with the patient about how each of them experiences the silence and how they might understand it together? Here it is crucial that the therapist is familiar with and able to tolerate silence, that is, that he can handle not just wordless contact but also an absence of contact, so that it is not the therapist's own needs, emotional arousal or current imbalance that dictates an intervention and thus breaks a silence that may have been fruitful for the patient.

Projective Identification

The concept of projective identification can contribute to a more nuanced understanding of transference and countertransference and to a more subtle psychotherapeutic handling of what plays out in the therapeutic relationship, especially in work with more disturbed patients. The complex psychological processes that the concept captures suggest that the therapist should not only adopt a psychotherapeutic stance to the patient and his or her actions in the therapeutic space but also to his own subjective experiences and reactions in the interaction with the patient; thus, the therapist should meet, observe and reflect on him/herself as 'the other patient' in the therapeutic space (Bollas 1987:202).

From its introduction by Klein in (1946) until today, the concept has been interpreted in so many different ways that it is at risk of losing all useful meaning. Klein (1946:160f) uses it primarily to refer to a defence mechanism and to (infant) phantasies of getting rid of unbearable or unintegratable parts of the self by projecting them into others (primarily the mother), while in later interpretations (Ogden 1979) it is also—and primarily—used about complex interpersonal processes between patient and therapist, which contain therapeutic potentials for the therapist who understands and is able to handle the phenomenon when it occurs in the therapeutic space. Kleinian psychoanalysts use projective identification to refer to a primitive psychological functioning level (the paranoid schizoid position in Klein's theory), but they also see it as containing a development potential for reaching a higher and more mature functioning level (the depressive position in Klein's theory) (cf. Jørgensen 2009:262ff).

There continues to be some disagreement about whether projective identification should be understood solely as an intrapsychic (one-person) phenomenon (cf. Tansey and Burke 1989:44f) or as a series of more interpersonal (two-person) processes (cf. Ogden 1979, 1982), including to what extent the therapist's therapeutic handling of the involved processes should be seen as an integrated part of the phenomenon or should be described separately. In addition to the fact that the concept is often used to mean different things and the lack of even a fairly accurate definition, there are further problems associated to the current understanding of projective identification: it is in some cases not sufficiently distinct from projection (however, see below) and, to some extent, from transference and countertransference. In some cases the therapist's subjective contribution to the phenomenon when it occurs in the therapeutic relationship is not sufficiently considered, as it is predominantly or solely viewed as a phenomenon pertaining to the patient, and finally, it is primarily used as a descriptive concept that may capture complex interpersonal processes but does not in itself hold any power of explanation. In extension of this, it should be noted that projective identification may in some cases come from the therapist, as he or she, more or less unconsciously, positions and seeks to process parts of him/herself within the patient.

An Interpersonal Phenomenon

As Kernberg (1992:159), among others, has pointed out, part of the confusion concerning the precise definition of projective identification arises because of a failure to distinguish between different patient groups or because of insufficient recognition of the impact of the patient's degree of structural organization (cf. distinction between conflict and deficit pathology, see later) on how the projective identification becomes manifest. In less severe psychopathology projective identification plays a much smaller role (or is completely insignificant) in the therapeutic relationship, and the psychological material that goes into the projective identification is far less primitive and considerably easier to handle. In the present context, the term is mainly used to refer to interactional processes between patient and therapist when patients have more severe personality disorders, mostly because projective identification largely plays out in relation to people with a psychological defence that is organized around splitting, which is primarily seen in persons with more severe personality pathology. In that context, the concept can help to establish a useful bridge between intrapsychic and relational phenomena, including contributing to generating creative thoughts for use in the therapeutic space (cf. Ogden 1982:11).

From a dynamic relational perspective projective identification refers to a complex interpersonal phenomenon where initially unbearable (unintegratable) parts of the patient's self are evacuated and projected into the therapist. At the same time, the patient acts and communicates—verbally and nonverbally—in the interaction with the therapist in ways that increase the likelihood of triggering psychological processes in the therapist that cause him or her temporarily and to varying degrees to experience and identify with a role (complete with related acts and so on) that in key aspects corresponds to or mirrors the patient's projected self-parts and mental states. These interpersonal processes and psychological processes in the therapist contain valuable information about the patient's inner liv and difficulties as well as therapeutic potential.

Via projective identification the patient is able (temporarily) to get rid of and achieve psychological distance to the projected affects and self-parts while maintaining contact with them through his or her contact with the therapist. This lets the patient handle the projected affects and self-parts 'inside the therapist', where they are at an emotionally safe distance and do not give rise to unmanageable inner conflicts. The projected affects may, for example, include anger, anxiety, shame or envy. Similarly, desires for sexual contact, an urge to break contact and seek isolation (loneliness, emptiness), confidence in the treatment, diffuse inner turmoil and bizarre thinking about the self or others may be projected into the therapist. As a consequence, the patient's perception of the therapist (and the patient's own self) is, to varying degrees, coloured or even distorted by the projected elements: 'Why are you so angry with me?' (where, initially, the patient was angry with the therapist, but the anger was then placed inside the therapist where the patient begins to process it); 'You're just waiting for an excuse to terminate the therapy' (where it is initially the patient who feels the urge to terminate a therapy process that makes her feel insecure because it brings her into contact with unknown and dangerous parts of herself).

Projective identification differs from the more mature projection in two important ways. One, is that—as mentioned earlier—it is typically organized around (often extensive) splitting, while projection is often based in a defence that is generally more mature and largely centred on repression (Kernberg 1992:159f). And two, it involves maintaining much closer emotional, and often also specific, contact with the projected material in the form of specific interactions with the person or persons who is/are the target for the projected aspects—an interaction that also often evokes experiences and mental states in the affected other(s) that match the projected material (see, however, Spillius 2012). To the extent that the other (the therapist) receives and contains the projected material, that may help reduce the patient's experience of being alone. The patient's perception of parts of the self being so unbearable, intolerable, unacceptable or destructive that they have to be kept hidden from view is moderated. In the projection, repressed experiences and self-parts are projected into others, following which the person distances him/herself both emotionally (feeling disgust, outrage and so on) and in concrete physical terms to the persons or groups that are the target of the projected material.

In extension of the above, Ogden (1979:362f) has argued quite convincingly that projective identification should be understood as serving several functions simultaneously:

- A *defence mechanism*, where the patient (imagines that she) gets rid of or achieves a psychological distance from mental states that she cannot contain and parts of the self that she cannot reconcile (integrate) with other parts of the self. The patient attempts to attain or maintain an inner psychological balance by rejecting parts of the self or certain mental states that are perceived as threats to the self or as incompatible with other parts of the self. As a defence mechanism, the projective identification can include both the patient's internal psychological reality (phantasy) and specific interactional processes in the therapeutic space (external reality in the form of the patient's and the therapist's behaviour).
- A *mode of communication*, where the interaction between the patient's actions in the therapeutic space and the therapist's readiness to react in different ways and experience a wide range of mental states evokes action urges, emotions and other mental states in the therapist that in key regards resemble or mirror the patient's projected self-parts and mental states. These are experiences, self-parts and mental states that the patient for various reasons is unable to verbalize but unconsciously (via nonverbal communication) contributes to evoking in the therapist (cf. the therapist's emotional and interactional responsiveness). The projective identification may thus contribute to evoking a feeling of being understood or having something in common with the therapist, which simultaneously enables the therapist to gain insight into key aspects of the patient's inner universe.
- An *object relationship,* a way of being in contact and interact with the other (the therapist) who is only partially psychologically separate from the self. The boundary between self and other becomes porous, and it can be difficult to discern exactly what belongs to the self versus the other, that is, whether the therapist's subjective experiences and mental states at a given time mirror similar experiences and mental states in the patient that he or she has evacuated and projected into the therapist.
- And—as discussed below—a *pathway for psychological change* in the patient, where the patient's unbeatable self-parts and mental states are psychologically processed and transformed (digested, detoxed, enriched with meaning) by the therapist and may subsequently be returned to patient—taken back by the patient—in a form that the patient can better contain and integrate into the self.

The complex internal and relational processes associated with projective identification underscore how important it is that the therapist meets what happens in the therapeutic relationship with a psychotherapeutic stance rather than, mindlessly and without reflection, letting relational processes unfold in the therapeutic space without paying much attention to them.

Largely Unconscious Processes

In some contexts, projective identification is presented as a more or less conscious and intentional process, where the patient almost as if by magic shifts affects or mental states from herself to the therapist. Such a view must be considered untenable and as reflective of a simplistic one-person understanding of the interactional processes and the unconscious communication between patient and therapist that the concept endeavours to capture. It is an unconscious or non-conscious communication that is not based in traditional psychoanalytic notions of a dynamic unconscious constituted and driven by repressed past experiences. Via the patient's actions (verbal and nonverbal communication) in the interaction with the therapist, emotions and other mental states are induced in the therapist, who in key regards mirrors the patient's experience and self. The evoked mental states in the therapist will inevitably be coloured by his or her personality and psychological structures and thus take on different expressions and be processed differently than in the patient (see also the section on resonance). The latter feature is what allows for the development of the patient's ability to contain and process the projected self-parts and mental states. Similarly, it increases the likelihood that the therapist identifies with a role, with its related behavioural tendencies, that he or she was unconsciously assigned in the patient's actualized internal object relations—via the patient's conscious and unconscious actions in the interaction with the therapist.

As mentioned, projective identification can play a role in the psychotherapeutic interaction especially in therapy with patients with more severe psychological disorders (personality disorders), where the patients generally do not use the therapeutic relationship primarily as a way to achieve a better understanding of themselves and their difficulties, but rather to evacuate or get rid of unbearable or unintegrated elements of their internal psychological reality; the therapist and the therapy are used as a 'waste bin' or a storage space for parts of the self and certain mental states (Moser 2001:113). Patients with more severe personality disorders rarely have the necessary psychological resources to verbalize and think nuanced thoughts about intense mental states, incompatible parts of the self and complex psychological and interpersonal processes. The verbal language is not just used to communicate meaning via the explicit content of the verbal communication but also to act with, and it may (on an unconscious level) evoke certain mental states and unverbalized experiences in the therapist. The patient's ability to form and use mental representations of mental states and self-parts is limited, which generally means that the nonverbal communication and the countertransference, including the projective identification in the interaction between patient and therapist, become the main sources for understanding the patient and an important focal points of the psychotherapeutic work.

Precisely because this relies on largely unconscious communication, it may be difficult for the therapist to register when the interaction with the patient is influenced by projective identification, and often he will only become aware of it after some time, after he has been caught up in acting out a behaviour that reflects elements of the patient's projected self-parts. A potential indication of projective identification may be that the patient explicitly says, perhaps accusingly, that the therapist has a particular feeling towards her, has a specific perception of her or has reacted to the patient in a manner that the therapist does not recognize. Or if the therapist registers that he has emotions, action urges or other mental states that he does not normally experience, does not recognize or does not perceive as a part of himself or of his normal self-perception. Normally, this mostly plays out in the therapeutic space, but it may also involve experiencing reactions to or coming into contact with elements of the work with the patient outside the therapeutic space, such as suddenly thinking of the patient or of specific episodes in a therapy session, or that the work with the patient flows into his dreams or mental state after a session.

Containing and Processing Projected Material

The therapist has to be ready to contain the experiences that are evoked in connection with projective identification. He or she has to be ready to experience the mental states and engage in the form of object relationship that the patient unconsciously invites. The latter may involves temporarily identifying with and experiencing in vivo both what it is like to be the patient in his or her activated object relationship or implicit relational knowledge and what is associated with the patient's internal internalized objects, including the position as 'the other' in the patient's recurring interpersonal patterns. In relation to this, Racker (1968:159f) writes about concordant and complementary identification, were the therapist may develop a sense of how the patient (concordant identification) and significant others (complementary identification) in the patient's life often feel and have felt, have felt they were treated and have acted in their mutual interaction. The therapist's resonance and way of responding to the projective identification is an important part of the countertransference and may serve as the basis of a deeper empathic understanding of the patient, provided the therapist is able to register, reflect on and decode how his own subjective experiences and reactions in the interaction with the patient contain valuable information about the patient's (unconscious) inner life and difficulties.

The psychotherapeutic stance thus involves making oneself available as a container for the patient's projected self-parts and avoiding to act on any urges to defend oneself against experiencing these unbearable self-parts and painful mental states (urges to reject or throw the patient's projections back to the patient), for example by acting on the need immediately to understand and interpret everything the patient says and does or by explicitly denying to the patient that one contains the mental states or action urges that the patient expresses that she believes one contains (cf. Ogden 1979:366). The therapist should allow the patient to use him or her as a projected storage space for parts of the patient's self (aggression, confidence in the therapy and the future, ability to think and understand and so on). He should allow himself to feel what the patient feels (but often with reduced intensity), which over time may give the patient an opportunity to internalize the therapist's more mature and balanced approach to and processing of the projected self-parts, emotions and other mental states. Wilfred Bion speaks of the patient's internalization of the therapist's alpha function (capacity for symbolization, reflection, ability to tolerate powerful affects and so on) and 'reverie' (psychological processing), where raw sensations and mental states—so-called beta elements—are converted into a form where they can be made the object of thinking and embedded in meaning-making narratives (Weiss 2007:182f).

Especially in therapy with more severely disturbed patients it can be a very demanding task to contain and process the harrowing experiences and potentially overwhelming mental states that may at times fill the therapeutic space; hence, especially less experienced therapists should have access to regular supervision and a chance to 'unload' and share their experiences from the therapeutic work with others. A therapist who is flooded with affects, impulses and other overwhelming mental states, where the ability to contain and regulate own reactions and to think can be seriously compromised, will not be able to help his patients; instead, he risks exacerbating their pathology, for example through reactions that confirm the patient's perception that the self is impossible for others to contain and of experiences affects as being dangerous, forbidden, disorganized and unbearable.

The projected material—the mental states that are activated in the therapist—should be verbalized in a form and embedded in a coherent, validating and meaning-making narrative where it becomes possible for the patient, so to speak, to take back the projected material or to contain and acknowledge the concerned self-parts and mental states in him/herself. That becomes a possibility when the therapist makes himself and his inner world, his capacity for psychological processing, available for the patient and contains and lets himself be used by the patient. In this process, the therapist continuously alternates between, on the one hand, going with the flow of current interpersonal processes and mental states in the therapeutic space and, on the other hand, taking a step back and applying an analytical, reflected perspective to the self-same processes and using them as a way to understand the patient, his or her difficulties and how they play out in vivo in the therapeutic space, here and now.

However, if the therapist struggles to contain and allow himself to experience what the patient is experiencing and what is happening in the therapeutic relationship, he may inadvertently reject the patient's projected self-parts and mental states ('no, I'm not angry', 'I don't recognize that at all') in ways that throw the patient's projected self-parts back to her in an unprocessed form, which risks destabilizing her further (increased anxiety level and so on) and exacerbate her already urgent sense of dealing with unbearable experience on her own. In doing so, the therapist would also confirm that the patient's experiences, self-parts and mental states are indeed unbearable, unacceptable, scary, destructive and so on (cf. Gorkin 1987:64). The psychotherapeutic approach to handling and using the projective identification is thus closely related to the therapist's balanced ability to manage countertransferences and opens new opportunities for understanding the patient's transference, including the nature of the internal object relations and mental states that dominate the patient's inner life and interactions with others. However, this is only possible if the therapist is able to handle coming into contact with his or her own (and others') regressive experiences, mental states and self-parts (Weiss 2007:191). When the therapist comes into contact with these regressive experiences, he should strive to meet them with curious interest and as a potential source of information about the patient, himself and the current therapy process rather than as a basis for judging or condemning himself for having these experiences.

A young woman with a borderline personality disorder has for several years had a series of largely sexual relationships with varying married men and men that she, for various reasons, never establishes any deeper emotional, let alone binding, contact with. In addition, since she was quite young, she has experienced her mother being very critical of men and warning her against having sex with men as this, in the mother's opinion, would inevitably expose her to harm and hurt, just as the mother, for various reasons, saw it as an important task to protect her daughter from rape by making sure that she in no way appeared sexually provocative. At the beginning of a session she says that she has recently initiated a new relationship with a married man. She says that she is very much in love with him, and she feels that he understands her on a level that she has never experienced in any relationship with a man before (apart from her relationship with the therapist). After a relatively short time, during which the therapist on a specific behavioural level has merely asked a few open, clarifying questions about this new relationship and about the emotional experiences her relationship with this man has given the patient, she attacks him for what she perceives is his sceptical attitude towards her new 'boyfriend'.

In her experience, the therapist does not believe that this relationship is different from her previous relationships with men or that it can develop into a lasting relationship, where he would leave his wife in order to be with the patient. She finds that the therapist says to her that she should avoid becoming swallowed up by a symbiotic relationship where she would pay a high price for a form of contact and an experience that there is a man who wants her. This makes her very angry, in part because she sees the therapist's reaction as a sign that he does not believe in her and does not believe that she is able to establish a relationship that is good for her. On the other hand, by her own statement, she is quite convinced that this relationship is 'completely different' from her previous ones, and that no one can make her give up the relationship. Initially, the therapist is surprised by this sudden attack from the patient, as he was not aware of having expressed any scepticism, let alone any moral concerns, about the patient's new relationship, although he is aware that deep down, he is thinking, 'Oh no, she seems about to repeat the same pattern where she engages in a sexual relationship with (what appears to be) an unattainable man that probably has no real future potential, and which probably—like previous similar situations—is going to make her feel disappointed and exploited and cause her to break off the relationship' (Kattlove 2016).

What is playing out in the therapeutic space here can be seen in relation to an internal conflict in the patient between, on the one hand, her strong need for contact that she, for various reasons, repeatedly seeks to satisfy by having relationships with married men, whom she in all likelihood cannot 'have' in the traditional sense, and who soon make her feel betrayed or abandoned, and, on the other hand a beginning awareness that she is repeating a recurring pattern that is destructive to herself and a desire for a different kind of relationship based on a deeper emotional, longer-lasting and not exclusively sexual contact. This conflict is further complicated by the fact that her mother's warnings against sexual relations are activated every time she engages in a new relationship with a man. However, she is not (yet) able to contain or integrate the two sides of this conflict with its related emotions. Unconsciously, she handles the conflict by projecting her doubts about whether the current relationship is in fact going to be different than her many previous relationships with married men—including the risk that she is exploited sexually by a man who simply wants to have sex with her and who is not interested in having her or 'seeing' her besides that, and the recognition that this may be (once again) a dead end into the therapist.

This means that she can hold on to her desire to engage in the relationship with this man, with all the related notions (phantasies, hopes, dreams) that 'he is completely different than all the other men I've met before—he understands me and sees me in a totally different way.' Once her doubts have been projected into the therapist, and she attacks it in the therapist—attacking the therapist for what she perceives as his lack of faith in her love and her ability to establish a viable relationship with a man—it becomes easier for her to hold on to the idea that 'this time it's different.' In the here-and-now she can get rid of the doubt and the internal conflict and ambivalence associated with being about to embark on yet another mainly sexual relationship with a married man. At the same time, she is able to maintain contact with this part of herself and try to deal with it or go into dialogue with it by addressing it—from a safe distance—inside the therapist (provided the therapist receives and is able to contain it). Superficially, the internal conflict may appear to be resolved, as one position or one side of it has been placed in and is in part lived out by the therapist, while the patient now only has to contain the other side.

The therapist handles the projective identification by first expressing that he is a little surprised by this intense attack from the patient, but that he can understand that she would be angry with him if she perceived his reaction to her story about her new boyfriend as a sign that he flatly rejects that his new relationship can be different than her previous relationships with men before he has really heard much about this new man and how she perceives him. On the other hand, the therapist is aware that he did have this doubt as soon as she told him about her new boyfriend, and that he felt an urge to try to convince her not to engage in this relationship, because he thought it would lead to her feeling abandoned and exploited again. He felt an urge to protect her. Thus, even though the therapist feels certain that he did not explicitly express this doubt and the urge to protect the patient, he has felt it—a doubt that one might assume mirrors a similar doubt in the patient. Hence, the therapist says to the patient that he actually did feel this doubt and an urge to act on it, which he perceived as an urge to protect her; he follows this up by briefly describing how he may have both a belief and a hope that this time will be different for her. At the same time (in light of the patient's previous similar relationships), he may also have doubts or be uncertain about whether it is realistic, and whether she is about to repeat a destructive relational pattern. He says to the patient that it can be difficult right now to determine which of the two assessments is more apt. Afterwards the therapist asks the patient whether she can recognize the two perspectives on what is happening in her relationship with the new man. She does, which is an important first step towards being able to contain and integrate the two self-parts. She also gets upset as she comes into contact with her own doubt and lack of—or at best fragile—confidence that she will ever be able to establish a lasting, equal relationship with a man—a sadness that she was also able to keep at bay as long as her doubt and uncertainty were deposited with the therapist.

11.6 Attuning to the Patient's Level of Functioning

It would hardly be fair to claim that the descriptions of and reflections on the psychotherapeutic stance that have been presented here are equally relevant to all types of therapeutic work with any group of patients. However, they are, to varying degrees, relevant to most patient categories and especially in long-term psychotherapeutic work with medium- and high-severity disorders in adolescents and adults. This is the case regardless of the specific therapy model, although some (who do not apply a dynamic-relational mindset) will disagree with this claim to some extent. However, all patients do not need the same specific implementation of the psychotherapeutic stance, and it is in fact a key point in the psychotherapeutic stance that the therapist should continuously attune his or her specific behaviour and approach to the individual patient's level of pathology, resources, current state and needs, just as the patient's dominant attachment style (is it mostly secure or insecure, is it fairly stable and organized, or is it disorganized?), tendency to over- or under-regulate emotions and other mental states, defence organization and whether the patient's pathology is predominantly internalizing or externalizing may have a bearing on the specific way the therapist should meet and relate to the patient in various contexts. In extension of this point it may be relevant before initiating a therapy course to assess the individual patient's general ego-strength, attachment style, mentalizing capacity and personality organization (structural functioning level) and to design the general therapeutic strategy and specific aspects of one's basic therapeutic stance accordingly. Although our formalized psychiatric diagnostic systems and elements of the prevailing diagnostic psychiatric practice can certainly be criticized on many points, a thorough diagnostic evaluation of the individual patient is always an important part of the foundation for the individual treatment plan (Jørgensen 2015).

Generally, patients with reduced or fragile mentalizing capacity and ego-strength, attachment disorder (severe relational difficulties, including difficulties with engaging in a therapeutic alliance), medium-to high-severity personality disorders and general deficits in their personality organization (mainly deficit pathology, cf. Killingmo 1989) will have a greater need for a predominantly supportive, empathically validating, active and structuring therapist who helps them build a sense of meaning and coherence, while patients with less severe pathology, a relatively higher level of personality organization (mainly conflict pathology, cf. Killingmo 1989) and a basic ability to engage in a therapeutic alliance with the therapist may benefit from a more explorative, confrontational and less actively structuring (slightly more emotionally withdrawn and interpretive) therapist with a focus on uncovering (unconscious material) and verbalizing meaning and links the patient's current difficulties, processes in the therapeutic relationship here and now (transference) and past events and experiences. It is, however, important to bear in mind that these very general guidelines are far from always applicable with the individual patient, and that the therapist must always evaluate what is the optimal strategy and specific implementation of the psychotherapeutic stance in relation to the individual patient at a given time in the therapy.

Relationship Before Technique

In work with more severe psychopathology there will often be prolonged periods where it is more important to establish and maintain a good therapeutic relationship that may correct the patient's negative perceptions of self and others than to implement certain (more explorative, insight-generating) interventions (Balint 1968:170), although these two levels of the therapeutic process cannot be completely separated, and it may often be necessary for the therapist to intervene in order to develop and maintain a good and sustainable therapeutic relationship, including repairing ruptures in the therapeutic alliance. Certain elements of long-term dynamic-relational psychotherapy (Jørgensen 2009) have the capacity to promote the development of internal structure in the patient and may thus, in an individually attuned form, be applied in therapy with most patients with medium- or high-severity personality-related disorders, including with the goal of developing the patient's ability to see, take a step back from and thinking about recurring patterns in his or her own experiences, mental states and actions and the ability to see own actions and recurring relational patterns as reactions to or in context with current internal or external dynamics. This may involve the use of dynamic chain analyses to analyse, in great detail, the specific course of these patterns and how they may be dynamically linked to earlier experiences in the patient's life, where the patient's current behaviours emerged as originally (to varying degrees) adaptive attempts to manage difficult experiences or conflicts but have now become dysfunctional and automated reactions. In this analysis, the patient is gradually helped to see his or her own share in and thus the potential for changing recurring maladaptive relational patterns (cf. Rudolf 2005:157f).

The psychotherapist must always strive to strike an appropriate balance between validating (support) and more challenging (confrontation, curious invitations to reflection and so on) and transformative interventions, just as he or she should continuously adjust this balance in light of the patient's current state and needs, including how the patient responds to the implemented interventions. The cognitive therapist (Young et al. 2003:92) says that the therapeutic stance should generally be centred on what he calls empathic confrontation or empathic reality-testing (of the patient's beliefs about reality). The therapist should both seek to empathize with and understand the background for the patient's (disturbed) perceptions of self and the world—based on the patient's previous experiences—and confront the patient with the possibility that these beliefs or perceptions may be wrong or, at least, simplistic and incompatible with current reality and that they lead to recurring maladaptive patterns in the patient's interactions with the world. As part of the latter activity the cognitive therapist invites the patient to take part in a shared investigation of the validity of (the objective evidence for) her automatic thoughts in order to initiate a dialogue between the patient's healthy (rational) and disturbed (irrational) sides.

Similarly, the behavioural therapist Linehan (1993:221f) writes that the therapist has to strike a balance between, on the one hand, validating the patient's maladaptive (symptom) behaviour as being understandable from the patient's perspective—as a (maladaptive) attempt to sole perceived problems—and, on the other hand, focusing on the need to change the patient's behaviour and personality. In striking this balance, it is important that the need for change is not communicated in a way that is perceived as invalidating by the patient, that is, as an indication that the therapist perceives the patient as being 'wrong'. The therapist has to remain focused, hold on to the need for change and the pursuit of longer-term goals and maintain the psychotherapeutic focus of the conversation, while also remaining flexible and nurturing and continuously adapting his or her strategy to the patient's current state and needs (Linehan 1993:108f). In this effort, it will often be necessary for the therapist to attune the internal balance between, on the one hand, holding back, listening and being receptive and, on the other hand, actively structuring and maintaining the shared attention on particular themes in the patient's material based on the individual patient's current state (functioning level) and needs. The therapist must continuously strive to balance these different tasks and concerns in the therapeutic space.

References

Akhtar, S. (2013). *Psychoanalytic listening: Methods, limits and innovations*. London, England: Karnac.

Balint, M. (1968[1994]). *Grundbristen* [The basic flaw]. Copenhagen, Denmark: Hans Reitzels Forlag.

Bateman, A., & Fonagy, P. (2016). *Mentalization-based treatment for personality disorders: A practical guide*. Oxford, England: Oxford University Press.

Bollas, C. (1987). *The shadow of the object*. New York, NY: Columbia University Press.

Bordin, E. (1979). The generalizability of the psychoanalytic concept of the working alliance. *Psychotherapy: Theory, Research, and Practice, 16,* 252–260.

Bruschweiler-Stern, N., Lyons-Ruth, K., Morgan, A. C., Nahum, J. P., Sander, L. W., & Stern, D. N. (2010). *Change in psychotherapy: A unifying paradigm*. The Boston Change Process Study Group. New York, NY: Norton.

Caligor, E., Kernberg, O. F., & Clarkin, J. F. (2007). *Handbook of dynamic psychotherapy for higher level personality pathology*. Washington, DC: American Psychiatric Publishing.

Caspar, F., & Holtforth, M. G. (2009). Responsiveness eine entscheidende Prozessvariable in der Psychotherapie [Responsiveness—A pivotal process variable in psychotherapy]. *Zeitschrift für Klinische Psychologie und Psychotherapie, 38*(1), 61–69.

Cremerius, J. (1979). Gibt es zwei psychoanalytische Techniken? [Are there two psychoanalytic techniques?] *Psyche*, *33*, 577–599.

Cushman, P., & Gilford, P. (2000). Will managed care change our way of being? *American Psychologist, 55,* 985–996.

Freud, S. (1957). The future prospects of psychoanalytic therapy. In J. Strachey (Ed. and Trans.), *The standard edition of the complete psychological works of Sigmund Freud* (Vol. 11, pp. 139–152). London, England: Hogarth (Original work published 1910).

Freud, S. (1958). Recommendations to physicians practising psycho-analysis. In J. Strachey (Ed. and Trans.), *The standard edition of the complete psychological works of Sigmund Freud* (Vol. 12, pp. 109–120). London, England: Hogarth (Original work published 1912).

Gelso, C. J. (2011). *The real relationship in psychotherapy: The hidden foundation of change*. Washington, DC: American Psychological Association.

Gorkin, M. (1987). *The uses of countertransference*. Northvale: Aronson.

Gullestad, S. E., & Killingmo, B. (2013). *Underteksten. Psykoanalytisk terapi i praksis* [Subtext. Psychoanalytic therapy in practice] (2nd ed.). Oslo, Norway: Universitetsforlaget.

Hayes, J. A., Gelson, C. J., & Hummel, A. M. (2011). Managing countertransference. Evidence-based psychotherapy relationships. In J. C. Norcross (Ed.), *Psychotherapy relationships that work: Evidence-based responsiveness* (2nd ed., pp. 239–260). New York, NY: Oxford University Press.

Heimann, P. (1950). On countertransference. In P. Heimann (Ed.), *About children and children-no-longer* (pp. 73–79). London, England: Routledge.

Høglend, P. (2014). Exploration of the patient-therapist relationship in psychotherapy. *American Journal of Psychiatry, 171,* 1056–1066.

Høglend, P., Amlo, S., Marble, A., Bøgwald, K.-P., Sørbye, Ø., Sjaastad, M. C., et al. (2006). Analysis of the patient-therapist relationship in dynamic psychotherapy: An experimental study of transference interpretations. *American Journal of Psychiatry, 163,* 1739–1746.

Høglend, P., Bøgwald, K.-P., Amlo, S., Marble, A., Ulberg, R., Sjaastad, M. C., et al. (2008). Transference interpretations in dynamic psychotherapy: Do they really yield sustained effects? *American Journal of Psychiatry, 165,* 763–771.

Jacobsen, C. H., & Mortensen, K. V. (2017). *Supervision af psykoterapi og andet behandlingsarbejde. Almen og psykodynamisk supervisionsteori* [Supervision of psychotherapy and other treatment work. General and psychodynamic supervision theory]. Copenhagen, Denmark: Hans Reitzels Forlag.

Jørgensen, C. R. (2002). *Psykologien i senmoderniteten* [Psychology in late modernity]. Copenhagen, Denmark: Hans Reitzels Forlag.

Jørgensen, C. R. (2008). *Identitet. Psykologiske og kulturanalytiske perspektiver* [Identity. Psychological and culture analysis perspectives]. Copenhagen, Denmark: Hans Reitzels Forlag.

Jørgensen, C. R. (2009). *Personlighedsforstyrrelser. Moderne relationel forståelse og behandling af borderlinelidelse* [Personality disorders. Modern relational understanding and treatment of borderline disorder] (2nd ed.). Copenhagen, Denmark: Hans Reitzels Forlag.

Jørgensen, C. R. (2012). *Danmark på briksen. Et psykologisk perspektiv på Danmark og danskerne i det senmoderne* [Denmark on the therapist's couch. A psychological perspective on Denmark and Danes in later modernity]. Copenhagen, Denmark: Hans Reitzels Forlag.

Jørgensen, C. R. (2014). *ADHD. Bidrag til en kritisk psykologisk forståelse* [ADHD. Contributions to a critical psychological understanding]. Copenhagen, Denmark: Hans Reitzels Forlag.

Jørgensen, C.R. (2015). Psykiatrisk diagnostik i dynamisk psykologisk lys. [Psychiatric diagnostics from a psychodynamic perspective]. In: Brinkmann, S. & Petersen, A. (eds.). *Diagnoser. Perspektiver, kritik og diskussion*. Aarhus: Klim, 319–41

Kattlove, S. (2016). Acknowledging the 'analyst as a person': A developmental achievement. *Journal of the American Psychoanalytic Association, 64,* 1207–1216.

Kernberg, O. F. (1992). *Aggression in personality disorders and perversions*. New Haven, CT: Yale University Press.

Kiesler, D. J. (1996). *Contemporary interpersonal theory & research: Personality, psychopathology, and psychotherapy.* New York, NY: Wiley.

Killingmo, B. (1989). Conflict and deficit: Implications for technique. *International Journal of Psychoanalysis, 70,* 65–79.

Klein, M. (1946). Notes on some schizoid mechanisms. *International Journal of Psycho-Analysis, 27,* 99–110.

Klöpper, M. (2014). *Die Dynamik des Psychischen. Praxishandbuch für das Verständnis der Beziehungsdynamik*. Stuttgart, Germany: Klett-Cotta Verlag.

Knox, S., Butler, M. C., Kaiser, D. J., Knowlton, G., & Hill, C. E. (2017). Something to laugh about: Humor as a characteristic of effective therapists. In L. G. Castonguay & C. E. Hill (Eds.), *How and why are some therapists better than others?* (pp. 285–306). Washington, DC: American Psychological Association.

Körner, J. (2013). Deuten [Interpreting]. In R. Sannwald, M. Schulte-Markwort, & F. Resch (Eds.), *Psychotherapeutische Fertigkeiten* (pp. 37–53). Göttingen, Germany: Vandenhoeck & Ruprecht.

Küchenhoff, J. (2010). Der Wandel psychoanalytischer Therapiekonzepte. Klinischer Herausforderungen und theoretischer Fortschritt [The transformation of psychoanalytic therapy concepts. Clinical challenges and theoretical advances]. In K. Münch, D. Munz, & A. Springer (Eds.), *Die Psychoanalyse im Pluralismus der Wissenschaften* (pp. 83–109). Gießen, Germany: Psychosozial-Verlag.

Lemma, A. (2003). *Introduction to the practice of psychoanalytic psychotherapy*. New York, NY: Wiley.

Levenson, H. (1995). *Time-limited dynamic psychotherapy: A guide to clinical practice*. New York, NY: Basic Books.

Linehan, M. M. (1993). *Cognitive behavioral treatment of borderline personality disorder*. New York, NY: Guilford.

Luborsky, L. (1984). *Principles of psychoanalytic psychotherapy: A manual for supportive-expressive treatment*. New York, NY: Basic Books.

Lyons-Ruth, K. (1999). The two-person unconscious: Intersubjective dialogue, enactive relational representation, and the emergence of new forms of relational organization. *Psychoanalytic Inquiry, 19*(4), 576–617.

Maroda, K. J. (1994). *The Power of countertransference*. New York, NY: Jason Aronson.

McWilliams, N. (2004). *Psychodynamic psychotherapy: A practitioner's guide*. New York, NY: Guilford.

Mertens, W. (2015). *Psychoanalytische Behandlungstechnik. Konzepte und Themen psychoanalytisch begründeter Behandlungsverfahren* [Psychoanalytic treatment technique. Concepts and themes of psychoanalytically motivated treatment methods]. Stuttgart, Germany: Kohlhammer.

Mitchell, S. A. (1997). *Influence and autonomy in psychoanalysis*. Hillsdale, MI: Analytic Press.

Mitchell, S. A. (2000). *Relationality: From attachment to intersubjectivity*. Hillsdale, MI: Analytic Press.

Moser, U. (2001). What is a bongaloo, daddy? Übertragung, Gegenübertragung, therapeutische Situation. Allgemein und am Beispiel 'früher Störungen' [What is a bongaloo, daddy? Transference, countertransference, therapeutic situation, in general and with reference to 'early disorders']. *Psyche, 55,* 97–136.

Muran, J. C., Safran, J. D., & Eubanks-Carter, C. (2010). Developing therapist abilities to negotiate alliance ruptures. In J. C. Muran, & J. P. Barber (Eds.), *The therapeutic alliance: An evidence-based guide to practice* (pp. 341–355). New York, NY: Guilford.

Nacht, S. (1962). The curative factors in psychoanalysis. *International Journal of Psychoanalysis, 43,* 206–211.

Ogden, T. H. (1979). On projective identification. *International Journal of Psychoanalysis, 60,* 357–373.

Ogden, T. H. (1982). *Projective identification and psychotherapeutic technique*. London, England: Karnac.

Ogden, T. H. (2016). *Reclaiming unlived life: Experiences in psychoanalysis*. London, England: Routledge.

OPD Task Force. (2008). *Operationalized Psychodynamic Diagnosis OPD-2*. Cambridge, MA: Hogrefe.

Racker, H. (1968). *Übertragung und Gegenübertragung* [Transference and countertransference]. Munich, Germany: Reinhardt Verlag.

Rønnestad, M. H., & Skovholt, T. M. (2013). *The developing practitioner: Growth and stagnation of therapists and counselors*. London, England: Routledge.

Rosa, H. (2016). *Resonanz. Eine Soziologie der Weltbeziehung* [Resonance. A sociology of the relationship to the world]. Berlin, Germany: Suhrkamp Verlag.

Rosa, H. (2018). *Unverfügbarkeit* [Inaccessibility]. Wien, Austria: Residenz Verlag.

Rudolf, G. (2005). *Strukturbezogene Psychotherapie. Leitfaden zur psychodynamischen Therapie struktureller Störungen* [Structural psychotherapy. Guidelines for psychodynamic therapy for structural disorders]. Stuttgart, Germany: Schattauer Verlag.

Safran, J. D. (2017). The unbearable lightness of being: Authenticity and the search for the real. *Psychoanalytic Psychology, 34,* 69–77.

Safran, J. D., & Muran, J. C. (2000). *Negotiating the therapeutic alliance: A relational treatment guide*. New York, NY: Guilford.

Sandler, J., Dare, C., & Holder, A. (1992). *The patient and the analyst*. London, England: Karnac.

Sassenfeld, A. (2015). *Relationale Psychotherapie. Grundlagen und klinische Prinzipien* [Relational psychotherapy. Basics and clinical principles]. Gießen. Germany: Psychosozial-Verlag.

Spillius, E. (2012). A brief review of projective identification in American psychoanalytic literature. In E. Spillius & E. O'Shaughnessy (Eds.), *Projective identification: The fate of a concept* (pp. 245–264). London, England: Routledge.

Stern, D. N. (2004). *The present moment in psychotherapy and everyday life*. New York, NY: Norton.

Stern, D. N., Sander, L. W., Nahum, J. P., Harrison, A. M., Lyons-Ruth, K., Morgan, A. C., et al. (1998). Non-interpretive mechanisms in psychoanalytic therapy: The something more than interpretation. *International Journal of Psychoanalysis, 79,* 903–921.

Sullivan, H. S. (1954). *The psychiatric interview*. New York, NY: Norton.

Sultanoff, S. M. (2013). Integrating humor into psychotherapy: Research, theory, and the necessary conditions for the presence of therapeutic humor in helping relationships. *The Humanistic Psychologist, 41,* 388–399.

Tansey, M. J., & Burke, W. F. (1989). *Understanding countertransference: From projective identification to empathy*. Hillsdale, MI: Analytic Press.

Thomä, H., & Kächele, H. (1985). *Lehrbuch der psychoanalytischen Therapie. 1. Grundlagen* [Handbook of psychoanalytic therapy. 1. Basics]. Berlin, Germany: Springer.

Tuckett, D. (2005). Does anything go? Towards a framework for the more transparent assessment of psychoanalytic competence. *International Journal of Psychoanalysis, 86,* 31–49.

Ulberg, R., Høglend, P., Marble, A., & Johansson, P. (2012). Women respond more favorably to transference intervention than men. *Journal of Nervous and Mental Disease, 200,* 223–229.

Valentine, L., & Gabbard, G. O. (2014). Can the use of humor in psychotherapy be taught? *Academic Psychiatry, 38,* 75–81.

Wachtel, P. L. (2008). *Relational theory and the practice of psychotherapy*. New York, NY: Guilford.

Weiss, H. (2007). Projektive Identifizierung und Durcharbeiten in der Gegenübertragung – ein mehrphasiges Modell [Projective identification and working-through in the countertransference—A multi-stage model]. In C. Frank & H. Weiss (red.) *Projektive Identifizierung. Ein Schlüsselkonzept der psychoanalytischen Therapie* (pp. 179–202). Stuttgart, Germany: Klett-Cotta Verlag.

Weiss, H. (2009). *Das Labyrinth der Borderline-kommunikation. Klinische Zugänge zum Erleben von Raum und Zeit*. Stuttgart, Germany: Klett-Cotta Verlag.

Weiss, H. (2015). Überlegungen zum agora-klaustrophoben dilemma des borderline-patienten. *Psyche, 69,* 916–935.

Winnicott, D. W. (1949). Hate in the countertransference. *International Journal of Psychoanalysis, 30,* 69–74.

Winnicott, D. W. (1971). *Playing and reality*. New York NY: Tavistock.

Yeomans, F. E., Clarkin, J. F., & Kernberg, O. F. (2002). *A primer of transference-focused psychotherapy for the borderline patient*. New York, NY: Aronson.

Young, J. E., Klosko, J. S., & Weishaar, M. E. (2003). *Schema therapy: A practitioner's guide*. New York, NY: Guilford.

Zwiebel, R. (2007). *Von der Angst Psychoanalytiker zu sein* [On the fear of being a psychoanalyst]. Stuttgart, Germany: Klett-Cotta Verlag.

Zwiebel, R. (2013). *Was macht einen guten Psychoanalytiker aus? Grundelemente professioneller Psychotherapie* [What makes a good psychoanalyst? Basic elements of professional psychotherapy]. Stuttgart, Germany: Klett-Cotta.

Chapter 12
Conclusion

> A physician has not now attained the highest degree of training of which he is capable when he knows the best and the most recent remedies and is practised in applying them [...] he also has to posses an eloquence adapted to every individual ... (Nietzsche 1886/1996:116f).

As outlined in Part I of the present book, there is fairly convincing scientific evidence by now that most patients with most psychological disorders have fairly good outcomes with psychotherapeutic treatment. Psychotherapy works, even though the share of patients who do not benefit or who have actually deteriorated post-treatment is still too big, and we need more knowledge about what characterizes the patients who fail to benefit from psychotherapy, and why they do not benefit. At the same time, recent meta-analyses of psychotherapeutic efficacy studies show that, broadly speaking, there are no clinically significant differences in the effectiveness of widely approved psychotherapeutic methods. That is a fairly remarkable finding, considering how much attention has been—and still is—devoted to individual therapeutic methods/techniques and their specific effects, including how many resources we continue to allocate to studying and comparing (evidence-basing) the effectiveness of specific therapeutic methods and on developing what is touted as new, revolutionizing methods for the treatment of specific disorders, which in practice rarely differ decisively from existing methods. Overall, the countless RCTs have not found clinically significant differences in the effectiveness of the different methods for the treatment of specific disorders—despite their widely approved status as the methodological gold standard for psychotherapeutic efficacy research and their overwhelmingly predominant focus on specific treatment methods aimed at specific disorders and thus on the impact of specific technical efficacy factors on treatment effect.

Similarly, no systematic correlation has been found between therapists' adherence to a standardized treatment method and treatment outcome, just as differences in therapists' specific technical competence (how competent they are in their implementation of a specific therapeutic method) also does not seem to have a major impact on treatment outcome. By all indications, the RCTs and thus much of the empirical psychotherapy research are thus focusing on the wrong issue, in the sense that even though psychotherapists should naturally be trained in the use of one or more of the

C. R. Jørgensen, *The Psychotherapeutic Stance*,
https://doi.org/10.1007/978-3-030-20437-2_12

scientifically validated treatment methods, and although innovative new therapeutic methods (which appear far less often than one might think) should naturally be tested, the choice of specific therapeutic method appear to have very limited impact on treatment outcome, as long as we are speaking of widely approved therapeutic methods, and the therapist chooses a treatment method and a strategy that matches the character of the individual patient's difficulties.

On the other hand, several large-scale studies have found considerable differences in average treatment outcomes between individual therapists. Generally, some therapists are clearly more effective than others, judging from the patients' typical therapy outcomes. This cannot be explained with reference to the specific therapeutic method the individual therapists subscribes to and must be presumed to use in their therapeutic work, and we need more knowledge about what specifically characterizes and explains the superior treatment outcomes achieved by 'master therapists'—both with a view to improving our understanding and so that we might direct our attention at the right aspects in our selection and training of prospective psychotherapists. Similarly, a number of meta-analyses of efficacy studies suggest that factors associated with the individual therapist are at least as important (and often more important) for any differences in treatment outcomes as the choice of specific therapeutic method. Thus, it seems clear that we need to look to something other and more than the applied therapeutic method, something related to the therapist, to explain the differences in treatment outcomes. This is the case, although few (de facto virtually no) efficacy studies are designed to optimize our ability to capture the potential role of therapist factors on treatment effectiveness.

Viewed in a wider historical and cultural context, psychotherapy appears as a unique cultural practice for understanding and curing what we define as psychological disorders. It is a practice with close ties to the modern sciences that help confer legitimacy and authority on officially certified psychotherapists (typically with a background in a medical or academic psychological degree)—an authority that may in itself contribute positively to their treatment outcomes (cf. the impact of expectancy factors on treatment outcome). Psychotherapists draw on a collection of scientifically validated theories on, among others, psychopathology, developmental psychology, personality psychology and, not least, clinical psychology and a number of specific treatment theories with related intervention methods. However, psychotherapy is about more than scientific theory and specific methodology. It is also a unique way of meeting, thinking about, relating to and interacting with the persons one works together with in the therapeutic space. Psychotherapy involves a unique dynamic-relational or other form of psychological thinking and conceptual model that the individual therapist then translates into a specific stance towards the individual patient, him/herself, the interaction between patient and therapist and everything that plays out in the therapeutic space.

Psychotherapy Combines Technical-Scientific and Personal Dimensions

Psychotherapy thus represents a special combination of, on the one hand, technical scientific elements and, on the other hand, a much more personal dimension, where psychotherapists are very much themselves, make themselves available and use themselves in their work (cf. Zwiebel 2004:862f). Therapists put (parts of) themselves, their own persons and their subjectivity into play and at stake in their therapeutic work. Psychotherapy is one of the professional fields, if not the professional field, whose practitioners most draw on themselves as persons, on their subjectivity (Kite 2016:1157). In practice, it can be difficult to distinguish between the technical and personal dimensions of psychotherapy, as it is always the specific therapist who translates a given standardized treatment method into actual therapeutic work. The specific implementation of a therapeutic method has to respect the individual patient's particular issues, current state and needs (exactly when and exactly how a given intervention should be used in work with a specific patient and so on)—a task that calls for judgment, empathic skills, responsiveness, social competences and an ability to be emotionally present that go far beyond what is included in our standardized treatment methods and thus relies on the therapist's more personal qualities to a high degree. Very broadly speaking, psychotherapeutic work involves that the therapist (1) identifies the core of the patient's difficulties and how they are manifested in specific symptoms and behaviour, (2) assesses what is happening in the patient, in him/herself and in the therapeutic relationship here and now and, on that basis, (3) determines what is the best and most helpful strategy and intervention in this particular context. These are all elements that draw on both theoretical and empirical knowledge and technical and personal competences in the therapist.

If we accept the premise that psychotherapy is far from a mere technical endeavour where a presumably random and replaceable therapist is tasked with providing an, ideally, objective implementation of a standardized method for the treatment of a specific disorder that has presumably been identified (diagnosed) in the patient, and that it is in fact a far more complex process that involves and relies on more personal qualities in the individual therapist, then it is less surprising that, all the research efforts notwithstanding, we have been unable to find major differences in the effectiveness of our well-reputed therapeutic methods. We should there focus our attention more on other aspects of the psychotherapeutic work than the specific treatment technique, especially on the competent therapist's more personal qualities and on what characterizes the psychotherapeutic stance beyond the general characteristics of working with psychotherapy.

Abandoning the Medical Model of Therapy

Overall, this suggests that we should abandon the prevailing medical understanding of psychotherapy with its tendency towards a far too one-sided focus on specific techniques for the treatment of specific disorders or, at least, achieve a better balance between this and a more dynamic-relational model of therapy. The previous pages have outlined a number of problems in the simplistic medical understanding of psychotherapy, including that:

1. There are no indications that the choice of specific therapeutic method/technique has the key impact on treatment outcome that the medical model of therapy claims and which it rests on. Although it is essential that the psychotherapist is trained in and masters one or more of our approved (coherent and scientifically

founded) therapeutic methods, the specific efficacy factors associated with a specific method by all indications have less impact on treatment outcome than the common efficacy factors that relate more to the individual therapist's personal qualities and general therapeutic competences and will be present in most successful treatment processes. We should not resort to a primitive either/or all-or-nothing thinking, where only evidence-based manualized treatment techniques or, alternatively, only common non-technical elements of the psychotherapeutic are taken seriously. Therapeutic technique, factors in the therapeutic relationship and the therapist's more personal qualities are closely interrelated aspects of the psychotherapeutic work. However, especially in therapy with more severe psychological disorders and in psychotherapeutic work that goes beyond the ambition of alleviating mild symptoms as quickly as possible (mild symptom disorders), we need to abandon the medical model of therapy and devote more attention to what characterizes the psychotherapeutic stance and to the common therapeutic factors, including factors in the therapeutic relationship and factors related to the individual therapist.

2. Psychological disorders are far from being the clearly defined or natural categories that they are implicitly assumed to be in both our authorized diagnostic systems and the medical understanding of psychotherapy, which weakens a key element in the foundation of the medical model of therapy, RCTs and the evidence trend in empirical efficacy research: that it is conceivably possible to identify or, eventually, to develop specific methods for the treatment of specific psychological disorders, as they are conceptualized by our categorical psychiatric diagnostic systems. This includes the notion that our officially authorized diagnoses would be able to capture all the aspects that are of real importance for the individual patient's difficulties, and that we can therefore generally assume that all patients with a given diagnosis need roughly the same standardized treatment (cf. the uniformity myths in psychotherapy research). Psychological disorders cannot readily be reduced to a finite number of specific and clear-cut diagnoses with the assumption that all patients sharing a diagnosis have the same problem with the same aetiology, just as the individual patient's personality organization, defence mechanisms, life circumstances and general functioning level should always be included in the assessment of which treatment to offer any particular patient (Steinert and Leichsenring 2017:57). It is far from all patients with a given diagnosis who need the same treatment, and hence, the ambition of developing specific methods for the treatment of specific disorders is only meaningful in a very limited sense, and then only on a more general level in the form of general therapeutic principles.

3. The strong focus on manualizing and standardizing specific therapeutic methods and efforts to secure an evidence base for them has caused us to focus our attention at the wrong element in our otherwise profoundly important effort to understand the core of psychotherapy and core efficacy factors and to improve psychotherapeutic treatments for people with psychological disorders. We

have not devoted nearly enough attention to the more personal qualities in the individual therapist and on factors in the therapeutic relationship, which appear to be absolutely crucial for the therapeutic process and treatment outcome, especially in the work with patients with more severe psychological disorders.

Considering how parts of our late modern Western societies operate—how we try to categorize, understand and manage problems by classifying reality in clear-cut categories (which typically reduce the complexity of reality considerably, for better and worse) and developing specific technical solutions to specific problems, it may seem like common sense, perhaps especially for technocrats and administrators who tend to see it as their prime purpose to optimize the use of society's resources (typically via increasingly tight control and rational management principles), to transfer conceptual models and research designs that proved successful in the somatic healthcare system and medical research to the field of psychiatry and psychological disorders with related treatment methods. The problem is that this is not possible without a huge simplification of the complexity of reality, which comes with consequences that have the potential to undermine psychotherapeutic work and lead to poorer treatment results. This risk is especially urgent if it involves the call for therapists to be trained in and restricted to implementing certain standardized methods for the treatment of patients with a given disorder, while our common ability to think and understand the complexity of psychological disorders is eroded, and it means that we are no longer going to offer the individual patient a choice between different therapeutic methods. No therapeutic method is effective with all patients, and there is no indication that we will ever develop a specific treatment method that is effective for even most patients. The very notion that this is inherently possible springs from an understanding of the core of psychotherapy that is at best simplistic.

The call for standardized and evidence-based treatments in the public healthcare system rests on a sensible core in the sense that we naturally need to strive to offer everyone the best possible treatment, regardless where they live. The standardization of treatments and the call for training new psychotherapists in specific evidence-based treatment methods can probably help raise the base standards of the treatments that are offered, also outside the most high-profile treatment institutions. However, when this call for standardization, evidence-based methods and the preparation of very detailed clinical guidelines goes too far, one might get the impression that it is not only driven by rational concerns but also by a (sometimes unconscious) urge for control and certainty in combination with a lack of trust in the individual psychotherapist's professional competence and judgment. Here it should be remembered that the quality of psychotherapeutic work can far from be reduced to whether therapists embrace and have completed formal training in an evidence-based method or follow standardized guidelines. The widespread rhetoric calling for psychotherapeutic treatment to be evidence-based frames the strategies that have been launched to improve psychotherapeutic treatments as allegedly knowledge-based. It is, however, debatable whether that is always the case, and there is a risk that an unreflected implementation of so-called evidence-based treatment methods requiring the use of certain treatment methods is not going to improve the treatments on offer but will rather undermine the important competences that are associated with qualified professional assessments in the individual case (Thomassen 2015:67). The end-result may be that we use significant resources without achieving the desired positive effect on treatment outcomes, because the implemented strategy rests on a flawed basis and on a flawed understanding of what is the core of good and effective psychotherapy.

Psychological theories, clinical guidelines and standardized treatment methods will always play an important role in informing the therapist, but they can never tell the therapist exactly what to do in specific situations. Good theories (here, the focus is especially on dynamic-relational and psychoanalytic theories in a broad sense) can help enhance the therapist's eye for the complexity of reality and help him or her achieve a more nuanced understanding of the individual patient, but they cannot prescribe specific solutions to clinical challenges. For a novice (and insecure) therapist, this may feel frustrating, and one may feel the urge to look for and lean strongly on specific instructions for what to do. Although that is understandable, there are no shortcuts: we have to acknowledge that such a strategy reflects a professionally untenable reduction of the complexity of the psychotherapeutic work, especially when working with patients with more severe and more complex psychological disorders. Although the inexperienced therapist may thus enjoy having a treatment manual and standardized clinical guidelines to rely on, in the long term this is not a viable strategy. A competent psychotherapist will gradually have to be able to move on from these standardized approaches to psychotherapy with a focus on specific technical interventions.

The previous pages have sought to argue that we need to abandon the medical model of psychotherapy in favour of what has been called a dynamic-relational understanding of psychotherapy. In part, this involves attempting to understand the patient's symptoms and disturbed behaviour as meaningful expressions of internal psychological and relational dynamics in the patient's life in each individual case, not as more or less arbitrary and meaningless manifestations of various types of specific (biochemical or other) deficits in the patient's psyche or brain. Also, the core elements of the psychotherapeutic stance, which acts as a kind of general framework for the psychotherapeutic work has been presented and specified. Compared to the medical model of therapy, the dynamic-relational model represents a different view of human psychology and a very different approach to the psychotherapeutic work, where common therapeutic factors, therapist factors and elements of the therapeutic relationship have a far more prominent position. The therapist's way of meeting, relating to and responding to the patient in the therapeutic relationship and in the therapeutic space, in part beyond specific techniques (but only in part, since the psychotherapeutic stance, the therapeutic relationship and the therapist's responsive use of specific interventions and treatment models are intimately interlinked), are considered crucial elements of the therapeutic process.

The Psychotherapeutic Space as a Counter-Image to Contemporary Culture

Although it may, as mentioned earlier, be difficult to speak about 'the psychotherapeutic culture' as a clear-cut, homogenous and well-defined phenomenon, most well-trained psychotherapists rely on set of norms and humanistically oriented values (including a common ethic), that are more or less shared across any more specific theoretical or technical professional disagreements. This means that they meet and seek to understand and help their patients in ways that are unique to the psychotherapeutic space and to the psychotherapeutic process. In that sense, the psychotherapeutic culture can be said in some regards to be in fairly stark contrast to some parts of our contemporary culture. What therapists do, and the norms and values that they represent in their psychotherapeutic work—what happens in the therapeutic space—may serve as a counter-image to some of the aspects of contemporary culture, which are presumably involved in causing excessive stress and developmental deficits in human psychology, and as such have, to varying degrees, contributed to the development of some of the psychological disorders the psychotherapist encounters in his or her patients, although, of course, this should not mislead us to embrace primitive notions that psychological disorders are exclusive the product of factors pertaining to society or contemporary culture. Of course, the picture is far more complicated than that.

We may point to a number of aspects where the psychotherapeutic culture and the psychotherapeutic space, including the psychotherapeutic stance, as it has been presented in the preceding pages, may serve as a counter-image to parts of our contemporary culture. Here, it is interesting to consider whether the fact that psychotherapy as a cultural practice represents a counter-image to prevailing tendencies in large parts of contemporary culture and offers the patient an opportunity to have and build experiences that may otherwise be difficult to achieve, in itself contains some of the common therapeutic efficacy factors and thus part of the basis of the effectiveness of psychotherapy.

- In a restless and accelerating culture, where many people have an everyday life that is dominated by a growing perceived workload, and where the prevalence of reported stress is growing, the therapeutic space, by contrast, is characterized by inviting the patient to slow down, pause and take the time to examine what may be behind his or her perceived difficulties. Rather than reproducing the patient's previous solution strategies once more, which typically revolve around taking action or coming up with a quick fix, the patient is invited to look inward, to think thoughts and to try to understand him/herself and his or her problems. Psychotherapy offers a space for reflection and represents an awareness that human development processes take time, sometimes quite a long time if the person is dealing with complex problems that have developed over many years. The psychotherapeutic space stimulates psychological development processes, which is something quite different from forcing these, often very fragile processes, which would typically end in developmental deficits and further mental anguish.
- It could be claimed that late modern Western culture is becoming increasingly oriented towards the here-and-now—that we focus increasingly on living in the moment—while our historical awareness, including our understanding of how history contributes to shaping our current life, both culturally and in our individual lives, is growing ever weaker. Our sense of time is narrowing, and it takes less and less time before events and insights are considered old and thus obsolete and pointless. On both an individual and a cultural level, we are oriented towards

the future, while it is regarded as a losing strategy to be stuck in the past, as if deciding to leave the past behind is always sufficient to actually move beyond it. The psychotherapeutic space represents a very different view of history in some regards, by presuming that it is far from always possible to leave the past behind without, at least, having examined it more closely and tried to learn from it. Instead of gazing almost desperately to the future ('let's look forward, now') and deny the role of the past, we pause and look back—in some cases far back into the patient's history—with a view to strengthening the patient's understanding of him/herself and the basis of his or her difficulties—a strategy that may over time weaken history's determining influence on the patient's current and future life without ever quite eliminating it.

- In a highly individualistic culture, where most people are socialized to be independent, take charge of their life, be in control, be decisive and strive to realize their own perception of the good life, the therapeutic culture rests on a slightly different and somewhat more nuanced idea about the human condition: that as human beings, we are not only—let alone always—strong autonomous individuals; we can also be both physically and mentally fragile, we may all wind up in situations where we lose our independence, and ultimately, we all die. The therapeutic space provides a room for getting into contact with and show another human being (the therapist) that one is also dependent on others, might feel weak, fragile, exposed and wrong, and that one far from always has the high degree of control over oneself and one's life that one might expect from oneself and tries to convey to the world. Behind the shiny, steely facade things might look very different, and the therapeutic space offers a setting for revealing and examining that without having to do so alone or being met with contempt, demands to 'pull it together' and so on. The psychotherapeutic space does not require decisiveness and control but invites being, introspection and self-reflection with a view to developing greater agency and better self-regulation.
- While it could be argued that at least parts of the late modern Western culture are characterized by a striking focus on superficial (virtual) contacts, including on the number of contacts (social network and so on) rather than their quality, the focus in the psychotherapeutic space by contrast is on establishing a close emotional, psychological and, in some cases, long-term contact between patient and therapist. In this context, the focus is not on the number of contacts but on their quality, just as it is a contact characterized by a high degree of confidentiality where the patient can be assured that what she says and reveals in the therapeutic space is not subsequently going to be shared with a large number of people across different forums and platforms. In this regard too, the therapeutic space can be said to stand out from at least parts of contemporary culture, which seems to have eliminated almost all boundaries in its sharing of (pseudo-) intimacy and profoundly personal information.
- Finally, much of late modern culture is characterized by a struggle for attention, by mutual competition and by a fairly instrumental (anti-mentalizing) approach to the self and one's own body—in an eternal quest for self-optimization and the realization of (often unrealistic) heroic ego-ideals (expectations of success, of

happiness)—which may prepare the ground for pathological self-loathing, shame and self-destructiveness when one fails in one's attempts at living up to contemporary and in many cases unrealistic (internalized) ideals. In this regard too, the psychotherapeutic space represents a counter-image to powerful trends in contemporary culture. For one hour a week or more, the patient has the therapist's full and undivided attention in an egalitarian relationship between equals, with a basic structure that involves no competition, and where the patient does not have to do anything to earn the therapist's presence or his or her dedication to focus on the patient rather than him/herself. The therapist takes an interest in the patient as a human being, in his or her subjective experiences and difficulties with a view to the shared main task, which is to understand the dynamic psychological and relational meaning of the patient's symptoms and maladaptive behaviour. The psychotherapeutic stance means that the therapist only to a very limited extent focuses on how the patient's problems might fit into established (diagnostic) categories and instead seeks to help patient achieve a greater and more nuanced understanding of him/herself, which in the long term is the opposite of an instrumental approach to the patient's self, body and psyche.

Precisely because the psychotherapeutic space is thus out of step with and reflects different norms and values than the prevailing norms and values in contemporary culture, one should be prepared that it may be under continuous threat from administrators—perhaps allied with politicians and professionals from related field, with whom the psychotherapist competes for society's scarce resources—who do not understand (nor can be expected to understand, unless we help them) what is so unique about the psychotherapeutic space/psychotherapeutic treatment and who therefore demand greater efficiency (for example in the form of demands for less costly short-term therapy) or otherwise try to adjust (typically in a negative direction) the conditions for the psychotherapeutic work, which in various ways depends on public funding. In private practice, where the patients pays for their own therapy, the psychotherapeutic space is better protected against measures from administrators and other outsiders.

We may therefore need to defend the psychotherapeutic space against these potentially destructive calls for increased efficiency and transparency, including demands from a documentation and evaluation culture that is out of control, where patients are asked to evaluate their treatment, the therapist and their benefit from the treatment at such short intervals that it is virtually meaningless, considering that it takes time, especially in work with more severe disorders, to form a sustainable therapeutic alliance, and that therapeutic results are far from always reflected in lower scores on standardized symptom scales within a short span of time.

Finally, the therapist needs to be aware that he or she has also grown up in and is, to varying degrees, socialized into operating under the same expectations, norms, values, ideals and concepts of reality that prevail in contemporary culture, and which contributed to shape the psychological disorders the patients present. In light of that, we should continuously ask ourselves what norms, values and ideals—what ideas about the good life and reality in general—we represent in our meeting with our patients, often unwittingly. That requires a considerable cultural awareness of main trends in contemporary culture and of the impact of prevailing cultural expectations and logics on oneself and one's way of interacting with others, one's way of meeting one's patients.

We have to be able to take a step back from what might generally be taken for granted, as indisputable aspects of reality, when they manifest in the patients' life, self-understanding and pathology and make them the object of critical reflection, both in relation to ourselves (to avoid uncritically representing and reproducing them in our interaction with the patients) and together with the patients. Is it reasonable that a patient who has suffered severe neglect during her upbringing and now struggles to handle everyday life is expected—and expects of herself—to undergo job assessment and training or complete an education programme within the normal timeframe because 'everyone needs to be able to provide for themselves and should not be a burden to society'? Or should we rather insist that such a patient needs long-term therapy and extensive support from her local council or others for a time to be able to lead an independent life in the long term? Most people want to provide for themselves and be what they perceive as normal, but not everybody can manage it, certainly not without help. There is an almost endless number of similar questions that could be raised; the key point is that we actually ask them and, in each case, consider on a professional basis what is required, and what might be helpful for this particular individual, without being governed by rigid notions about what reality is or rather should be according to the prevailing trends in contemporary culture at any given time.

12.1 Training and *Bildung*: Cultivating Professional Skills and Personal Qualities

> If you had a good friend badly in need of therapeutic help, and I gave you the name of a therapist who was a Diplomate in Clinical Psychology, with no other information, would you send your friend to him? Of course not. You would want to know what he is like as a person and a therapist, recognizing that there are many with diplomas on their walls who are not fit to do therapy [or] lead a group [...] We must face the fact that in dealing with human beings, a certificate does not give much assurance of real qualification (Rogers 1990:364f).

> ... there are conspicuous dangers attendant [...] To avoid a split between what men consciously know because they are aware of having learned it by a specific job of learning, and what they unconsciously know because they have absorbed it in the formation of their characters by intercourse with others, becomes an increasingly delicate task... (Dewey 1916:29f).

As discussed on the previous pages, the therapist's more personal qualities and ability to maintain the psychotherapeutic stance, also under pressure, is of key importance in the dynamic-relational model of psychotherapy. That also means that any peculiarities and psychological disorders that the individual therapist might have, including significant deficits in his or her relational skills, emotional sensitivity and ethical compass, can have severe consequences for the therapeutic process and thus for the patients (cf. Kite 2016:1157ff). This underscores the need for a qualified and systematic selection of prospective psychotherapists and for some form of continuous monitoring of psychotherapists' mental health, especially in relation to psychotherapeutic work with more at-risk and severely disturbed patients, who do not always have the necessary resources to speak up for themselves in relation to therapists who violate their boundaries or otherwise act with incompetence. How this should be realized, more specifically, including what criteria should be applied in the selection of students for psychotherapeutic training, and who should oversee it, is naturally a complicated matter, and there are no easy answers. That does not, however, diminish their relevance.

In light of that, it is remarkable how relatively little attention has been devoted to the therapist's personality, character, judgment and other more personal qualities in the literature and, not least, in empirical research. A number of more qualitatively oriented attempts to uncover and describe what characterizes particularly competent master therapists may, however, expand out understanding of some of the more personal qualities that must be assumed to contribute positively to the therapeutic work (see Chap. 7), just as there are a few empirical studies (including Henry et al. 1990; Henry et al. 1993a, b) that identify some of the more personal therapist characteristics that appear to make an unambiguously negative contribution to the course and outcome of psychotherapy. A correlation has also been identified between therapists' interpersonal competence and treatment outcome.

In contrast to therapists who have primarily learned a static set of guidelines, standardized methods and procedures, and who operate with technical rationality (cf. Schön 1987), exceptional practitioners demonstrate a form of knowing and reflection-in-action that is much more dynamic and which reflects an almost artistic creativity and a real ability to (re)think. It is an ability to apply available knowledge and acquired methods in a way that is attuned to the given patient, and which is able to respond to the unique and the unexpected (cf. Schön 1987:35), which other therapists may dream of and strive to develop, but which few can ever fully achieve. Efforts to define explicitly what master therapists' knowing-in-action more specifically involves is an important first step towards making it an integral element in the training of prospective therapists and seeking to convey these skills to others. Similarly, attempts to identify what it involves, more specifically, to adopt a psychotherapeutic stance, may contribute to making the development of a psychotherapeutic stance a more highly prioritizes aspect of psychotherapeutic training.

Selection of Candidates for Psychotherapeutic Work

There is reason to assume that not all the physicians, psychologists and persons from other professions who wish to practice psychotherapy, and who believe they have the personal qualities for the job, actually have or could reasonably be expected to develop the personal qualities necessary for being competent psychotherapeutic practitioners (cf. Rønnestad and Skovholt 2013:157f). A few will probably be able to become fairly effective psychotherapists with little formalized education or training, while most, with education, training and supervision would be able to improve from fairly mediocre (insecure, rigid, non-responsive in their contact with the patient and so on) to very good therapists. Finally, we should expect that there is a group of people with ambitions of becoming psychotherapists who would not be able to improve much, regardless of how much education, training and supervision they undergo, and who would never rise to become even reasonably competent psychotherapists (cf. Hill and Knox 2013:801). The latter group should be filtered out, to the extent it is possible, and should not undergo training as psychotherapists or practice psychotherapy.

Precisely because the therapist's more personal qualities and role in the psychotherapeutic process are so crucial for the course and outcome of treatment, as discussed in the previous chapters, psychotherapeutic training should not only focus on the patient and his or her difficulties, but also on the therapist's own psyche and relational dynamics. The individual therapist's own reaction patterns and internal dynamics, as they manifest themselves in the therapeutic space and in the interaction with the patient, need to be addressed in psychotherapeutic training. The therapist's self-insight and ability to register and control his or her urge to act out countertransferences, capacity for reflection-in-action and ability to take a step back from and reflect on what is playing out in him/herself and in the therapeutic relationship right now as a basis for a balanced intervention are crucial psychotherapeutic competences, both in order to prevent escalated negative processes in the therapeutic space and in order to maximize the patient's access to corrective experiences in the therapeutic relationship. Hence, the development of the therapist's psychotherapeutic stance, not just towards the patient, but also towards him/herself and his or her own subjective experiences and reactions in the therapeutic space, is a key element in psychotherapeutic training.

The development of psychotherapeutic skills is related not only to the acquisition of mainly cognitive and specific technical skills but also to the development of emotional (empathy, sensitivity, tolerance) and social (relational skills, ability to register and heal ruptures in the alliance) skills. Developing one's capacity for self-regulation and self-reflection, self-insight and, not least, general personal psychological maturity is also of great importance. Despite the remarkable lack of research in this areas, there is some evidence that training novice therapists, including psychology students in basic relational and conversation skills (theoretical instruction, demonstration, hands-on exercises and feedback to these and so on) can be effective (Hill and Knox 2013:776f).

Our knowledge about how this training subsequently affects treatment outcomes for the patients of the therapists who underwent training is limited, however (Hill and Knox 2013:781f, Binder 1993), just as it has so far proven difficult to document clear effects of formalized training of more experienced therapists. Experienced therapists' participation in workshops, training courses and other individual training offers that do not involve working on the specific implementation of the conveyed skills in practice thus seems to have a fairly limited impact on their therapeutic work, just as there is, so far, virtually no evidence that experienced therapists' participation in these courses are subsequently translated into improved patient outcomes, although the therapists report that they are satisfied with the courses (Hill and Knox 2013:792ff). Generally, however, we have remarkably limited knowledge about the concrete, including the longer-term and less specific effects of formalized therapeutic training and supervision in terms of their ability to improve the therapist's treatment outcomes, ability to manage difficult situations in the therapeutic space (ruptures in the alliance, intense affects, countertransferences and so on) and ability to work with a wider range of patients, including patients with more severe pathology. Here it should be remembered that it is far from simple to examine the more complex outcomes of psychotherapeutic training, in part because therapists typically increase both their caseload and the complexity of the cases they take with growing competence and experience, which may complicate any direct comparisons with their own results at earlier stages in their career and with other therapists who have less experience and/or training.

While some of the more specifically technical aspects of the psychotherapeutic work can thus to some extent be learned via formalized education and clinical training, it is unlikely that the more personal aspects that go into the psychotherapeutic process, including the capacity for a responsive use of specific techniques, can be developed or learned via formalized education. It could be argued that there is a need to include a greater element of general personal development and *bildung* in the education of psychotherapists. This involves something other and more than teaching standardized knowledge and developing specific competences (which may appear to lend themselves to being documented) for solving specific problems, which can readily be formulated as very specific learning objectives, a practice that is increasingly embraced by our universities as they are increasingly controlled and infected by new public management logics. In extension of the discussion of the psychotherapeutic stance over the previous chapters, certain aspects of more general learning, development and *bildung* can be proposed (see also Chap. 10) that it would probably be beneficial to include in the education of future psychotherapists, including, among others, the folllowing (see, e.g., Råbu and McLeod 2016; Levitt and Piazza-Bonin 2017):

- Reflected ethical awareness.
- Capacity for independent, context-sensitive and critical thinking, including critical reflection on professional authority figures or positions that claim to have found the truth and hold the answers to what is the only or the best evidence-based treatment.
- Professional responsibility and integrity, which may in part be important for resisting the concrete consequences of the administrators' and others' lack of trust in or ignorance about (and possibly manifested in attacks on) one's professional competence or the psychotherapeutic space.
- Professional curiosity, openness, doubt and good judgment; the ability to ask questions without the need for immediate answers or action.
- Knowledge of and understanding for people from different (sub)cultures and social classes; openness to other perspectives on reality than one's own.
- A basic ability to think in dynamic-relational and psychological terms, including mentalizing capacity.
- Self-insight and ability to take a step back from and reflect critically on what norms, values and ideals one represents in the meeting with others, including one's patients.

In this discussion, it is potentially problematic that our university programmes, including especially the medical and psychological professional programmes, mainly focus on developing the students' cognitive (theoretical) understanding, while it is implicitly assumed that the necessary emotional and social skills are either already present or will emerge more or less automatically in prospective psychotherapists, independent of the formal training, perhaps during fairly simple clinical training that is part of the formalized programme or potential subsequent additional training in psychotherapy. This will probably happen in most of the students who later choose to become psychotherapists, but essentially, we do not know if it will. There is no systematic monitoring of this aspect, and to the extent that most of the prospective psychotherapist actually do develop the necessary skills, we would have to say that they do so despite and not because of what is (not) done to strengthen these skills as an integrated part of the degree programme. Again, one might ask, of course, whether it would even be practically possible to establish this kind of monitoring system. What specific criteria should we use to evaluate whether a person has adequate therapeutic skills for practicing psychotherapy? (however, see, e.g., Tuckett 2005; Israelstam 2011; Centre for Outcome Research and Effectiveness, UCL). It is of course also not without problems to set up learning or competence goals for a training programme if it is not possible to specify and formulate a related set of criteria to determine whether the goals are met. Persons who are trained to provide supervision of psychotherapists' work are probably in the best position to assess the individual therapist's therapeutic skills, but as Jacobsen and Mortensen (2017:139f), among others, have pointed out, so far, we lack common, explicit criteria for when a supervisor may approve a supervision course and thus legitimize a therapist's therapeutic competence. In relation to this issue, we should expect that it would be less complicated to identify cases where the person clearly failed to develop the necessary psychotherapeutic competences, including the ability to establish and maintain a psychotherapeutic stance, compared to what it would take to formulate in positive terms what characterized sufficient psychotherapeutic competence, including, not least, specific criteria for evaluating whether it is present in a specific therapist (cf. Jacobsen and Mortensen 2017:146ff). Similarly, it will be somewhat easier to define more basic psychotherapeutic skills than the more complex psychotherapeutic skills and more personal qualities that are often necessary in longer-term psychotherapy with patients with severe psychological disorders.

In addition, acceptance into one of the degree programmes in medicine and psychology (including in Denmark) requires exceptionally high marks from upper secondary school, which means that only young people who have learned to perform at the highest cognitive-academic level will make it into one of the lines of study that have traditionally been the main entrance to practicing psychotherapy in public-sector institutions. Although a good intellect and good cognitive-academic skills are important conditions for earning a university degree and, later, for working with psychotherapy, they are not in themselves a guarantee for similarly well-developed social and emotional skills, a well-developed moral-ethical compass or the ability to empathize with and contain people from other (sub)cultures who have a very different background from one's own, which are crucial qualifications for practicing psychotherapy.

Overall, the programmes that in practice have to build the professional foundation for psychotherapeutic work have a considerable cognitive slant (in their enrolment criteria, content and examination formats), which may mean that some persons who would perhaps have been better suited for another field may be trained as psychotherapists, while someone who has an obvious talent for psychotherapeutic work may find it unreasonably difficult to get formalized training in psychotherapy at the highest level. We may of course hope that the labour market (and supervisors) in practice regulate and compensate for these challenges, in the sense that individuals without the necessary emotional and social skills are not hired for positions where they work with psychotherapy, while individual with exceptional skills for working with psychotherapy who fail to be accepted into one of the two relevant degree programmes finder other paths into the profession (for example via a medium-duration programme in nursing or social work). However, there is no guarantee that this actually happens, and one might speculate that, especially in more rural areas where perhaps the field of qualified applicants is smaller, individuals may be employed to work as psychotherapists who are not sufficiently qualified.

Balancing Theoretical-Declarative and Procedural Knowledge

Psychotherapeutic skills rest largely on four pillars: scientific knowledge, a measure of technical competence, personal qualities and the ability to establish and maintain a psychotherapeutic stance. The scientific knowledge is largely descriptive and serves in part as the basis of the therapist's capacity for systematically observing, understanding and explaining issues pertaining to the patient and processes in the therapeutic space, just as it involves descriptive knowledge about therapeutic methods, efficacy factors and so on (Körner 2015:17f). Therapists may draw on psychological theory as a kind of third object outside the dyadic therapeutic relationship, which offers a stable foundation for their way of listening to, reflecting on and understanding what the patient communicates, and what plays out in the therapeutic space. Further, theoretical knowledge can help underpin the therapist's working model and professional practice (Zwiebel 2012:54). The therapist's technical competence refers to the therapist's ability to act, to implement acquired therapeutic methods and thus apply scientific theory (knowledge) in practice, including the ability to act with professional competence in specific situations, where the therapist is, to varying degrees, involved as a person (cf. the countertransference) (Körner 2015:17f). This ability to act competently and translate descriptive knowledge into practical skills in the work with the individuals patient is closely related to the ability to adopt a psychotherapeutic stance and can therefore not always be fully distinguished in practice (Körner 2015:26). Generally speaking, we can identify at least three models for the training of psychotherapists, each of which comes with various pros and cons (cf. Buchholz 2017:14f). One is a model that has as its primary focus to give prospective psychotherapists a research-based education and prepare them for a research career. Here, the main emphasis is on theory, empirical findings and how they may be applied in practice, just as there is a higher priority on developing a research ethic than a professional ethic. Specific psychotherapeutic training is not, or only to a very limited extent, included in the formalized training, and it is largely up to the individual student to acquire this after graduation.

Another model is one that in many regards is quite different, where the main focus from the outset is on professional practice, training in examination and therapeutic methods and acquiring clinical experience, while knowledge of and training in implementing various research methods is secondary and features at a later stage in the programme.

Finally, there is a third model, which can be said to position itself in between the former two, where the goal is to train both research and practical therapeutic skills in ways where the two fields engage in a mutual dialogue and serve as fruitful mutual correctives to one another. Ideally, the latter model would provide the best conditions for the necessary integration of the theoretical-technical and personal aspects of psychotherapeutic work. The current Danish degree programme in psychology is positioned somewhere in between the first and the third models, where knowledge of research methods and empirical research findings has, however, become a significantly higher priority in recent decades. This development may be viewed in part as a necessary corrective to the clear shortcomings in this area in the past, while the development of practice skills and of a professional ethic receives fairly little attention and is largely something the individual has to take in hand after graduation if the person's goal is to practice psychotherapy. This is not unproblematic but is largely dictated by budget constraints, as Denmark allocates far less funding to the study of psychology than, for example, the other Nordic countries and in practice leave it up to the individual psychologist and his or her future employer to arrange for training in psychotherapeutic skills and completing formalized additional training in psychotherapy. Moreover, it should be noted that a research career and a career as a practicing psychotherapist call for very different talents and skills, which are not necessarily found in the same person, meaning that individuals who have the talent for a research career do not necessarily have the talent for becoming a good psychotherapist or a good teacher of prospective psychotherapists, and vice versa.

Receiving formal education and theoretical and methodological schooling and reading a book such as the present one, are only the first, albeit an important, step towards developing a fundamental psychotherapeutic stance in their therapeutic work and developing basic psychotherapeutic competences. It is, however, crucial that psychotherapists subsequently, particularly in the early stages of their career, work in a professional environment that places a strong emphasis on the psychotherapeutic stance, the dynamic-relational understanding and thinking in psychological terms about the patients' difficulties, about the interaction between patients and therapists and—not to forget or repress—about the interaction between therapists and what happens in their own organization. Working with psychotherapy in a strong psychotherapeutic environment is thus very important for developing psychotherapeutic skills.

The American anthropologist Jean Lave argued that learning is far from reducible to an internalization or acquisition of cognitive declarative knowledge. This view applies particularly to education aimed at tasks that also involve more craft-based skills, such as psychotherapy (Lave and Wenger 1991). What a person has to learn or develop in order to work with psychotherapy cannot simply be limited to specific competences or skills that can be captured by specific learning objectives or conveyed via textbooks, just as it also is not confined to something that a teacher knows and can simply pass on in the form of theoretical declarative knowledge, even if that may help lay a stable foundation for psychotherapeutic practice. As a minimum it also involves a way of thinking, acting and interacting in psychotherapeutic practice; it is a form of partially tacit procedural knowledge, which is 'situated in a community of practice' (Lave and Wenger 1991:94), and which the individual therapist primarily learns via what Lave and Wenger (1991:89f) have called 'legitimate peripheral participation' in a psychotherapeutic community of practice. When a less experienced therapist becomes part of a psychotherapeutic environment and, to varying degrees, participates in the practice of more experienced therapists—initially from a more protected position with less responsibility (one is not assigned the most severely disturbed patients, one is not left alone with the responsibility for patients and so on)—one gradually forms a (only partially conscious explicit) impression of what it is one does, and how one thinks, speaks and acts in the psychotherapeutic space and in the psychotherapeutic culture. One acquires the psychotherapeutic stance. Over time, one develops one's own voice in one's own specific realization of the psychotherapeutic stance and incorporates dynamic-relational thinking.

This kind of knowledge and learning involves all aspects of the learner as a person and is thus based on something other and more than intended teaching; it is a form of learning-in-practice—learning via participation in a psychotherapeutic practice—that goes beyond the acquisition of propositional knowledge. That may in principle serve as the basis for taking a critical look at our formalized academic education programmes and their heavy emphasis on cognitive knowledge and tendency to revolve largely around teaching situations that are very different from the situations where the learners will later need to function in practice (Lave and Wenger 1991:32). In a sense, the students become expert at handling learning situations and passing the related formal, often abstract exams without necessarily developing a similar grasp of how the acquired theoretical knowledge is translated to practice. In this discussion it is important, however, to avoid falling into a primitive either/or mindset (see the section on Aristotle, Chap. 9). Competent psychotherapeutic practice requires both firm scientific knowledge about human psychology, psychopathology and psychotherapeutic method (acquired through formalized education) and training/acquisition of the psychotherapeutic stance and the psychotherapeutic way of thinking and acting in clinical practice.

As Binder and Henry (2010:298ff), among others, have pointed out, we need to distinguish between, on the one hand, theoretical-declarative knowledge about key psychotherapeutic skills, for example knowledge about ruptures in the alliance and negative interpersonal processes, and, on the other hand, procedural knowledge and the ability to use psychotherapeutic skills competently in practice, for example by registering and handling ruptures in the alliance and negative processes in the therapeutic space here and now in a constructive way. Formalized education and training will increase the student's theoretical declarative knowledge, which will typically be reflected in the student's ability to reproduce this knowledge in a formalized (typically written) exam format, but that does not in itself ensure that the student is able to convert this knowledge into competent action in clinical practice, although naturally, the two contexts are not completely unrelated. Lave and Wenger (1991:105f) distinguish between 'talking about' and 'talking within' a specific practice, where we may, on the one hand, learn something with a view to expressing declarative knowledge ('talking about'/or writing about, for example at an exam)—Lave also speaks of the 'exchange value' of learning, which in some cases is unrelated to the practice where it is to be used. On the other hand, one may acquire and develop procedural knowledge with a view to acting competently in clinical practice; Lave refers to this as the 'use value' of learning, which is in part catalysed in different learning environments and via different learning forms, and which is not similarly suitable for testing in our classical exam formats.

Being Embedded in a Firmly Rooted Psychotherapeutic Practice Community

Although declarative knowledge with a basis in science is absolutely essential for competent action in clinical practice, we must thus be aware that learning to talk about psychotherapy and psychotherapeutic skills is not the same as learning to act competently in the actual psychotherapeutic practice that the declarative knowledge and the theoretical scientific language addresses or refers to. It is not in itself sufficient for the student to acquire a wide range of scientific theories and knowledge about empirical findings and research methods and to learn to speak in certain ways and use certain concepts and to demonstrate (reproduce) this ability in formalized exam situations (cf. Lave and Wenger 1991:91). The student should also learn to convert this knowledge to competent psychotherapeutic work in clinical practice. With regard to that, the student's/novice therapist's gradual integration into a supportive and competent psychotherapeutic community of practice is crucial. Similarly, it is not in itself sufficient for the novice therapist to acquire the declarative knowledge about the psychotherapeutic work that is described in a treatment manual. He or she must also learn to convert this knowledge into competent and responsive action in the work with the individual patient; the declarative knowledge must be converted into procedural knowledge (knowing-in-action) that can be applied flexibly in the work with a diverse range of patients (cf. Binder 1999). Generally, on the other hand, it will also not be in any way sufficient for a person without former theoretical academic schooling to complete some form of practical psychotherapeutic training and begin to work with psychotherapy in a community of practice of some sort. In summary, the development of psychotherapeutic skills can be said to consist of a progression of steps, ideally involving continuous variation between theoretical schooling and clinical work:

- Theoretical schooling/education, development of a strong professional foundation in the form of scientific knowledge from the main disciplines of psychology and knowledge about psychopathology. This includes learning key dynamic-relational concepts and learning how to think in dynamic-relational terms with the inclusion of specific clinical issues/examples and not just abstract presentations of complex theory (declarative knowledge).
- Encountering the work of experienced psychotherapists (see them work) and initial training in basic clinical skills, conversation training.

- Embeddedness in a psychotherapeutic environment/community of practice where the psychotherapeutic stance and psychotherapeutic thinking and interaction forms are a top priority—first independent work with psychotherapy, beginning with less demanding patients and less complex disorders and preparation to the negative interpersonal processes and ruptures in the alliance that inevitably occur, especially in the work with more severely disturbed patients.
- Continuous supervision/feedback to own psychotherapeutic work from more experienced colleagues. This requires that the therapist openly and honestly presents his or her treatment challenges to the supervisor and is able to use the supervisor's feedback as a basis for reflecting on his or her own therapeutic work, including how his or her more personal dynamic-relational characteristics may influence the psychotherapeutic process.
- Gradually working with more demanding patients and more complex disorders under less close supervision, perhaps begin to act as a supervisor to less experienced colleagues.

The optimal setting for developing a psychotherapeutic stance and psychotherapeutic skills is thus a psychotherapeutic environment where all or most of the staff embody the psychotherapeutic stance in their thinking, being and approach to their work. It is a professional environment and a treatment culture with a high degree of mutual trust and a sense of security, with established settings, including a formalized space for supervision, where the therapist can verbalize and receive qualified professional feedback to help him or her think about both personally and professionally difficult aspects of the therapeutic process and does not, for various reasons, feel compelled to keep these concerns to him/herself or to try to resolve serious challenges related to his or her psychotherapeutic treatment courses alone. The most fruitful psychotherapeutic environment is one that is characterized by a basic consensus on a humanistic worldview, model of pathology and fundamental therapeutic principles, as internal disagreements between rigid representatives of fundamentally different psychotherapeutic approach might lead to confusion, internal conflicts and a lack of coherence in the therapeutic work, which can be stressful, especially for younger therapists and their patients. Incompatible approaches to the patient and the therapeutic work in a psychotherapeutic institution will often be destructive to the handling of shared psychotherapeutic tasks.

Working with psychotherapy requires that the therapist is professionally embedded in a professional community and an organization that is able to offer containment and support when difficult situations arise in the therapeutic process; this involves providing the time and space for shared psychotherapeutic reflection on the problems that arise, in contrast to the urge to implement quick solutions in the form of specific and rash actions. That applies to young and experienced therapists alike but in particular to the work with severely disturbed patients. The ability to maintain a stable psychotherapeutic stance and good treatment outcomes is thus not only a question of the presence of certain characteristics in the individual therapist, but also requires the therapist to be embedded in a well-functioning organization that is based on a profound understanding of the psychotherapeutic work, which permeates the entire organization, including the leadership, and which is able to protect the individual therapist and the psychotherapeutic space.

On the other hand, a psychotherapeutic culture can be severely compromised and ultimately destroyed by organizational management strategies driven by unreflected public-management thinking, where the fear—or ideological liberalist perceptions—that public-sector institutions are inefficient and operating with incompetence because they are not subject to the same competition pressures as private production companies, seek to manage treatment, education and other public-sector institutions through the continuous monitoring of simplistic quantitative performance measures (cf. Crouch 2015:106ff; Maio 2014). In treatment institutions, for example, this happens in the form of focusing on waiting lists for assessment or treatment, number of closed patient cases or number of patient contacts, without the crucial nuanced awareness of the quality of the proffered treatment, adaptation of the treatment to the individual patient and treatment outcomes in addition to very simplistic measures such as patient satisfaction. Quality assurance is reduced to what can be standardized, quantified and evaluated by simple means. Psychotherapeutic quality is reduced to a requirement for the individual therapist and clinic or institution to complete training courses in and embracing treatment methods that, for various reasons, are approved as being evidence-based, even though we know that the choice of specific treatment method, by all indications, is less important than the individual therapist's more personal qualities (cf. Part I of the present book).

When this type of management and efficiency thinking is mindlessly transferred from industrial manufacturing to public-sector treatment institutions, power or decision-making competence will typically be concentrated in the budget and financial office, whose staff and managers do not necessarily have the necessary understanding for the substance of the psychotherapeutic work (or have been in administration for so long that they have gradually forgotten, or whose worldview has become dominated by internalized public-management logics), while highly qualified psychotherapists lose power and influence over their own working life, as they are subjected to and, to varying degrees, internalize an economic mindset that is focused on efficiency and on which services produce the highest rate of payment to their economically struggling institution. To the extent that this management logic overburdens the therapists (stress) and leads them to offer their patients therapeutic treatment that is far from optimal (too brief, dictated by requirements for standardization and so on) and which is in conflict with their professional identity, the result over time may be a sense of cynicism and opportunism in the individual therapists in an attempt to protect themselves against further stress and burnout, which ultimately undermines the space for empathy and psychotherapeutic thinking.

Psychotherapists have a moral ethical responsibility to the individual patient and to what should, from a professional point of view be done for the patient that cannot be suspended or trumped by budget considerations or adherence to standardized guidelines for 'best' or evidence-based practice. If that happens, it may be a step towards cynicism and the erosion of the therapist's empathy. Specific and effective performance in the form of initiating standardized procedures ('I do my job the way I've been told to') may take centre stage, while anti-mentalizing and overly specifically minded action-oriented attitudes may take hold and threaten to undermine the psychotherapeutic work, including the institution's identity as an organization that is based on driven by psychotherapeutic thinking. On the other hand, psychotherapists' work must always be framed by a realistic understanding of the given conditions for the treatment, which typically also include an organizational and economic reality that is not readily open to change, and which they therefore have to work with, as best they can. Generally, the management organization and dominant inherent logics of an institution may thus have crucial impact on the psychotherapeutic work and on the way in which new psychotherapists are socialized into thinking about and understanding the psychotherapeutic work and the psychotherapeutic stance.

Even in a professionally fruitful environment, however, qualities such as personal maturity, inner calm, clear potentials (founded early in life) for developing emotional sensitivity, empathy, tolerance, social-relational competences and well-developed conceptualization skills for empathizing with very different individuals' very different lives and experiences must be present within the individual therapist as a basis for developing, over time, into a competent psychotherapist. Besides, we must always remember that it takes time and patience, including clinical experience in the form of many (supervised) course of psychotherapy with a diverse range of patients and problems—the patient is the therapist's best teacher (cf. Rønnestad and Skovholt 2013:153)—and possibly undergoing therapy oneself to become a competent therapist and develop a fundamental psychotherapeutic stance that is perceived as a natural and integrated part of one's way of meeting one's patients, the challenges they present and what plays out in the therapeutic space.

References

Binder, J. L. (1993). Is it time to improve psychotherapy training? *Clinical Psychology Review, 13,* 301–318.

Binder, J. L. (1999). Issues in teaching and learning time-limited psychodynamic psychotherapy. *Clinical Psychology Review, 19,* 705–719.

Binder, J. L., & Henry, W. P. (2010). Developing skills in managing negative process. In J. C. Muran & J. P. Barber (Eds.), *The therapeutic alliance: An evidence-based guide to practice* (pp. 285–304). New York, NY: Guilford.

Buchholz, M. (2017). Zur Lage der professionellen Psychotherapie. Nach DSM-5, Neurohype und RCT-Dominanz [On the status of professional psychotherapy. After DSM-5, neurohype and RCT dominance]. *Forum der Psychoanalyse, 33*(3): 289–310.

Crouch, C. (2015). *The knowledge corrupters: Hidden consequences of the financial takeover of public life*. Cambridge, England and Malden, MA: Polity Press.

Dewey, J. (1916). *Democracy and education: An introduction to the philosophy of education*. New York, NY: Macmillan.

Henry, W. P., Schacht, T. E., & Strupp, H. H. (1990). Patient and therapist introject, interpersonal process, and differential therapy outcome. *Journal of Consulting and Clinical Psychology, 58,* 768–774.

Henry, W. P., Schacht, T. E., Strupp, H. H., Butler, S. F., & Binder, J. L. (1993a). Effects of training in time-limited dynamic psychotherapy: Mediators of therapists' responses to training. *Journal of Consulting and Clinical Psychology, 61,* 441–447.

Henry, W. P., Strupp, H. H., Butler, S. F., Schacht, T. E., & Binder, J. L. (1993b). Effects of training in time-limited dynamic psychotherapy: Changes in therapist behavior. *Journal of Consulting and Clinical Psychology, 61,* 434–440.

Hill, C. E., & Knox, S. (2013). Training and supervision in psychotherapy. In M. Lambert (Ed.), *Bergin and Garfield's handbook of psychotherapy and behavior change* (6th ed., pp. 775–812). New York, NY: Wiley.

Israelstam, K. (2011). The interactive category schema of candidate competence: An Australian experience. *International Journal of Psychoanalysis, 92,* 1279–1313.

Jacobsen, C. H., & Mortensen, K. V. (2017). *Supervision af psykoterapi og andet behandlingsarbejde. Almen og psykodynamisk supervisionsteori* [Supervision of psychotherapy and other treatment work. General and psychodynamic supervision theory]. Copenhagen, Denmark: Hans Reitzels Forlag.

Kite, J. V. (2016). The fundamental ethical ambiguity of the analyst as person. *Journal of the American Psychoanalytic Association, 64*(6), 1153–1171.

Körner, J. (2015). *Psychotherapeutische Kompetenzen. Ein Praxismodel zu Kompetenzprofilen in der Aus- und Weiterbildung* [Psychotherapeutic competences. A practice model for competence profiles in basic and continuin education]. Berlin, Germany: Springer Verlag.

Lave, J., & Wenger, E. (1991). *Situated learning: Legitimate peripheral participation.* Cambridge, England: Cambridge University Press.

Levitt, H. M., & Piazza-Bonin, E. (2017). The professionalization and training of psychologists: The place of clinical wisdom. *Psychotherapy Research, 27,* 127–142.

Maio, G. (2014). *Geschäftsmodell Gesundheit. Wie der Markt die Heilkunst abschafft* [Business model 'health'. How the market is abolishing the healing arts]. Frankfurt am Main, Germany: Suhrkamp Verlag.

Nietzsche, F. (1996). *Human, all too human: A book for free spirits.* Cambridge, England: Cambridge University Press (Original work published 1886).

Råbu, M., & McLeod, J. (2016). Wisdom in professional knowledge: Why it can be valuable to listen to the voices of senior psychotherapists. *Psychotherapy Research* (ahead of print). https://doi.org/10.1080/10503307.2016.1265685.

Rogers, C. R. (1990). *The Carl Rogers reader.* London, England: Constable.

Rønnestad, M. H., & Skovholt, T. M. (2013). *The developing practitioner: Growth and stagnation of therapists and counselors.* London, England: Routledge.

Schön, D. A. (1987). *Educating the Reflective Practitioner.* San Francisco, CA: Jossey-Bass Publishers.

Steinert, C., & Leichsenring, F. (2017). *Psychodynamische Psychotherapie in Zeiten evidenzbasierter Medizin.* Göttingen, Germany: Vandenhoech & Ruprecht.

Thomassen, O. J. (2015). Muligheter for profesjonell kritikk [Opportunities for professional critique]. In B. A. Hennum, M. Pettersvold, & S. Østrem (Eds.), *Profesjon og kritikk* (pp. 63–81). Bergen, Norway: Fagbokforlaget.

Tuckett, D. (2005). Does anything go? Towards a framework for the more transparent assessment of psychoanalytic competence. *International Journal of Psychoanalysis, 86,* 31–49.

Zwiebel, R. (2004). Der Analytiker als Anderer: Überlegungen zum Einfluß der Person des Analytikers in der analytischen Praxis [The analyst as 'other': Thoughts on the influence of the analyst's personality in the analytical practice]. *Psyche, Zeitschrift für Psychoanalyse, 58,* 836–868.

Zwiebel, R. (2012). Von der Schwierigkeit Psychoanalytiker zu werden und zu bleiben [On the difficulty of being and remaining a psychoanalyst]. In C. E. Walker, H. Blass, R. Paul, & M. Teising (Eds.), *Die Psychoanalytische Haltung* (pp. 53–69). Frankfurt am Main, Germany: Congress-Organisation Geber & Reusch.

MIX
Papier aus verantwortungsvollen Quellen
Paper from responsible sources
FSC® C105338
FSC
www.fsc.org

If you have any concerns about our products,
you can contact us on
ProductSafety@springernature.com

In case Publisher is established outside the EU,
the EU authorized representative is:
Springer Nature Customer Service Center GmbH
Europaplatz 3, 69115 Heidelberg, Germany

Printed by Libri Plureos GmbH
in Hamburg, Germany